江苏大学英文教材基金资助出版
江苏大学数学科学学院留学本科生教学项目

CALCULUS FOR MEDICINE AND PHARMACY

医用高等数学

主编

范兴华
（Fan Xinghua）   江苏大学

彭 凌
（Peng Ling）   湖南医药学院

程悦玲
（Cheng Yueling）   江苏大学

陈 燕
（Chen Yan）   江苏大学

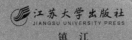

江苏大学出版社
JIANGSU UNIVERSITY PRESS

镇江

图书在版编目(CIP)数据

医用高等数学 = Calculus for Medicine and
Pharmacy：英文 / 范兴华等主编. —镇江：江苏大学
出版社，2022.8
ISBN 978-7-5684-1735-8

Ⅰ. ①医… Ⅱ. ①范… Ⅲ. ①医用数学－英语 Ⅳ.
①R311

中国版本图书馆 CIP 数据核字（2022）第 155003 号

医用高等数学

Calculus for Medicine and Pharmacy

主　编/范兴华　彭　凌　程悦玲　陈　燕
责任编辑/张小琴
出版发行/江苏大学出版社
地　　址/江苏省镇江市京口区学府路 301 号（邮编：212013）
电　　话/0511-84446464（传真）
网　　址/http：//press.ujs.edu.cn
排　　版/镇江文苑制版印刷有限责任公司
印　　刷/江苏凤凰数码印务有限公司
开　　本/787 mm×1 092 mm　1/16
印　　张/19.75
字　　数/661 千字
版　　次/2022 年 8 月第 1 版
印　　次/2022 年 8 月第 1 次印刷
书　　号/ISBN 978-7-5684-1735-8
定　　价/60.00 元

如有印装质量问题请与本社营销部联系（电话：0511-84440882）

PREFACE

As the changes of mathematical study, calculus has been widely used in the medical field in order to better the outcomes of both the science of medicine as well as the use of medicine as treatment. There has been a strong movement towards the inclusion of additional mathematical training throughout the world for future researchers in medicine and pharmacy.

This textbook is aimed at undergraduate foreign students of medicine and pharmacy in China. The book makes an effort to guide students, particularly of medicine and pharmacy, through the core concepts of calculus and to help them understand how those concepts apply to their lives and the world around them. It emphasizes the important role of calculus in the medicine and pharmacy sciences. Most of the contents have been practiced at Jiangsu University. The material is well-suited for self-study, as we know from experience.

The book is intended for the first semester of study. It covers the traditional single variable calculus course as well as probability and statistics. Emphasis is put on calculus since it serves as the base of probability theory. There are eight chapters in the textbook. The very first chapter talks about function, about which students have been familiar with. Topics that follow are traditional contents of differential calculus and the basic concepts of integral, as well as probability and statistics: limits, derivatives, additional derivative topics, graphing and optimization, integration, applications of integration, probability and statistics.

Chapters in this book consist of three main parts. Sections discuss new material, interspersed with a handful of Practice. Working on these two-or-three-minute exercises will help to master

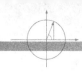

the material and provide a break from reading by doing something more active. Exercises are arranged behind each section, on average 10 per section. For about half of the exercises, answers are given in the Answer section. The last part of each chapter is devoted to summary and review of the chapter.

The textbook is written in an easy to read manner that students can use to follow-up on material taught in class. Graphs are used extensively in both the text and exercises. Key terms, key concepts, and key equations at the end of each chapters, and the index for the text are very helpful for referencing information.

The material can be arranged to teach or learn in 80 class hours. It can be used as the textbook for the required courses of all majors in medical schools. Lectures can pay emphasis on either integration or probability.

We would like to acknowledge the contribution of many people to the conception and completion of this book. Lu Dianchen and Qian Lijuan have greatly influenced our careers. Gao Jing and Wu Yuhai gave us some advices. Zhang Qi and Liu Qin read parts of the manuscript and offered helpful suggestions. We gratefully acknowledge the team at Jiangsu University Press for their support of this work. Finally, we would like to thank our families and our parents for their love and support.

Fan Xinghua, Peng Ling,

Cheng Yueling, Chen Yan

December, 2021

CONTENTS

Chapter 1   Functions

⁘ Introduction

The fundamental objects that we deal with in calculus are functions. This chapter prepares the way for calculus by discussing the basic ideas concerning functions and their graphs. We stress that a function can be represented in different ways: by an equation, in a table, by a graph, or in words.

1.1   Lines in the Plane

The invention of Cartesian coordinates in the 17th century by René Descartes (Latinized name: Cartesius) revolutionized mathematics by providing the first systematic link between Euclidean geometry and algebra. The modern Cartesian coordinate system in two dimensions is defined by an ordered pair of perpendicular lines, a single unit of length for both axes, and an orientation for each axis.

1.1.1   Coordinates on the Line

One dimensional cartesian coordinate system depends on the real number line.

1.1.1.1   Real number line

In mathematics, the real line, or real number line is the line whose points are the real numbers. That is, the real line is the group **R** of all real numbers, viewed as a geometric space, namely the Euclidean space of dimension one. Numbers are ordered on the real number line so that if $a < b$, then a is to the left of b.

We choose a point O of the line (the origin), a unit of length, and an orientation for the line. An orientation chooses which of the two half-lines determined by O is the positive, and which is negative; we then say that the line "is oriented" (or "points") from the negative half towards the positive half. Then each point P of the line can be specified by its distance from O, taken with a "+" or "−" sign depending on which half-line contains P.

Every real number, whether integer, rational, or irrational, has a unique location on the line. Conversely, every point on the line can be interpreted as a number in an ordered continuum which includes the real numbers (Figure 1.1). The number is then called the coordinate of the point and we usually refer the number as a point. We write the coordinate of the point inside a pair of round parentheses, for instance, $P(3)$.

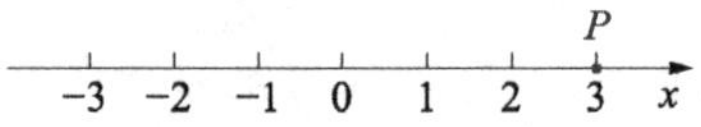

$$
\begin{array}{cccccccc}
& & & & & & P & \\
\hline
-3 & -2 & -1 & 0 & 1 & 2 & 3 & x
\end{array}
$$

Figure 1.1

Your Practice 1.1 Draw a real number line. Locate the points $A(-3)$, $B(-2)$, $C\left(\dfrac{1}{2}\right)$, $D(3)$.

1.1.1.2 Absolute value

In mathematics, the absolute value (or modulus) $|x|$ of a real number x is the non-negative value of x without regard to its sign, namely, $|x|=x$ for a positive x, $|x|=-x$ for a negative x, and $|0|=0$. For example, the absolute value of 3 is 3, and the absolute value of -3 is also 3. The absolute value of a number x may be regarded as its distance from the origin and can be represented as

$$
|x| = \begin{cases} x, & \text{if } x \geqslant 0, \\ -x, & \text{if } x < 0. \end{cases}
$$

The absolute value of the difference of two real numbers is the distance between them, that is, the ***distance*** between the two points $P_1(x_1)$ and $P_2(x_2)$ on the real line is then $|x_2 - x_1| = \sqrt{(x_2 - x_1)^2}$.

We will frequently need to solve equations containing absolute values, for which the following property is useful. Assume $b \geqslant 0$, the equation $|a|=b$ is equivalent to $a=b$ if $a \geqslant 0$, and to $-a=b$ if $a<0$.

Example 1.1 Solve $\left|\dfrac{3}{2}x-1\right| = \left|\dfrac{1}{2}x+1\right|$.

Solution Either $\dfrac{3}{2}x-1 = \dfrac{1}{2}x+1$, $x=2$,

or $\dfrac{3}{2}x-1 = -\left(\dfrac{1}{2}x+1\right)$, $\dfrac{3}{2}x-1 = -\dfrac{1}{2}x-1$, $2x=0$, $x=0$.

Therefore, the solutions are $x=2$ or $x=0$. #

Your Practice 1.2 Solve $|x-9|=2$.

1.1.1.3 Sets

A set is a well defined collection of distinct objects. The objects that make up a set can be anything: numbers, people, letters of the alphabet, other sets, and so on. The objects in a set are called elements. Every element of a set must be unique. Sets are conventionally denoted with capital letters. Sets A and B are equal if and only if they have precisely the same elements.

There are two ways of describing or specifying the members of a set. The first is by extension, that is, listing each member of the set. An extensional definition is denoted by enclosing the list of members in curly brackets:

$$C=\{4, 2, 1, 3\}, D=\{\clubsuit, \diamondsuit, \heartsuit, \spadesuit\}.$$

In words, C is the set whose members are the first four positive integers. D is the set of playing card suits.

The other is by using set-builder notation, through which, for instance, the set F of the ten smallest integers that are two less than perfect squares can be denoted:

$$F=\{n^2-2 \mid n \text{ is an integer, and } 0 \leqslant n \leqslant 10\}.$$

In this notation, the vertical bar " $\mid$ " means "such that", and the description can be interpreted as "F is the set of all numbers of the form n^2-2, such that n is a whole number in the range from 0 to 10 inclusive". Sometimes the colon "$:$" is used instead of the vertical bar.

1.1.1.4　Intervals

In mathematics, a (real) interval is a set of real numbers with the property that any number that lies between two numbers in the set is also included in the set. For example, the set of all numbers x satisfying $0 \leqslant x \leqslant 1$ is an interval which contains 0 and 1, as well as all numbers between them. Other examples of intervals are the set of all real numbers, the set of all negative real numbers, and the empty set.

The interval of numbers between a and b, including a and b, is often denoted $[a, b]$. The two numbers are called the endpoints of the interval. In countries where numbers are written with a decimal comma, a semicolon may be used as a separator, to avoid ambiguity.

To indicate that one of the endpoints is to be excluded from the set, the corresponding square bracket can be either replaced with a parenthesis, or reversed. For example, the interval $[a, b)$ indicates that the right endpoint is to be excluded from the set; the interval (a, b) indicates the right endpoint and the left endpoint are to be excluded from the set.

In both styles of notation, one may use an infinite endpoint to indicate that there is no bound in that direction. Specifically, one may use $-\infty$ or $+\infty$ (or both). For example, $(0, +\infty)$ is the set of all positive real numbers, and $(-\infty, +\infty)$ is the set of real numbers. Table 1.1 shows different representations of intervals.

Table 1.1

Interval notation	Inequality notation	Line graph
$[a, b]$	$a \leqslant x \leqslant b$	
$[a, b)$	$a \leqslant x < b$	
$(a, b]$	$a < x \leqslant b$	
(a, b)	$a < x < b$	

Continued

Interval notation	Inequality notation	Line graph
$(-\infty, b]$	$x \leqslant b$	←———————●→ x 　　　　　　　b
$(-\infty, b)$	$x < b$	←———————○→ x 　　　　　　　b
$[a, +\infty)$	$a \leqslant x$	———————●————→ 　　　　a　　　　x
$(a, +\infty)$	$a < x$	———————○————→ 　　　　a　　　　x

Your Practice 1.3 Draw the intervals $(-2, -1)$, $(1, 2]$, $[3, 4]$, and $[5, +\infty)$.

Example 1.2 Solve inequalities.

(1) $|2x - 5| < 3$.

(2) $|3x - 4| \geqslant 2$.

Solution (1) We rewrite $|2x - 5| < 3$ as

$$-3 < 2x - 5 < 3.$$

Adding 5 to all three parts, we obtain

$$2 < 2x < 8.$$

Dividing the result by 2, we find

$$1 < x < 4.$$

The solution is therefore the set $\{x \mid 1 < x < 4\}$. In interval notation, the solution can be written as the open interval $(1, 4)$.

(2) To solve $|3x - 4| \geqslant 2$, we go through the following steps:

either $\qquad\qquad 3x - 4 \geqslant 2, 3x \geqslant 6, x \geqslant 2,$

or $\qquad\qquad 3x - 4 \leqslant -2, 3x \leqslant 2, x \leqslant \dfrac{2}{3}.$

The solution is the set $\left\{x \,\middle|\, x \geqslant 2 \text{ or } x \leqslant \dfrac{2}{3}\right\}$, or in interval notation $\left(-\infty, \dfrac{2}{3}\right] \cup [2, +\infty)$. 　　　　#

1.1.2　Cartesian Coordinates in the Plane

Using the Cartesian coordinate system, geometric shapes (such as curves) can be described by Cartesian equations: algebraic equations involving the coordinates of the points lying on the shape.

1.1.2.1　Cartesian coordinates in the plane

To form a Cartesian or rectangular coordinate system, we select two real number lines—one horizontal and one vertical, and let them cross through their origins as indicated in Figure 1.2.

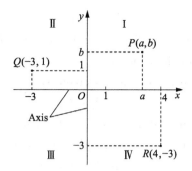

Figure 1.2

The lines are commonly referred to as the x and y-axes where the x-axis is taken to be horizontal, oriented from left to right and the y-axis is taken to be vertical, oriented from bottom to top. The point where the axes meet is taken as the origin for both, thus turning each axis into a number line. For a given point P, a line is drawn through P perpendicular to the x-axis to meet it at a and a second line is drawn through P perpendicular to the y-axis to meet it at b. The value of a is called the x-coordinate or abscissa and the value of b is called the y-coordinate or ordinate. The Cartesian coordinates of a point are usually written in parentheses and separated by commas, as in $P(a, b)$ or $Q(-3, 1)$.

The coordinate axes divide the plane into four parts called quadrants, which are numbered counter clockwise from I to IV.

Your Practice 1.4 Draw the points in the Cartesian plane with coordinates $(1, 2)$, $(-2, 2)$, $(3, -2)$, $(-1, -2)$.

1.1.2.2 Graphing equations

We now can visualize equations of two unknowns. Let the solutions of an equation to be the coordinates of a point. Then the solution set makes a group of points in the plane. For example, the graph of the equation $x^2 + y^2 = 1$ is the unit circle centered at the origin. Here we apply the distance in the plane: the distance between the points $P_1(x_1, y_1)$ and $P_2(x_2, y_2)$ on the plane is

$$|P_1 P_2| = \sqrt{(x_2 - x_1)^2 + (y_2 - y_1)^2},$$

which is the analogy of the distance on the real number line.

1.1.3 Linear Equations

We will frequently encounter situations in which quantities are linearly related, that is, these quantities satisfy a linear equation. For example, when a weight is attached to a helical spring made of some elastic material (and the weight is not too heavy), the length y of the spring will be linearly related to the weight x:

$$y = y_0 + kx. \tag{1.1}$$

This is known as Hook's law. Here, y_0 denotes the length of the spring when no weight is attached to it. The change in length $y - y_0$, is said to be proportional to the attached weight, and we write

$$y - y_0 \propto x$$

or, after introducing the proportionality factor k, $y - y_0 = kx$, yielding Equation (1.1) after adding y_0 to both sides of the equation.

The standard form of a linear equation is given by

$$Ax + By = C,$$

where A, B, and C are constants (A and B are not both zero), x and y are variables. Since the equation describes proportionality, the graph of a linear equation is a straight line, and any line in a Cartesian coordinate system is the graph of an equation of this form.

1.1.4 Equations of Lines

If we know two points $P_1(x_1, y_1)$ and $P_2(x_2, y_2)$ on a straight line, then the slope of the line is

$$m = \frac{y_2 - y_1}{x_2 - x_1}, \quad x_1 \neq x_2. \tag{1.2}$$

This is illustrated in Figure 1.3. The slope measures the steepness of a line. The vertical change $y_2 - y_1$ is often called the rise, and the horizontal change is often called the run. The slope may be positive, negative, zero, or undefined.

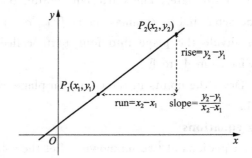

Figure 1.3

We illustrate in Figure 1.4 two special cases: vertical lines and horizontal line. A horizontal line has slope zero while vertical lines have no slope.

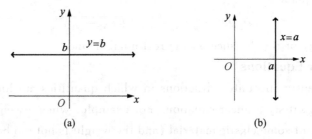

Figure 1.4

Two points (or one point and the slope) are sufficient to determine the equation of a straight line. If you are given two points or one point and the slope, the point-slope form of a straight line can be used to write down its equation.

$$y - y_0 = m(x - x_0),$$

where m is the slope and (x_0, y_0) is a point on the line.

The most frequently used form of a line equation is the slope-intercept form

$$y = mx + b,$$

where m is the slope and b is the y-intercept, which is the point of intersection of the line with the y-axis; it has coordinates $(0, b)$.

Example 1.3　A line has slope 4 and passes through the point $(3, 8)$. Find an equation of the line in point-slope form, slope-intercept form, and standard form.

Solution　Let $m = 4$ and $(x_0, y_0) = (3, 8)$. Substituting them into the point-slope form $y - y_0 = m(x - x_0)$.

Point-slope form: $y - 8 = 4(x - 3)$,　　　　　　　　　　　(add 8 to both sides)

$$y = 4(x - 3) + 8.$$　　　　　　　　　　　(simplify)

Slope-intercept form: $y = 4x - 4$.　　　　(subtract 4x from both sides then add 4)

Standard form: $-4x + y + 4 = 0$.　　　　　　　　　　　　　#

Example 1.4　Find an equation for the line that passes through the two points $(-3, 2)$ and $(-4, 5)$.

Solution　The slope of the line is

$$m = \frac{y_2 - y_1}{x_2 - x_1} = \frac{5 - 2}{-4 - (-3)} = \frac{3}{-1} = -3.$$

Using the point-slope form with $(-3, 2)$, we find

$$y - 2 = -3[x - (-3)],$$

that is,

$$y = -3x - 7.$$

We can also use the other point $(-4, 5)$, and obtain the same result.　　　　#

Your Practice 1.5　A line has slope -3 and passes through the point $(-2, 10)$. Find an equation of the line in point-slope form, slope-intercept form, and standard form.

Example 1.5　Determine the slope and the y-intercept of the line $3y - 2x + 9 = 0$.

Solution　We solve for y: $3y = 2x - 9$ and thus $y = \frac{2}{3} - 3$. We can now read off the slope $m = \frac{2}{3}$ and the y-intercept $b = -3$.　　　　　　　　　　　　#

Example 1.6　Sketch a graph of

$$y = 2x - 1.$$

Solution　Recall that two points are sufficient for a straight line. We select two specific values of x and then determine the corresponding y values. We let $x = 0$ and 1 for simplicity. Then the y-values are -1 and 1, respectively, as shown in Table 1.2.

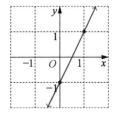

Figure 1.5

Table 1.2

x	0	1
y	-1	1

Then we locate the points $(0, -1)$ and $(1, 1)$. Connecting them we get the straight line as in Figure 1.5.   #

Your Practice 1.6 Sketch a graph of $y = x + 1$. Find the x-intercept and the y-intercept.

Exercise 1.1

1. Use interval notation to write the solution set of the inequality.

(1) $-4x + 21 < 1$;

(2) $x(x - 9) \leqslant 0$;

(3) $|9x + 4| \geqslant 14$.

2. Use interval notation to write the solution set of the inequality.

(1) $2x + 5 < 0$;

(2) $x(x - 3) \geqslant 0$;

(3) $|3x - 4| \leqslant 5$.

3. Sketch a graph of the following equations in a rectangular coordinate system.

(1) $3x + 2y = 12$;

(2) $4x + 5y = 20$;

(3) $y = 3 + 4x$.

4. Find the slope and y-intercept of the graph for the following equations.

(1) $y = 2x + 3$;

(2) $2y = 3 + 4x$;

(3) $4x + y = 8$.

5. Write the slope-intercept form of the equation of the line in Figure 1.6.

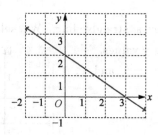

Figure 1.6

6. Write an equation of the line with slope 6/7 and y-intercept $-9/2$, using the form of $Ax + By = C$.

7. Determine the equation in standard form for the line that satisfies the stated requirements.

(1) The line passing through $(2, 4)$ with slope 1/3;

(2) The line passing through $(-3, 1)$ with slope 2;

(3) The line passing through $(-2, 4)$ and $(-1, 6)$;

(4) The line passing through $(3, -1)$ and $(2, 4)$;

(5) The horizontal line through $(3, -1/2)$;

(6) The vertical line through $(-2, 7)$.

8. Given two points $(1, 2)$ and $(3, 5)$,

(1) Find the point-slope form of the equation of the line;

(2) Find the slope-intercept form of the equation of the line;

(3) Find the standard form of the equation of the line.

9. To convert the weight of an object from kilograms (kg) to pounds (lbs), we use the fact that a weight measured in kilograms is proportional to a weight measured in pounds, and that 1 kg corresponds to 2.20 lbs. Find an equation that relates weight measured in kilograms to weight measured in pounds. Use your answer to convert the following measure-

ments.

(1) 54 lbs;

(2) 130 lbs;

(3) 4. 8 kg;

(4) 83 kg.

10. To convert the volume of a liquid measured in ounces to a volume measured in liters, we use the fact that 1 liter equals 33. 81 ounces. Denote by x the volume measured in liters. Assume a linear relationship between these two units of measurements.

(1) Find the equation relating x and y;

(2) A typical soda contains 18 ounces of liquid. How many liters is it?

1.2 Concept of Function

Central to the concept of function is correspondence.

1.2.1 Basic Conception

You are familiar with correspondences in daily life. For example, to each person, there corresponds his/her age. To each radius r of a circle, there corresponds the area A. Table 1. 3 shows the correspondence of the human population (in millions) of the world to the time (Source: www. Worldometers. info).

Table 1. 3

Year	1960	1970	1980	1990	2000	2010	2020
Population	3034	3700	4458	5327	6143	6956	7784

The electrocardiogram from an Apple Watch in Figure 1. 7 shows the correspondence of the electrical signal level on the time.

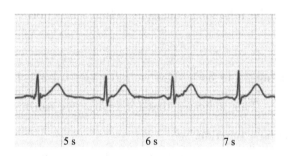

Figure 1. 7

One of the most important aspects of any science is the establishment of correspondences among various types of phenomena. Once a correspondence is known, predictions can be made. A medical researcher would like to know the correspondence between heart disease and obesity; a psychologist would like to predict the level of performance after a subject has repeated a given number of times; a cost analyst would like to predict costs for various levels of output in a manufacturing process; and so on.

What do all of these examples have in common? Each describes the matching of elements from one set with the elements in a second set. The definition of the term function will explain.

Definition 1. 1

A function is a correspondence rule between two sets such that for each element in the first set S there is exactly one corresponding element in the second set T.

The first set S is called the **domain** of the function. The set of corresponding elements in the second set is called the **range**. A symbol that represents an arbitrary number in the domain of a function $f(x)$ is called an **independent variable**. A symbol that represents a number in the range is called a **dependent variable**. Figure 1.8 shows the definition.

The function $f(x)$ is like a transformer that translates the domain set into the range set. Each time a given member of the domain set goes through the function transformer, it always produces the same member in the range set. For each member of the domain set, there must be only one corresponding member in the range set.

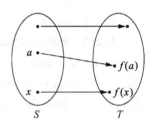

Figure 1. 8

The domain set and range set can be expressed as pairs $(x, f(x))$. Those pairs make the graph of the function. Graphs of functions only have one value for y for each x value. We typically construct graphs with the input values along the horizontal axis and the output values along the vertical axis.

Functions specified by equations

If in an equation of two variables x and y, we can get exactly one output y for each x, then the equation defines a function.

Example 1. 7 Can the following equations define a function?

(1) $4y-3x=8$；

(2) $y^2-x^2=9$.

Solution (1) Adding $3x$ to both sides we have $4y=8+3x$. Dividing both sides by 4 then we get $y=2+\dfrac{3}{4}x$. This indicates that for each x we can have one and only one y. Thus this equation define a function.

(2) Obviously, letting $x=0$, we have $y^2=9$, then $y=3$ or -3. This indicates that for an x there are two ys. Thus this equation can not define a function.   #

Your Practice 1. 7 Can the following equations define a function?

(1) $3y-2x=3$；

(2) $y^2-x^4=9$.

1.2.2 Function Notation

We see that the equation $y=x^2+1$ defines a function. Let $f(x)$ be the function specified by it：

$$f: y=x^2+11. \tag{1.3}$$

To make the outputs more informative, the outputs from the f function will be called $f(x)$ instead of y.

Now, when we plug 5 into the f function, instead of saying $y=26$, we say $f(5)=26$. This tells us that we used the f function and 5 was our input—much more informative! Also, now instead of having to say the f function is x^2+1, we can simply write $f(x)=x^2+1$. Again, these are basically the same as $y=x^2+1$.

This way of writing $f(x)$ instead of y is called **function notation** and is going to be used throughout maths and science classes from now on.

Example 1.8   Let $f(x)=2x+1$, find $f(3)$.

Solution   Remember that the independent variable just plays like a place holder. To find the function value at 3, you just replace x with 3.
$$f(x)=2x+1,$$
$$f(3)=2\times3+1=6+1=7.$$
Therefore, $f(3)=7$. ♯

Your Practice 1.8   Let $f(x)=\dfrac{12}{x-2}$, find $f(6)$.

Your Practice 1.9   Let x and h be real numbers and $g(x)=x^2$. Which of the following is true?

(1) $g(x+h)=x^2+h$;

(2) $g(x+h)=x^2+h^2$;

(3) $g(x+h)=(x+h)^2$.

1.2.2.1 Domain

The domain of a function $f(x)$ is the set of all values for which the function is defined.

Example 1.9   Find the domains of

(1) $f(x)=\dfrac{12}{x-2}$;

(2) $g(x)=1-x^2$;

(3) $h(x)=\sqrt{1-x}$.

Solution   (1) $f(x)$ is defined when the denominator is nonzero, that is $x-2\neq0$. Thus the domain of $f(x)$ is $(-\infty, 2)\cup(2,+\infty]$.

(2) $g(x)$ is defined for every real number, that is to say, the domain of g is $(-\infty, +\infty)$.

(3) We know that only a positive number or zero can be taken the square root. So $h(x)$ is meaningful when $1-x\geqslant0$, i. e. $x\leqslant1$. Thus the domain of h is $(-\infty, 1]$. ♯

Your Practice 1.10   Find the domain of the function specified by the equation $y=\sqrt{4-x}$.

Another way to identify the domain and range of functions is by using graphs. Because the domain refers to the set of possible input values, the domain of a graph consists of all

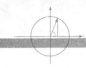

the input values shown on the x-axis. The range is the set of possible output values, which are shown on the y-axis.

Example 1.10　The graph of a function is shown in Figure 1.9.

(1) Find the values of $f(1)$ and $f(4)$.

(2) What are the domain and range of f?

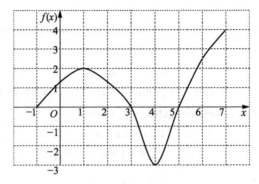

Figure 1.9

Solution　The graph of a function f is the set of points which satisfy the equation $y = f(x)$. That is, the point (x, y) is on the graph of f if and only if $y = f(x)$. To find $f(1)$, we locate the point on graph of $f(x)$ with x-coordinate 1, read the y-coordinate. The value of the y-coordinate is the function value. We then have $f(1) = 2$ and $f(4) = -3$.

The leftmost point on the curve has x-coordinate -1 and the rightmost has 7. The lowest point has y-coordinate -3 and the highest has 4. Therefore, the domain is the closed interval $[-1, 7]$ and the range is $[-3, 4]$.　　　　　　　#

1.2.2.2　Vertical line test

Functions are a special breed of equation. Not every equation gets to be a function. Multiple inputs can have the same output, but one input cannot lead to multiple outputs. Each input must have a unique output.

Example 1.11　Let

$$f(x) = \begin{cases} -3, & \text{if } x \leqslant 1, \\ x+2, & \text{if } x > 1. \end{cases}$$

Is this a function?

Solution　If $x > 1$, then the second rule applies and the graph of f lies on the $f(x) = x+2$. If $x \leqslant 1$, then the first rule applies and the graph of f lies on the line $f(x) = -3$. And x only belong to $x \leqslant 1$ or $x > 1$. So, f is a function.　　　　　　#

Your Practice 1.11　Let

$$g(x) = \begin{cases} 4, & \text{if } x \leqslant 3, \\ 2x-7, & \text{if } x \geqslant 2. \end{cases}$$

Determine whether g is a function.

If we are looking at a graph of an equation, we can test whether or not it is a function with the **vertical line test**. For any x-value, if this imaginary vertical line that we drag across the graph ever touches the graph in more than one spot, it is not a function, but if it does not, it is a function.

Example 1. 12   Is the curve in Figure 1. 10 the graph of a function?

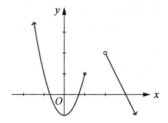

Figure 1. 10

Solution   This is a function because for any x-value we pick, there is only one spot on the line that goes with that value.   #

Example 1. 13   Is the curve in Figure 1. 11 the graph of a function?

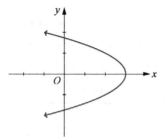

Figure 1. 11

Solution   It is not a function because for any x-value right in the middle, there are actually two different spots on the line that go with it. It is therefore not a function.   #

Your Practice 1.12   Are the curves in Figures 1. 12 and 1. 13 the graph of a function?

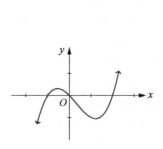

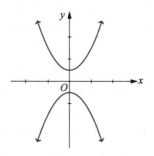

Figure 1. 12   Figure 1. 13

1.2.2.3   Piecewise defined functions

Functions whose definitions involve more than one rule are called piecewise-defined functions. For example,

$$|x| = \begin{cases} -x, & \text{if } x < 0, \\ x, & \text{if } x \geqslant 0. \end{cases}$$

Example 1. 14   The taxi fare of Zhenjiang is 10 Yuan for the first three kilometers,

2.7 Yuan and 3 Yuan per additional kilometer for the travel distance longer than 3 kilometres and 16 kilometres respectively. Write a piecewise definition of the charges $C(x)$ for a customer who travels x kilometers. Then graph $C(x)$.

Solution If $0 < x \leqslant 3$ the customer is charged 10 Yuan . If $x > 3$ but $x \leqslant 16$, the customer is charged 10 Yuan for the first 3 kilometers plus the extra $2.7(x-3)$, that is $10 + 2.7(x-3) = 2.7x + 1.9$. If $x > 16$, the customer is charged $2.7 \times 16 + 1.9 = 45.1$ plus the extra 3 $(x-16)$, that is $45.1 + 3(x-16) = 3x - 2.9$.

We then set the formula

$$C(x) = \begin{cases} 10, & 0 < x \leqslant 3, \\ 2.7x + 1.9, & 3 < x \leqslant 16, \\ 3x - 2.9, & x > 16. \end{cases}$$

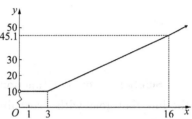

The graph is shown in Figure 1.14 which consists of three line segments with different slope $0, 2.7$ and 3 respectively.　　　　　　　　　　　　#

Figure 1.14

Your Practice 1.13 China Resources Gas Group Limited uses the rates shown in Table 1.4 to compute the annual cost of natural gas for residential customers. Write a piecewise definition for the cost of consuming x m³ of natural gas and graph the function.

Table 1.4

Price	Cost
2.69 Yuan per m³	the first 300 m³
2.93 Yuan per m³	the next 300 m³
3.66 Yuan per m³	all over 600 m³

1.2.3 Even and Odd Functions

A function f is even if its graph is symmetric with respect to the y-axis. This criterion can be stated algebraically as follows: f is even if $f(-x) = f(x)$ for all x in the domain of f. For example, the function $f(x) = x^2$ is even because

$$f(-x) = (-x)^2 = x^2 = f(x).$$

An even function has geometric significance. If we already have the graph of f for $x \geqslant 0$, we can obtain the entire graph simply by reflecting this portion about the y-axis.

A function f is odd if its graph is symmetric with respect to the origin. This criterion can be stated algebraically as follows: f is odd if $f(-x) = -f(x)$ for all x in the domain of f. For example, the function $f(x) = x^3$ is odd because

$$f(-x) = (-x)^3 = -x^3 = -f(x).$$

Likewise, if we have plotted the graph of f for $x \geqslant 0$, we can obtain the entire graph simply by rotating this portion through $180°$ about the origin.

Example 1.15 Determine whether each of the following function is even, odd, or neither even nor odd.

(1) $f(x) = x^2 - 1$;

(2) $g(x)=x+x^3$;

(3) $h(x)=x-x^2$.

Solution (1) Because

$$f(-x)=(-x)^2-1=x^2-1=f(x),$$

we find that f is an even function.

(2) Since

$$g(-x)=(-x)+(-x)^3=-x-x^3=-(x+x^3)=-f(x),$$

so g is odd.

(3) We find

$$h(-x)=-x-(-x)^2=-x-x^2.$$

Since $h(-x)\neq h(x)$ and $h(-x)\neq -h(x)$, we conclude that h is neither even nor odd.   #

1.2.4 Increasing and Decreasing Functions

Informally, we see that a function is increasing on an interval if its graph is rising from left to right over the interval and that a function is decreasing on an interval if its graph is falling from left to right over the interval.

Graphs of functions usually have rising and falling sections as we scan graphs from left to right. We all know that if something is increasing then it is going up and if it is decreasing it is going down. Referring to the graph of $f(x)=3x-x^3$ in Figure 1.15. We see that on the interval $(-\infty,-1)$, the graph of f is falling, $f(x)$ is decreasing. On the other hand, on the interval $(-1,1)$, the graph of f is rising, $f(x)$ is increasing. Finally, on the interval $(1,+\infty)$, the graph of f is falling, $f(x)$ is decreasing.

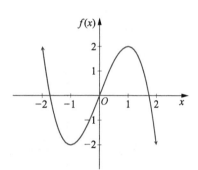

Figure 1. 15

We phrase the definition of increasing and decreasing functions.

> **Definition 1. 2**
>
> *A function $f(x)$ is called (strictly) increasing on I if*
> $$f(x_1)<f(x_2) \ whenever \ x_1<x_2 \ in \ I.$$
> *Similarly, it is called (strictly) decreasing on I if*
> $$f(x_1)>f(x_2) \ whenever \ x_1<x_2 \ in \ I.$$

An increasing or decreasing function is called **monotonic**.

The word "strictly" in the above definition refers to have a strict inequality ($f(x_1)<f(x_2)$ and $f(x_1)>f(x_2)$). We will often drop "strictly". If we have the inequality $f(x_1)\leqslant f(x_2)$ whenever $x_1<x_2$ in I, we call f nondecreasing. Similarly, if $f(x_1)\geqslant f(x_2)$ whenever $x_1<x_2$ in I, then we call f nonincreasing.

Figures 1.16 and 1.17 illustrate the definition of increasing and decreasing functions.

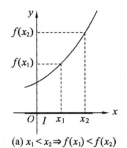

(a) $x_1 < x_2 \Rightarrow f(x_1) < f(x_2)$

Figure 1. 16

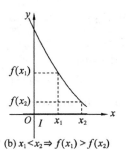

(b) $x_1 < x_2 \Rightarrow f(x_1) > f(x_2)$

Figure 1. 17

Exercise 1.2

1. The graph of the function f is shown in Figure 1. 18. Then

(1) $f(-2) =$ _____ ;

(2) $f(-1) =$ _____ ;

(3) $f(1) =$ _____ ;

(4) $f(2) =$ _____ .

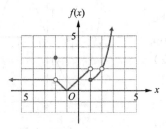

Figure 1. 18

2. The graph of the function f is shown in Figure 1. 19. Then

(1) $f(2) =$ _____ ;

(2) $f(-1) =$ _____ ;

(3) $f(0) =$ _____ ;

(4) $f(-3) =$ _____ .

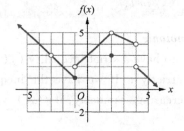

Figure 1. 19

3. Indicate whether each graph in Figures 1. 20, 1. 21 and 1. 22 defines a function.

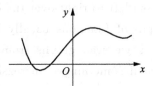

Figure 1. 20

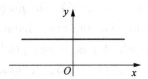

Figure 1. 21

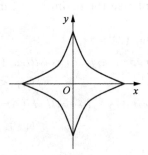

Figure 1. 22

4. Does the equation specify a function with independent variable x? If so, find the domain of the function. If not, find a value of x to which there corresponds more than

one value of y.

(1) $x(x+y)=4$;

(2) $x^3-y^2=0$;

(3) $x^2+4x-3=y$;

(4) $x=y^2$.

5. Find and simplify the expression if $f(x)=x^2-4$.

(1) $f(2h)$;

(2) $f(2)+f(h)$;

(3) $f(2+h)$;

(4) $f(2+h)-f(2)$;

(5) $\dfrac{f(x+h)-f(x)}{h}$.

6. Find the domain of $f(x)$.

(1) $f(x)=\dfrac{1}{\sqrt{5-x}}$;

(2) $f(x)=\dfrac{2}{3x+4}$;

(3) $f(x)=\sqrt{x^2-6x+5}$.

7. The area A and perimeter P of a rectangle with length L and width W are:

$$A=LW, \quad P=2L+2W.$$

The area of a rectangle is 25 square meters. Express the perimeter $P(W)$ as a function of the width W, and state the domain of this function.

8. Indicate whether each function shown in the graph in Figures 1.23, 1.24 and 1.25 is even or odd or neither odd nor even.

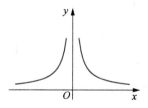

Figure 1.23

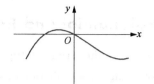

Figure 1.24

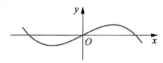

Figure 1.25

9. Determine algebraically whether the following function is even or odd or neither odd nor even.

(1) $f(x)=3x^2+4$;

(2) $g(x)=4x^3-5x$;

(3) $h(x)=3x^5-5x^2-6x+7$.

10. $f(x)=x^2+1$, $g(x)=x^3-3x$, $h(x)=3x^5+2x^3$.

Are the following products even or odd or neither odd nor even?

(1) $f(x)g(x)$;

(2) $g(x)h(x)$;

(3) $f(x)g(x)h(x)$.

11. The graph of a function is given in Figure 1.26. Determine the intervals on which the function increases and decreases.

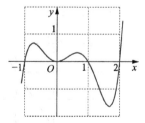

Figure 1.26

12. Determine whether the function $f(x)=3-4x$ is increasing or decreasing on $(-\infty,+\infty)$.

13. Determine whether the function $f(x)=\dfrac{2}{x}$ is increasing or decreasing on $(0,+\infty)$.

1.3 Polynomial and Rational Functions

We discuss the primary types of functions that occur in calculus and describe the process of using these functions as mathematical models of real-world phenomena.

1.3.1 Linear Functions and Straight Lines

Linear equations in two variables have (straight) lines as their graphs.

Definition 1.3

The function

$$f(x) = mx + b, \ m \neq 0$$

is called a linear function, or first-degree function. The function

$$f(x) = b$$

is called a constant function.

The linear function $f(x) = mx + b$ is the function that is specified by the linear equation $f(x) = mx + b$.

If a function is given by a formula and the domain is not stated explicitly, the domain is the set of all numbers for which the formula makes sense and defines a real number.

Graphs of functions are graphs $f(x)$ of equations $y = f(x)$. To graph functions, the values in the domain set correspond to the x-axis and the related values in the range set correspond to the y-axis.

Example 1.16 A characteristic feature of linear functions is that they grow at a constant rate. For instance, the following shows a graph of the linear function $f(x) = 2x - 1$ and a table of sample values (Figure 1.27 and Table 1.5). Notice that whenever x increases by 0.1, the value of $f(x)$ increases by 0.2. So $f(x)$ increases two times as fast as x. Thus the slope of the graph $y = 2x - 1$, namely 2, can be interpreted as the rate of change of y with respect to x. #

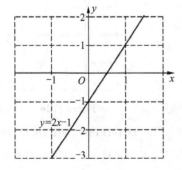

Figure 1.27

Table 1.5

x	$f(x) = 2x - 1$
1.0	1.0
1.1	1.2
1.2	1.4
1.3	1.6

Your Practice 1.14 Sketch the graph and find the domain and range of each function.

(1) $g(x) = -0.5x + 1$; (2) $h(x) = 3$.

Note The graph of a linear function is a straight line that is neither horizontal nor vertical. The graph of a constant function is a horizontal line.

1.3.2 Quadratic Functions

Curved antennas, such as the ones shown in Figure 1. 28, are commonly used to focus microwaves and radio waves to transmit television and telephone signals, as well as satellite and spacecraft communication. The cross-section of the antenna is in the shape of a parabola, which can be described by a quadratic function.

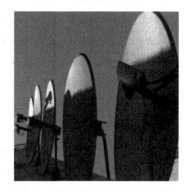

Figure 1. 28

Quadratic functions frequently model problems involving area and projectile motion. They provide a good opportunity for a detailed study of function behavior because it is less complex working with quadratic functions than working with higher degree functions.

Definition 1.4

If a, b and c are real numbers with $a \neq 0$, then the function
$$f(x) = ax^2 + bx + c$$
is a quadratic function and its graph is a parabola.

The domain of any quadratic function is the set of all real numbers.

We will discuss the graph sketching skills after the studying of derivatives. We just show the graph of a typical parabola in Figure 1. 29.

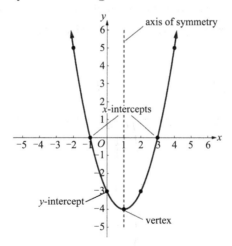

Figure 1. 29

The graph of a quadratic function is a U-shaped curve called a parabola. One important feature of the graph is that it has an extreme point, called the **vertex.** If the parabola opens up, the vertex represents the lowest point on the graph, or the minimum value of the quadratic function. If the parabola opens down, the vertex represents the highest point on the graph, or the maximum value. In either case, the vertex is a turning point on the graph. The graph is also symmetric with a vertical line drawn through the vertex, called the axis of symmetry.

An x-intercept of a function is also called a zero of the function. The x-intercepts of a quadratic function can be found by solving the quadratic equation $y=ax^2+bx+c=0$ for x, $a\neq0$. The quadratic formula is as follows.

If $ax^2+bx+c=0$, $a\neq0$, then

$$x=\frac{-b\pm\sqrt{b^2-4ac}}{2a}, \text{ provided } b^2-4ac\geqslant0.$$

1.3.3 Polynomial Functions and Rational Functions

Linear and quadratic functions are special cases of the more general class of *polynomial functions*. These functions consist of one or more terms of variables with whole number exponents (the whole numbers are positive integers and zero).

> **Definition 1.5**
>
> A *polynomial function is a function that can be written in the form*
> $$f(x)=a_nx^n+a_{n-1}x^{n-1}+\cdots+a_1x+a_0$$
> *for n a nonnegative integer, called the degree of the polynomial. The coefficients a_0, a_1, $\cdots$, a_n are real numbers with $a_n\neq0$. The domain of a polynomial function is the set of all real numbers.*

Still we will discuss the graph of any polynomial after studying the derivatives. Figure 1.30 shows graphs of representative polynomial functions of degrees 1 through 6. The figure suggests some general properties of graphs of polynomial functions.

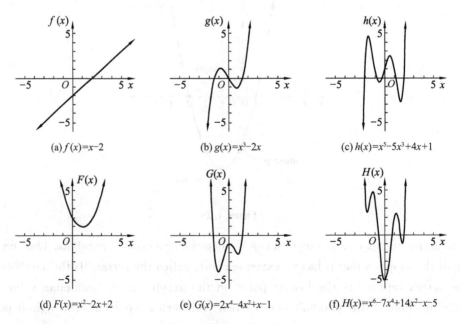

(a) $f(x)=x-2$

(b) $g(x)=x^3-2x$

(c) $h(x)=x^5-5x^3+4x+1$

(d) $F(x)=x^2-2x+2$

(e) $G(x)=2x^4-4x^2+x-1$

(f) $H(x)=x^6-7x^4+14x^2-x-5$

Figure 1.30

Notice that the odd-degree polynomial graphs start negative, end positive, and cross the x-axis at least once. The even-degree polynomial graphs start positive, end positive, and may not cross the x-axis at all. In all cases in Figure 1.30, the leading coefficient—that is, the coefficient of the highest-degree term—was chosen positive. If any leading coefficient had been chosen negative, then we would have a similar graph but reflected in the x-axis.

A polynomial of degree n can have, at most, n linear factors. Therefore, the graph of a polynomial function of positive degree n can intersect the x-axis at most n times. Note from Figure 1.30 that a polynomial of degree n may intersect the x-axis fewer than n times. An x-intercept of a function is also called a ***zero*** or ***root*** of the function.

1.3.3.1   Rational functions

Definition 1.6

The function

$$f(x) = \frac{n(x)}{d(x)}$$

is called a rational function, where $n(x)$ and $d(x)$ are polynomials.

Just as rational numbers are defined in terms of quotients of integers, rational functions are defined in terms of quotients of polynomials. The domain is the set of all numbers such that $d(x) \neq 0$. For example, $f(x) = \frac{x-2}{x+1}$ is a rational function. Figure 1.31 shows the graphs of some rational functions.

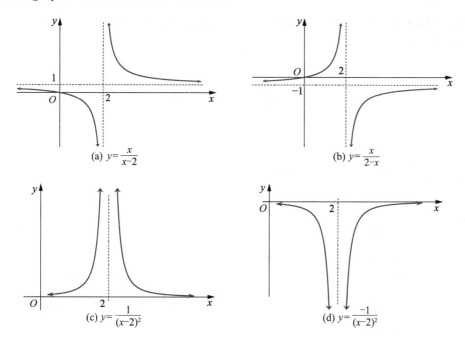

(a) $y = \dfrac{x}{x-2}$

(b) $y = \dfrac{x}{2-x}$

(c) $y = \dfrac{1}{(x-2)^2}$

(d) $y = \dfrac{-1}{(x-2)^2}$

Figure 1.31

1.3.3.2 Vertical asymptote

The graph of a rational function have breaks or holes at those x-values where it is undefined. The vertical line passing through the undefined point is called the vertical asymptote of the graph of the function. For example, $x=2$ is a vertical asymptote of the graph of the function $y=\dfrac{x}{x-2}$ and the function $y=\dfrac{x}{2-x}$ (Figure 1.31a). Graphing rational functions is aided by locating vertical and horizontal asymptotes first, if they exist.

If $d(a)=0$ but $n(a)\neq 0$, then the graph of the rational function $f(x)=\dfrac{n(x)}{d(x)}$ has a vertical asymptote at $x=a$. If $n(a)$ and $d(a)$ are both zero, then the graph of the rational function $f(x)=\dfrac{n(x)}{d(x)}$ may have a hole at $x=a$ rather than an asymptote.

1.3.3.3 Horizontal asymptotes

Next we move to the graph of $f(x)=\dfrac{x}{x-2}$ in Figure 1.31a. As x gets large—that is, as we move away from the origin along the x-axis in either direction—the corresponding y-values get closer and closer to 1. The graph approaches, but never coincides with the line $y=1$. We say that the graph has a horizontal asymptote at $y=1$.

When does a rational function $f(x)=\dfrac{n(x)}{d(x)}$ have a horizontal asymptote? It depends on the degrees of the polynomials $n(x)$ and $d(x)$. The degree of the numerator of $n(x)$ is less or equal to the degree of the denominator $d(x)$. In other words, the highest power of x in the numerator (1, in this case) is smaller than or the same as the highest power in the denominator.

Your Practice 1.15 Write down the equation of any vertical or horizontal asymptotes of the graphs in Figures 1.31b—d.

Exercise 1.3

1. Match the functions to the following graphs in Figures 1.32 and 1.33.

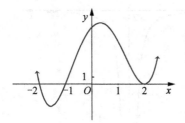

Figure 1.32

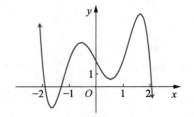

Figure 1.33

(1) $2-x(x-1)(x-2)(x^2+3x+2)$;

(2) $(x-2)^2(x^2+3x+2)$.

2. Graph the following functions.

(1) $f(x) = \begin{cases} 4-2x, & \text{if } x<1, \\ x-2, & \text{if } x\geqslant 1; \end{cases}$

(2) $f(x) = \begin{cases} x+2, & \text{if } x\geqslant 3. \\ 6-2x, & \text{if } x<3; \end{cases}$

(3) $h(x) = \begin{cases} 3x, & \text{if } 0\leqslant x\leqslant 30, \\ x+25, & \text{if } 30<x\leqslant 60, \\ 0.5x+60, & \text{if } x>60; \end{cases}$

(4) $h(x) = \begin{cases} 3x-1, & \text{if } 0\leqslant x\leqslant 2, \\ x+2, & \text{if } 2<x\leqslant 4, \\ -x+6, & \text{if } x>4. \end{cases}$

3. For polynomial function $f(x) = (x-1)^2(x^2+3x-4)$, find:

(1) the degree of the polynomial;

(2) all x-intercepts;

(3) the y-intercept.

4. Find the equation of any horizontal asymptote and/or vertical asymptote of the graph of function shown in Figure 1. 34.

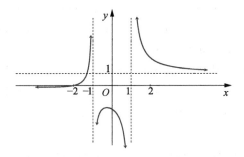

Figure 1. 34

5. A plant can manufacture at most 200 golf clubs per day. It makes 80 golf clubs per day for a total daily cost of $ 7647 and 100 golf clubs per day for a total daily cost of $ 9147.

(1) Assuming that daily cost and production are linearly related, find the total daily cost of producing x golf clubs.

(2) Interpret the slope and y-intercept of this cost equation.

6. In stable air, the air temperature drops about 3. 6 ℉ for each 1000-feet rise in altitude. If the temperature at sea level is 70 ℉. (1 feet≈0. 3048 m)

（1） Write a linear equation that expresses temperature T in terms of altitude in thousands of feet;

（2） At what altitude is the temperature 34 ℉ ?

7. At a price of $ 2. 28 per bushel, the supply of barley is 7500 million bushels and the demand is 7900 million bushels. At a price of $ 2. 37 per bushel, the supply is 7900 million bushels and the demand is 7800 million bushels.

(1) Find a price-supply equation of the form $p=mx+b$;

(2) find a price-demand equation of the form $p=mx+b$;

(3) find the equilibrium point;

(4) graph the price-supply equation, price-demand equation, and equilibrium point in the same coordinate system.

8. At a price of $ 1. 94 per bushel, the supply of corn is 9800 million bushels and the demand is 9300 million bushels. At a price of $ 1. 82 per bushel, the supply is 9400 million bushels and the demand is 9500 million bushels.

(1) Find a price-supply equation of the form $p=mx+b$;

(2) find a price-demand equation of the form $p=mx+b$;

(3) find the equilibrium point;

(4) graph the price-supply equation, price-demand equation, and equilibrium point in the same coordinate system.

Summary and Review

Important Terms, Symbols, and Concepts

- A Cartesian or rectangular coordinate system is formed by the intersection of a horizontal x-axis and a vertical y-axis at their origins. Each point in the plane corresponds to its coordinates—an ordered pair (a, b) determined by passing vertical and horizontal lines through the point. The abscissa or x coordinate a is the coordinate of the intersection of the vertical line and the x-axis, and the ordinate or y coordinate b is the coordinate of the intersection of the horizontal line and the y-axis.

- A linear equation in two variables is an equation that can be written in the standard form $Ax+By=C$, where A, B, and C are constants (A and B are not both zero), and x and y are variables.

- The graph of a linear equation in two variables is a line, and every line in a Cartesian coordinate system is the graph of an equation of the form $Ax+By=C$.

- A function is a correspondence between two sets of elements such that to each element in the first set there corresponds one and only one element in the second set. The first set is called the domain and the set of corresponding elements in the second set is called the range.

- If x is a placeholder for the elements in the domain of a function, then x is called the independent variable or the input. If y is a placeholder for the elements in the range, then y is called the dependent variable or the output.

- If in an equation in two variables we get exactly one output for each input, then the equation specifies a function. The graph of such a function is just the graph of the specifying equation. If we get more than one output for a given input, then the equation does not specify a function.

- The symbol $f(x)$ represents the element in the range of f that corresponds to the element x of the domain.

- If a function is specified by an equation and the domain is not indicated, we assume that the domain is the set of all inputs that produce outputs of real numbers. The vertical-line test can be used to determine whether or not an equation in two variables specifies a function.

- A function of the form $f(x)=mx+b$, where $m \neq 0$, is a linear function.

- A function of the form $f(x)=ax^2+bx+c$, where $a \neq 0$, is a quadratic function in standard form, and its graph is a parabola.

- A polynomial function is a function that can be written in the form
$$f(x)=a_nx^n+a_{n-1}x^{n-1}+\cdots+a_1x+a_0$$
for n a nonnegative integer called the degree of the polynomial. The coefficients a_0, $a_1, \cdots, a_n$ are real numbers with the leading coefficient $a_n \neq 0$. The domain of a

polynomial function is the set of all real numbers.

- The graph of a polynomial function of degree n can intersect the x-axis at most n times. An x-intercept is also called a zero or root.

- The graph of a polynomial function has no sharp corners and has no holes or breaks.

- A rational function is any function that can be written in the form

$$f(x) = \frac{n(x)}{d(x)}, \ d(x) \neq 0$$

where $n(x)$ and $d(x)$ are polynomials. The domain is the set of all real numbers such that $d(x) \neq 0$.

- A rational function can have vertical asymptotes [but not more than the degree of the denominator $d(x)$] and at most one horizontal asymptote.

- A function f is even if $f(-x) = f(x)$ for all x in its domain. Its graph is symmetric with respect to the y-axis.

- A function f is odd if $f(-x) = -f(x)$ for all x in its domain. Its graph is symmetric with respect to the origin.

- A function $f(x)$ is called (strictly) increasing on I if $f(x_1) < f(x_2)$ whenever $x_1 < x_2$ in I. Its graph is rising from left to right over the interval.

- A function $f(x)$ is called (strictly) decreasing on I if $f(x_1) > f(x_2)$ whenever $x_1 < x_2$ in I. Its graph is falling from left to right over the interval.

Important Formula

- If (x_1, y_1) and (x_2, y_2) are two points on a line with $x_1 \neq x_2$, then the slope of the line is $m = \dfrac{y_2 - y_1}{x_2 - x_1}$.

- The point-slope form of the line with slope m that passes through the point (x_0, y_0) is $y - y_0 = m(x - x_0)$.

- The slope-intercept form of the line with slope m that has y-intercept b is $y = mx + b$.

- The graph of the equation $x = a$ is a vertical line, and the graph of $y = b$ is a horizontal line.

Chapter 2　Limits

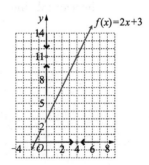

:: Introduction

How do algebra and calculus differ? In algebra, we solve equations for a particular value of a variable—a static notion. In calculus, we are interested in how a change in one variable affects another variable—a dynamic notion. In Chapter 2 we introduce the Limits, one of the key concepts to study calculus.

2.1　Concept of Limit

Newton and Leibnitz, the inventor of calculus, were very much aware of the importance of taking limits in their development of calculus. Limits help us to describe, in a precise way, the behavior of $f(x)$ when x is close, but not equal, to a particular value c. In this section, we develop informal and formal approaches to evaluating limits.

2.1.1　Intuitive Definition of Limits

For the calculus student, the precise definition is not of fundamental importance, but it is vital to have an intuitive understanding of the limit. We approach this understanding from graphical and analytical ways.

2.1.1.1　A graphical approach

We introduce the graphical approach analyzing behavior of the values of $f(x) = 2x + 3$ when x is close to 4. We begin by drawing a graph of f that includes the domain value $x = 4$ (Figure 2.1). In this figure, we are using a static drawing to describe a dynamic process. This requires careful interpretation. The thin vertical lines in Figure 2.1 represent values of x that are close to 4. The corresponding horizontal lines identify the value of $f(x)$ associated with each value of x. The graph in Figure 2.1

Figure 2.1

indicates that as the values of x get closer and closer to 4 on either side of 4, the corresponding values of $f(x)$ get closer and closer to 11.

Graphs are not as accurate as calculations. We report approximations to $f(x)$ at the values given in Table 2.1.

Table 2.1

x	$f(x)$	x	$f(x)$
3.9	10.8	4.1	11.2
3.99	10.98	4.01	11.02
3.999	10.998	4.001	11.002
3.9999	10.998	4.0001	11.0002

Both the graph and the table suggest that $f(x)$ eventually gets closer and closer to a specific value 11 as x approaches 4. We say that the limit of $f(x)$ as x approaches 4 is 11 and write

$$\lim_{x \to 4} f(x) = 11.$$

Note that $f(4) = 11$. That is, the value of the function at 4 and the limit of the function as x approaches 4 are the same. Graphically, this means that there is no hole or break in the graph of f at $x = 4$. This relationship can be expressed as

$$\lim_{x \to 4} f(x) = f(4) = 11.$$

Your Practice 2.1　Let $f(x) = x + 2$. Discuss the behavior of the values of $f(x)$ when x is close to 1.

We now present an informal definition of the important concept of a limit.

Definition 2.1 (Limits)

A function $f(x)$ has a limit L at c if $f(x)$ can be made arbitrarily close to L whenever x is sufficiently close to c (but not equal to c). We denote this by

$$\lim_{x \to c} f(x) = L$$

or

$$f(x) \to L \text{ as } x \to c.$$

If $\lim_{x \to c} f(x) = L$ where L is a finite number, we say that ***the limit exists*** and that $f(x)$ converges to L. If the limit does not exist, we say that $f(x)$ ***diverges*** as x tends to c.

Example 2.1　Find $\lim_{x \to 2} x^2$.

Solution　The graph of $y = x^2$ is shown in Figure 2.2. As x approaches 2 from the left, the point on the curve moves upwards the point $(2, 4)$. Then the corresponding y value of these points approaches 4. Similarly, when x approaches 2 from the right, the point on the curve moves downwards the point $(2, 4)$ and the corresponding y value approaches 4. Therefore we have $\lim_{x \to 2} x^2 = 4$.

We can also get the result from Table 2.2 where we compute values of x^2 for x close to 2 (but not equal to 2). In the left half of the table, we let x approach 2 from the left ($x < 2$); in the right half of the table, we let x approach 2 from the right ($x > 2$). As x

approaches 2 from both sides, the function value approaches 4. We conclude that

$$\lim_{x\to 2} x^2 = 4.$$

#

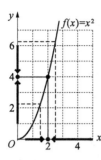

Figure 2.2

Table 2.2

x	x^2	x	x^2
1.9	3.61	2.1	4.41
1.99	3.9601	2.01	4.0401
1.999	3.996001	2.001	4.004001
1.9999	3.99960001	2.0001	4.00040001

You might ask, "why can't I just plug 2 into $y(x) = x^2$, since this would give me the correct answer, namely 4?" First, the definition of limits explicitly says that we are not allowed simply plug in the value c that x is supposed to approach. Second, $\lim_{x\to c} f(x) = f(c)$ is rather special, and we call such functions continuous at c (Continuity will be the topic of Section 2.3). Third, when we take the limit of $f(x)$ as $x \to c$, many times the function $f(x)$ is not defined at $x = c$. We give an example of this important case.

Example 2.2 Find $\lim_{x\to 3} \dfrac{x^2 - 9}{x - 3}$.

Solution We denote $f(x) = \dfrac{x^2 - 9}{x - 3}$, $x \neq 3$. Since the denominator of $\dfrac{x^2 - 9}{x - 3}$ is equal to 0 when $x = 3$, we exclude $x = 3$ from the domain of f. When $x \neq 3$, we can simplify the expression

$$f(x) = \frac{x^2 - 9}{x - 3} = \frac{(x-3)(x+3)}{(x-3)} = x + 3.$$

We can cancel the term $x - 3$, since assumed $x - 3 \neq 0$, that is $x \neq 3$. The graph of $f(x)$ is a straight line with one point deleted at $x = 3$ (Figure 2.3). We find

$$\lim_{x\to 3} \frac{x^2 - 9}{x - 3} = \lim_{x\to 3} (x + 3) = 6.$$

#

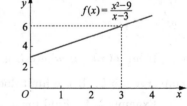

Figure 2.3

Your Practice 2.2 Find $\lim_{x\to 2} \dfrac{x^2 - 4x + 4}{x - 2}$.

2.1.1.2 One-sided limits

Example 2.3 Find $\lim_{x\to 0} \dfrac{|x|}{x}$ if possible.

Solution Let $f(x) = \dfrac{|x|}{x}$. The function $f(x)$ is defined for all real numbers except zero ($f(0) = \dfrac{|0|}{0}$ is undefined). We rewrite

$$f(x) = \frac{|x|}{x} = \begin{cases} 1, & \text{if } x > 0, \\ -1, & \text{if } x < 0. \end{cases}$$

A graph of $f(x)$ is shown in Figure 2.4. It illustrates the behavior of $f(x)$ for x near 0. Note that the absence of a solid dot on the vertical axis indicates that f is not defined when $x = 0$. When x is near 0 (on either side of 0), is $f(x)$ near one specific number? The answer is "No", because $f(x)$ is -1 for $x<0$ and 1 for $x>0$. Consequently, we say that $\lim\limits_{x \to 0} \dfrac{|x|}{x}$ does not exist. Neither $f(x)$ nor the limit of $f(x)$ exists at $x=0$.　♯

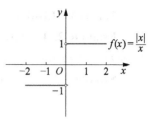

Figure 2.4

Your Practice 2.3　Find $\lim\limits_{x \to 1} \dfrac{x-1}{|x-1|}$ if possible.

In Example 2.3, we see that the values of the function $f(x)$ approach a specific number either from the left or from the right direction. So it is natural to refer to these values as "the limit from the left" and "the limit from the right". These experiences suggest that the notion of *one-sided limits* will be very useful in discussing basic limit concepts.

Definition 2.2 (One-sided Limit)

　　We call K the left-hand limit if $f(x)$ is close to K whenever x is close to, but to the left of c on the real number line, and write

$$\lim_{x \to c^-} f(x) = K.$$

We call L the right-hand limit if $f(x)$ is close to L whenever x is close to, but to the right of c on the real number line, and write

$$\lim_{x \to c^+} f(x) = L.$$

The notations $x \to c^-$ is read "x approaches c from the left" and means $x \to c$ and $x<c$, $x \to c^+$ is read "x approaches c from the right" and means $x \to c$ and $x>c$.

If no direction is specified in a limit statement, we will always assume that the limit is *two-sided or unrestricted*. Theorem 2.1 states an important relationship between one-sided limits and unrestricted limits.

Theorem 2.1 (Limit to Exist)

　　For a (two-sided) limit to exist, the limit from the left and the limit from the right must exist and be equal. That is,

$$\lim_{x \to c} f(x) = L \ if \ and \ only \ if \ \lim_{x \to c^-} f(x) = \lim_{x \to c^+} f(x) = L.$$

In Example 2.3, since

$$\lim_{x \to 0^+} \frac{|x|}{x} = 1 \ \text{and} \ \lim_{x \to 0^-} \frac{|x|}{x} = -1,$$

the function $f(x)$ has the left-hand limit -1 and the right-hand limit 1. Since the left-hand and right-hand limits are not the same, we say $\lim\limits_{x \to 0} \dfrac{|x|}{x}$ does not exist.

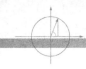

Calculus for Medicine and Pharmacy

2.1.1.3 Limits that do not exist

Example 2. 4 Given the graph of the function $f(x)$ in Figure 2. 5, discuss the behavior $f(x)$ for x near 1 and 2.

Solution We see from Figure 2. 5,

$$\lim_{x \to 1^-} f(x) = 3, \ \lim_{x \to 1^+} f(x) = 3.$$

So we say that $\lim_{x \to 1} f(x) = 3$.

$$\lim_{x \to 2^-} f(x) = 2, \ \lim_{x \to 2^+} f(x) = 5,$$

$$\lim_{x \to 2^-} f(x) \neq \lim_{x \to 2^+} f(x).$$

So $\lim_{x \to 2} f(x)$ does not exist.   #

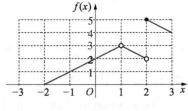

Figure 2. 5

Example 2. 5 Given the function

$$f(x) = \begin{cases} x+1, & \text{if } x<0, \\ 0, & \text{if } x=0, \\ x-1, & \text{if } x>0, \end{cases}$$

discuss the behavior of $f(x)$ for x near 0.

Solution It is shown in Figure 2. 6 that

$$\lim_{x \to 0^-} f(x) = \lim_{x \to 0^-} (x+1) = 1,$$

$$\lim_{x \to 0^+} f(x) = \lim_{x \to 0^+} (x-1) = -1.$$

Since $1 \neq -1$, the limit of $f(x)$ does not exist.   #

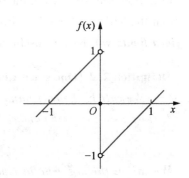

Figure 2. 6

2.1.2 Properties of Limits

Graphs are very useful tools for investing limits, especially if something unusual happens at the point in question. When functions are presented in analytically forms, it would not be practical to use the graphs every time to compute a limit. Fortunately, there are limit laws, which make computing limits much easier.

Theorem 2. 2 (Limit Laws)

Let $f(x)$ and $g(x)$ be two functions, and assume that

$$\lim_{x \to c} f(x) = L, \ \lim_{x \to c} g(x) = M,$$

where L and M are real numbers (both limits exist). Then

(1) $\lim_{x \to c} k = k$ for any constant k;

(2) $\lim_{x \to c} x = c$;

(3) (Constant rule) $\lim_{x \to c} k f(x) = k \lim_{x \to c} f(x) = kL$ for any constant k;

(4) (Sum rule) $\lim_{x \to c} [f(x) \pm g(x)] = \lim_{x \to c} f(x) \pm \lim_{x \to c} g(x) = L \pm M$;

(5) (Product rule) $\lim_{x \to c} [f(x) \cdot g(x)] = \lim_{x \to c} f(x) \cdot \lim_{x \to c} g(x) = LM$;

(6) (*Quotient rule*) $\lim\limits_{x \to c} \dfrac{f(x)}{g(x)} = \dfrac{\lim\limits_{x \to c} f(x)}{\lim\limits_{x \to c} g(x)} = \dfrac{L}{M}$ (*if* $M \neq 0$);

(7) (*Power rule*) $\lim\limits_{x \to c} [f(x)]^r = [\lim\limits_{x \to c} f(x)] = L^r$, *r is any real number* ($L > 0$ *for r even*).

Each law in Theorem 2.2 is valid if $x \to c$ is replaced everywhere by $x \to c^-$ or replaced everywhere by $x \to c^+$.

Proofs of these laws require the precise definition of the limit.

An algebraic approach

Many of the limits encountered in the calculus are routine and can be evaluated quickly with a little algebraic simplification, some intuition, and the properties of limits.

Example 2.6　Find $\lim\limits_{x \to 3} (x^2 + 3x)$.

Solution　$\lim\limits_{x \to 3} (x^2 + 3x) = \lim\limits_{x \to 3} x^2 + \lim\limits_{x \to 3} 3x$　(sum rule)

$\qquad\qquad\qquad = [\lim\limits_{x \to 3} x]^2 + 3 \lim\limits_{x \to 3} x$,　(power rule, constant rule)

so $\qquad\qquad\qquad \lim\limits_{x \to 3} (x^2 + 3x) = 3^2 + 3 \times 3 = 18$.　♯

Your Practice 2.4　Find $\lim\limits_{x \to 3} (x^2 - 4x + 3)$.

If $f(x) = x^2 + 3x$ and c is any real number, then, just as in Example 2.6,

$$\lim_{x \to c} f(x) = \lim_{x \to c} (x^2 + 3x) = c^2 + 3c = f(c).$$

So the limit can be found easily by evaluating the function value $f(x)$ at c. This simple method for finding limits is very useful, because there are many functions that satisfy the property

$$\lim_{x \to c} f(x) = f(c). \tag{2.1}$$

Either the polynomial function or the rational function satisfy Equation(2.1) as shown in the following theorem.

Theorem 2.3 (Limits of Polynomial and Rational Functions)

(1) *If* $p(x) = a_n x^n + a_{n-1} x^{n-1} + \cdots + a_0$ *is any polynomial function, then*

$$\lim_{x \to c} p(x) = p(c);$$

(2) *If* $r(x) = \dfrac{n(x)}{d(x)}$ *is any rational function with a nonzero denominator at* $x = c$, *then*

$$\lim_{x \to c} r(x) = r(c).$$

Example 2.7　Find

$$\lim_{x \to 1} \frac{2x^3 + 3x^2 + 1}{x^2 + 2x - 1}.$$

Solution　We will find

$$f(x) = \frac{2x^3 + 3x^2 + 1}{x^2 + 2x - 1}$$

is a rational function that is defined for $x=1$ (the denominator is not equal to 0 when we substitute $x=1$). Therefore, applying Theorem 2.2 to find the limit is to evaluate the function

$$\lim_{x\to 1}\frac{2x^3+3x^2+1}{x^2+2x-1}=f(1)=\frac{2\times 1^3+3\times 1^2+1}{1^2+2\times 1-1}=3.$$

\#

Example 2.8 Find

$$\lim_{x\to -1}\sqrt{2x^2+3}.$$

Solution We first write

$$\sqrt{2x^2+3}=(2x^2+3)^{1/2}.$$

Then we find

$$\lim_{x\to -1}2x^2+3=2(-1)^2+3=5.$$

Finally, according to the power rule in Theorem 2.2, we know that

$$\lim_{x\to -1}\sqrt{2x^2+3}=\sqrt{\lim_{x\to -1}(2x^2+3)}=\sqrt{5}.$$

\#

Your Practice 2.5 Find $\lim_{x\to 2}\sqrt{4x^2+1}$.

Example 2.9 Let

$$f(x)=\begin{cases}x^2+2, & \text{if } x<2,\\ x-1, & \text{if } x>2.\end{cases}$$

Find: (1) $\lim_{x\to 2^-}f(x)$; (2) $\lim_{x\to 2^+}f(x)$; (3) $\lim_{x\to 2}f(x)$; (4) $f(2)$.

Solution

(1) If $x<2$, $f(x)=x^2+2$, then

$$\lim_{x\to 2^-}f(x)=\lim_{x\to 2^-}(x^2+2)=2^2+2=6.$$

(2) If $x>2$, $f(x)=x-1$, then

$$\lim_{x\to 2^+}f(x)=\lim_{x\to 2^+}(x-1)=2-1=1.$$

(3) Since the one-sided limits are not equal, the whole limit $\lim_{x\to 2}f(x)$ does not exist.

(4) $f(2)$ does not exist because the definition of $f(x)$ does not assign a value to $f(x)$ for $x=2$, only for $x<2$ and $x>2$.

\#

Your Practice 2.6 Let

$$f(x)=\begin{cases}x^2+3, & \text{if } x<1,\\ -x+1, & \text{if } x>1.\end{cases}$$

Find: (1) $\lim_{x\to 1^-}f(x)$; (2) $\lim_{x\to 1^+}f(x)$; (3) $\lim_{x\to 1}f(x)$; (4) $f(1)$.

Exercise 2.1

Questions 1—5 are based on the graph (Figure 2.7) of the function $f(x)$. Estimate the indicated limits and function values.

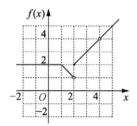

Figure 2.7

1. $f(-1)$.
2. $f(1)$.
3. (1) $\lim\limits_{x \to 0^-} f(x)$;
   (2) $\lim\limits_{x \to 0^+} f(x)$;
   (3) $\lim\limits_{x \to 0} f(x)$;
   (4) $f(0)$.
4. (1) $\lim\limits_{x \to 2^-} f(x)$;
   (2) $\lim\limits_{x \to 2^+} f(x)$;
   (3) $\lim\limits_{x \to 2} f(x)$;
   (4) $f(2)$.
5. (1) $\lim\limits_{x \to 4^-} f(x)$;
   (2) $\lim\limits_{x \to 4^+} f(x)$;
   (3) $\lim\limits_{x \to 4} f(x)$;
   (4) $f(4)$.

Use the graph (Figure 2.8) of the function $f(x)$ shown to estimate the indicated limits and function values in Questions 6—8.

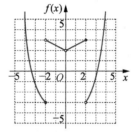

Figure 2.8

6. (1) $\lim\limits_{x \to -2^-} f(x)$;
   (2) $\lim\limits_{x \to -2^+} f(x)$;
   (3) $\lim\limits_{x \to -2} f(x)$;
   (4) $f(-2)$;
   (5) Is it possible to redefine $f(-2)$ so that $\lim\limits_{x \to -2} f(x) = f(-2)$? Explain.
7. (1) $\lim\limits_{x \to 0^-} f(x)$;
   (2) $\lim\limits_{x \to 0^+} f(x)$;
   (3) $\lim\limits_{x \to 0} f(x)$;
   (4) $f(0)$;
   (5) Is it possible to redefine $f(0)$ so that $\lim\limits_{x \to 0} f(x) = f(0)$? Explain.
8. (1) $\lim\limits_{x \to 2^-} f(x)$;
   (2) $\lim\limits_{x \to 2^+} f(x)$;
   (3) $\lim\limits_{x \to 2} f(x)$;
   (4) $f(2)$;
   (5) Is it possible to redefine $f(2)$ so that $\lim\limits_{x \to 2} f(x) = f(2)$? Explain.
9. Find each limit if it exists.
   (1) $\lim\limits_{x \to 4} 3x$;
   (2) $\lim\limits_{x \to 3} (2x+1)$;
   (3) $\lim\limits_{x \to 0} (x^2 - 4x + 2)$;
   (4) $\lim\limits_{x \to 2} (x^2 + 3x)$;

(5) $\lim\limits_{x \to -1} \dfrac{x}{x^2+5}$;

(6) $\lim\limits_{x \to -1} \dfrac{2x-4}{x^2+2x-1}$;

(7) $\lim\limits_{x \to 1} \sqrt{5x+4}$;

(8) $\lim\limits_{x \to 2} \sqrt{2x^2+3}$;

(9) $\lim\limits_{x \to 1} \sqrt[3]{2x^2+3x}$;

(10) $\lim\limits_{x \to -1} \sqrt[3]{x^2+x+3}$.

10. Let

$$f(x) = \begin{cases} 3+x^2, & \text{if } x \leqslant 0, \\ 1+x^2, & \text{if } x > 0. \end{cases}$$

Find:

(1) $\lim\limits_{x \to 0^-} f(x)$;

(2) $\lim\limits_{x \to 0^+} f(x)$;

(3) $\lim\limits_{x \to 0} f(x)$;

(4) $f(0)$.

11. Let

$$f(x) = \begin{cases} x+2, & \text{if } x \leqslant 0, \\ 2-x, & \text{if } x > 0. \end{cases}$$

Find:

(1) $\lim\limits_{x \to 0^-} f(x)$;

(2) $\lim\limits_{x \to 0^+} f(x)$;

(3) $\lim\limits_{x \to 0} f(x)$;

(4) $f(0)$.

12. Let

$$f(x) = \begin{cases} x+3, & \text{if } x < -1, \\ \sqrt{x+1}, & \text{if } x > -1. \end{cases}$$

Find:

(1) $\lim\limits_{x \to -1^-} f(x)$;

(2) $\lim\limits_{x \to -1^+} f(x)$;

(3) $\lim\limits_{x \to -1} f(x)$;

(4) $f(-1)$.

13. Let $f(x) = \dfrac{|x-1|}{x-1}$. Find:

(1) $\lim\limits_{x \to 1^-} f(x)$;

(2) $\lim\limits_{x \to 1^+} f(x)$;

(3) $\lim\limits_{x \to 1} f(x)$;

(4) $f(1)$.

14. Let $f(x) = \dfrac{x-3}{|x-3|}$. Find:

(1) $\lim\limits_{x \to 3^-} f(x)$;

(2) $\lim\limits_{x \to 3^+} f(x)$;

(3) $\lim\limits_{x \to 3} f(x)$;

(4) $f(3)$.

15. Let

$$f(x) = \begin{cases} \dfrac{x^2-9}{x+3}, & \text{if } x < 0, \\ \dfrac{x^2-9}{x-3}, & \text{if } x > 0. \end{cases}$$

Find:

(1) $\lim\limits_{x \to -3} f(x)$;

(2) $\lim\limits_{x \to 0} f(x)$;

(3) $\lim\limits_{x \to 3} f(x)$.

16. Let $f(x) = \dfrac{x^2-x-6}{x+2}$. Find:

(1) $\lim\limits_{x \to -2} f(x)$;

(2) $\lim\limits_{x \to 0} f(x)$;

(3) $\lim\limits_{x \to 3} f(x)$.

2.2 Infinite Limits

Evaluating the limit of a function at a point or evaluating the limit of a function from the right and left at a point helps us to characterize the behavior of a function around a given value. In this section, we will describe the behavior of functions that do not have finite limits.

2.2.1　Infinite Limits

Now we consider $f(x)=\dfrac{1}{x-1}$. From its graph (Figure 2.9) and Table 2.3, we note that as x approaches 1 from the right, the values of $f(x)$ are positive and become larger and larger; that is, $f(x)$ increases without bound. Mathematically, we say that the limit of $f(x)$ as x approaches 1 from the right is positive infinity. Symbolically, we express this idea as

$$\lim_{x\to 1^+}\frac{1}{x-1}=+\infty \text{ or } f(x)=\frac{1}{x-1}\to +\infty \text{ as } x\to 1^+. \tag{2.2}$$

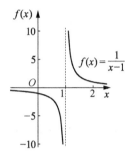

Figure 2.9

Table 2.3

x	$f(x)=\dfrac{1}{x-1}$	x	$f(x)=\dfrac{1}{x-1}$
0.9	-10	1.1	10
0.99	-100	1.01	100
0.999	-1000	1.001	1000
0.9999	-10000	1.0001	10000

Similarly, when x approaches 1 from the left, the values of $f(x)$ are negative and become larger and larger in absolute value; that is, $f(x)$ decreases through negative values without bound. We say that the limit of $f(x)$ as x approaches 1 from the left is negative infinity and denote

$$\lim_{x\to 1^-}\frac{1}{x-1}=-\infty \text{ or } f(x)=\frac{1}{x-1}\to -\infty \text{ as } x\to 1^-. \tag{2.3}$$

More generally, we define infinite limits as follows:

Definition 2.3 (Infinite Limits)

Infinite limits from the left: Let $f(x)$ be defined in an open interval (a, c).

(1) If the values of $f(x)$ increase without bound as x (where $x<c$) approaches the number c, then we say that the limit as x approaches c from the left is positive infinity and we write

$$\lim_{x\to c^-}f(x)=+\infty;$$

(2) If the values of $f(x)$ decrease without bound as x (where $x<c$) approaches the number c, then we say that the limit as x approaches c from the left is negative infinity and we write

$$\lim_{x\to c^-}f(x)=-\infty.$$

Infinite limits from the right: Let $f(x)$ be defined in an open interval (c, b).

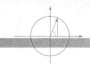

(1) *If the values of $f(x)$ increase without bound as x (where $x>c$) approaches c, then we say that the limit as x approaches c from the right is positive infinity and we write*

$$\lim_{x \to c^+} f(x) = +\infty;$$

(2) *If the values of $f(x)$ decrease without bound as x (where $x>c$) approaches c, then we say that the limit as x approaches c from the right is negative infinity and we write*

$$\lim_{x \to c^+} f(x) = -\infty.$$

Two-sided infinite limit: Let $f(x)$ be defined for all $x \neq c$ in an open interval containing c.

(1) *If the values of $f(x)$ increase without bound as x (where $x \neq c$) approaches c, then we say that the limit as x approaches c is positive infinity and we write*

$$\lim_{x \to c} f(x) = +\infty;$$

(2) *If the values of $f(x)$ decrease without bound as x (where $x \neq c$) approaches c, then we say that the limit as x approaches c is negative infinity and we write*

$$\lim_{x \to c} f(x) = -\infty.$$

Example 2.10   Find: (1) $\lim\limits_{x \to 0^-} \dfrac{1}{x}$; (2) $\lim\limits_{x \to 0^+} \dfrac{1}{x}$; (3) $\lim\limits_{x \to 0} \dfrac{1}{x}$.

Solution   We graph the function in Figure 2.10.

(1) The values of $\dfrac{1}{x}$ decrease without bound as x

approaches 0 from the left. We conclude that

$$\lim_{x \to 0^-} \frac{1}{x} = -\infty.$$

(2) The values of $\dfrac{1}{x}$ increase without bound as x

approaches 0 from the right. We conclude that

$$\lim_{x \to 0^+} \frac{1}{x} = +\infty.$$

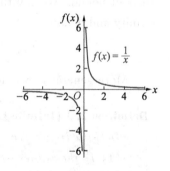

Figure 2.10

(3) Since $\lim\limits_{x \to 0^-} \dfrac{1}{x} = -\infty$ and $\lim\limits_{x \to 0^+} \dfrac{1}{x} = +\infty$, we conclude that $\lim\limits_{x \to 0} \dfrac{1}{x}$ does not exist.   #

It is important to understand that when we write statements such as $\lim\limits_{x \to c} f(x) = -\infty$ or $\lim\limits_{x \to c} f(x) = +\infty$, we are describing the behavior of the function, as we have just defined it. We are not asserting that a limit exists. For the limit of a function $f(x)$ to exist at c, it must approach a real number L as x approaches c. That is, if, for example, $\lim\limits_{x \to c} f(x) = -\infty$, we always write $\lim\limits_{x \to c} f(x) = -\infty$ rather than $\lim\limits_{x \to c} f(x)$ does not exist.

Your Practice 2.7   Let $g(x) = \dfrac{1}{2x-1}$. Construct tables for $g(x)$ as $x \to \dfrac{1}{2}^+$ and as

$x \to \frac{1}{2}^-$. Use these tables and infinite limits to discuss the behavior of $g(x)$ near $x = \frac{1}{2}$.

Your Practice 2.8   Find

$$\lim_{x \to 0} \frac{1}{x^2}.$$

Functions in the form of $f(x) = \frac{1}{(x-c)^n}$ have infinite limits as follows:

$$\lim_{x \to c} \frac{1}{(x-c)^n} = +\infty, \text{ if } n \text{ is a positive even integer;}$$

$$\lim_{x \to c^+} \frac{1}{(x-c)^n} = +\infty, \text{ if } n \text{ is a positive odd integer;}$$

$$\lim_{x \to c^-} \frac{1}{(x-c)^n} = -\infty, \text{ if } n \text{ is a positive odd integer.}$$

Facts about infinite limits

We present a few facts about infinite limits.

Facts About Infinite Limits

Given the functions $f(x)$ and $g(x)$,

$$\lim_{x \to c} f(x) = +\infty, \ \lim_{x \to c} g(x) = L$$

for some real numbers c and L,

(1) $\lim\limits_{x \to c} [f(x) \pm g(x)] = +\infty$;

(2) *if $L > 0$ then* $\lim\limits_{x \to c} [f(x)g(x)] = +\infty$;

(3) *if $L < 0$ then* $\lim\limits_{x \to c} [f(x)g(x)] = -\infty$;

(4) $\lim\limits_{x \to c} \dfrac{g(x)}{f(x)} = 0$.

Note   The above set of facts also holds for one-sided limits. They will also hold if $\lim\limits_{x \to c} f(x) = -\infty$, with a change of sign on the infinities in the first three parts.

2.2.2   Vertical Asymptote

Consider the dashed vertical line $x = 1$ in Figure 2.9. We point out that points on the graph of $\frac{1}{x-1}$ having x-coordinates very near to 1 are very close to the vertical line $x = 1$. That is, as x approaches 1, the points on the graph of $f(x)$ are closer to the line $x = 1$. The line $x = 1$ is called a vertical asymptote of the graph. We formally define a vertical asymptote as follows:

Definition 2.4 (Vertical Asymptote)

The vertical line $x = c$ is called a vertical asymptote for the graph of $y = f(x)$ if

$$f(x) \to +\infty \text{ as } x \to c^+ \text{ or } f(x) \to -\infty \text{ as } x \to c^-.$$

That is, if $f(x)$ either increases or decreases without bound as x approaches c from the right or from the left.

Now we introduce how we locate vertical asymptotes. If $f(x)$ is a polynomial function, then $\lim\limits_{x \to c} f(x)$ is equal to the real number $f(c)$ (Theorem 2.2, Section 2.1). So a polynomial function has no vertical asymptotes. Similarly, a vertical asymptote of a rational function can occur only at a zero of its denominator. Theorem 2.4 provides a simple procedure for locating the vertical asymptotes of a rational function.

> **Theorem 2.4 (Locating Vertical Asymptotes of Rational Functions)**
>
> If $f(x) = \dfrac{n(x)}{d(x)}$ is a rational function, $d(c)=0$ and $n(c)\neq0$, then the line $x=c$ is a vertical asymptote of the graph of $f(x)$.

If $f(x) = \dfrac{n(x)}{d(x)}$ and both $d(c)=0$ and $n(c)=0$, Theorem 2.4 does not apply.

Example 2.11 Let

$$f(x) = \frac{x^2}{x+1}.$$

Describe the behavior of $f(x)$ at each zero of the denominator. Use $+\infty$ and $-\infty$ when appropriate. Identify all vertical asymptotes.

Solution Let $n(x) = x^2$ and $d(x) = x+1$. We see that

$$d(x) = x+1 = 0$$

has one zero $x = -1$. We also see that

$$\lim_{x \to -1^-} \frac{x^2}{x+1} = -\infty \text{ and } \lim_{x \to -1^+} \frac{x^2}{x+1} = +\infty.$$

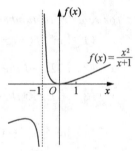

Since $d(-1)=0$ and $n(-1)=1\neq0$, according to Theorem 2.4, the line $x=-1$ is a vertical asymptote. The graph of $f(x)$ (Figure 2.11) shows the behavior at the vertical asymptote $x=-1$.   #

Figure 2.11

Your Practice 2.9 Let

$$f(x) = \frac{1}{(x+2)^2}.$$

Describe the behavior of $f(x)$ at each zero of the denominator. Use $+\infty$ and $-\infty$ when appropriate. Identify all vertical asymptotes.

Example 2.12 Let

$$f(x) = \frac{x^2+x-2}{x^2-1}.$$

Describe the behavior of $f(x)$ at each zero of the denominator. Use $+\infty$ and $-\infty$ when appropriate. Identify all vertical asymptotes.

Solution Let $n(x) = x^2+x-2$ and $d(x) = x^2-1$. Factoring the denominator, we see that

$$d(x) = x^2-1 = (x+1)(x-1)$$

has two zeros: $x=1$ and $x=-1$.

First we consider $x=-1$. Since $d(-1)=0$ and $n(-1)=-2\neq0$, according to

Theorem 2.4, the line $x=-1$ is a vertical asymptote.

Now we consider the other zero of $d(x)$, $x=1$. This time $n(1)=0$ and Theorem 2.4 can not be applied. We simplify $f(x)$ to find

$$\lim_{x\to 1} f(x) = \lim_{x\to 1} \frac{x^2+x-2}{x^2-1}$$
$$= \lim_{x\to 1} \frac{(x-1)(x+2)}{(x-1)(x+1)}$$
$$= \lim_{x\to 1} \frac{x+2}{x+1}$$
$$= \frac{3}{2}.$$

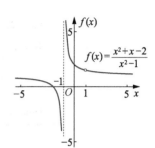

Since the limit exists as x approaches 1, $f(x)$ does not have a vertical asymptote at $x=1$. The graph of $f(x)$ (Figure 2.12) shows the behavior at the vertical asymptote $x=-1$ and also at $x=1$.   #

Figure 2.12

Your Practice 2.10　Let $f(x)=\dfrac{x-3}{x^2-4x+3}$. Describe the behavior of $f(x)$ at each zero of the denominator. Use $+\infty$ and $-\infty$ when appropriate. Identify all vertical asymptotes.

Exercise 2.2

1. The graph of the function f is shown in Figure 2.13. Find:

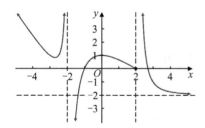

Figure 2.13

(1) $\lim\limits_{x\to -2^-} f(x)$;

(2) $\lim\limits_{x\to -2^+} f(x)$;

(3) $\lim\limits_{x\to -2} f(x)$;

(4) $\lim\limits_{x\to 2^-} f(x)$;

(5) $\lim\limits_{x\to 2^+} f(x)$;

(6) $\lim\limits_{x\to 2} f(x)$;

(7) identify any vertical asymptotes of the function.

2. The graph of the function f is shown in Figure 2.14. Find:

(1) $\lim\limits_{x\to 0^-} f(x)$;

(2) $\lim\limits_{x\to 0^+} f(x)$;

(3) $\lim\limits_{x\to 0} f(x)$;

(4) $\lim\limits_{x\to 6^-} f(x)$;

(5) $\lim\limits_{x\to 6^+} f(x)$;

(6) $\lim\limits_{x\to 6} f(x)$;

(7) identify any vertical asymptotes of the function.

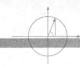

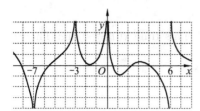

Figure 2. 14

3. Set up a table of values (Table 2. 4) to find $\lim\limits_{x\to 3}\dfrac{x-6}{(x-3)^2}$. Round to eight digits.

Table 2. 4

x	$\dfrac{x-6}{(x-3)^2}$	x	$\dfrac{x-6}{(x-3)^2}$
-0.1		0. 1	
-0.01		0. 01	
-0.001		0. 001	
-0.0001		0. 0001	

4. Set up a table of values (Table 2. 5) to find $\lim\limits_{x\to 0}\dfrac{x-1}{x^2(x+1)}$. Round to eight digits.

Table 2. 5

x	$\dfrac{x-1}{x^2(x+1)}$	x	$\dfrac{x-1}{x^2(x+1)}$
2. 9		3. 1	
2. 99		3. 01	
2. 999		3. 001	
2. 9999		3. 0001	

5. Evaluate each of the following limits. Identify any vertical asymptotes of the function $\dfrac{1}{(x-2)^3}$.

(1) $\lim\limits_{x\to 2^-}\dfrac{1}{(x-2)^3}$;

(2) $\lim\limits_{x\to 2^+}\dfrac{1}{(x-2)^3}$;

(3) $\lim\limits_{x\to 2}\dfrac{1}{(x-2)^3}$.

6. Evaluate each of the following limits. Identify any vertical asymptotes of the function $\dfrac{1}{(x-5)^4}$.

(1) $\lim\limits_{x\to 5^-}\dfrac{1}{(x-5)^4}$;

(2) $\lim\limits_{x\to 5^+}\dfrac{1}{(x-5)^4}$;

(3) $\lim\limits_{x\to 5}\dfrac{1}{(x-5)^4}$.

7. Determine the vertical asymptote of each function. If it does not exist, state that.

(1) $f(x)=\dfrac{2x-3}{x-5}$;

(2) $f(x)=\dfrac{x+4}{x-2}$;

(3) $f(x)=\dfrac{4x}{x^2-2}$;

(4) $f(x)=\dfrac{3x}{x^2-9}$;

(5) $f(x)=\dfrac{x+3}{x^2-x}$;

(6) $f(x)=\dfrac{x+2}{x^3+2x}$.

8. Given $f(x)=\dfrac{x^2+x-2}{(x-1)^3}$. Find each limit. Use $-\infty$ and $+\infty$ when appropriate. Identify any vertical asymptotes of the function.

(1) $\lim\limits_{x\to 1^-}f(x)$;

(2) $\lim\limits_{x\to 1^+}f(x)$;

(3) $\lim\limits_{x\to 1}f(x)$.

9. Given $f(x)=\dfrac{x^2+x-2}{(x-1)^2}$. Find each limit. Use $-\infty$ and $+\infty$ when appropriate. Identify any vertical asymptotes of the function.

(1) $\lim\limits_{x\to 1^-}f(x)$;

(2) $\lim\limits_{x\to 1^+}f(x)$;

(3) $\lim\limits_{x\to 1}f(x)$.

2.3 Continuity

We have noted some "nice" functions whose graph is a single unbroken curve. Such functions are called continuous. A firm understanding of continuous is essential for sketching and analyzing graphs. We will also see that continuity properties provide a simple and efficient method for solving inequalities.

2.3.1 Concept of Continuity

The graph shown in Figure 2. 15 represents a continuous function. Geometrically, this means that we can draw the graph without lifting your pencil. Thus there are no jumps in the graphs of a continuous function. That is, if we pick a point on the graph and approach it from the left and right, the values of the function approach the value of the function at that point. However, we can see that this is not true for function values near $x=c$ on the graph in Figure 2. 16 which is not continuous at that location. In Figure 2. 16, a jump occurs at $x=c$. In order to draw the graph, we must lift the pencil. The function in Figure 2. 15 is continuous, the function in Figure 2. 16 is discontinuous. Of course, this is not a definition, but it explains intuitively what we mean by a continuous function. To define continuity, we first explain what it means for a function to be continuous at the point $x=c$.

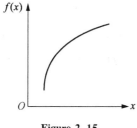

Figure 2. 15

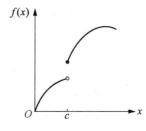

Figure 2. 16

Definition 2. 5 (Continuous at a Point)

  A function $f(x)$ is said to be continuous at $x=c$ if
$$\lim_{x \to c} f(x) = f(c).$$

In order to check whether a function is continuous at $x=c$, we therefore need to check the following three conditions.

Guideline for Checking Continuity at a Point

  A function $f(x)$ is continuous at $x=c$ if the following three conditions hold :
  (1) $f(c)$ is defined (that is, c belongs to the domain of f);
  (2) $\lim_{x \to c} f(x)$ exists (that is, left-hand limit equals to right-hand limit);
  (3) $\lim_{x \to c} f(x) = f(c)$ (that is, the numbers (1) and (2) are equal).

If any of these three conditions fails, the function is discontinuous at $x=c$.

Example 2.13   Show that $f(x)=x^2+2x-1$, $x\in\mathbf{R}$ is continuous at $x=1$.

Solution   We must check all three conditions.

(1) $f(x)$ is defined at $x=1$ since $f(1)=2$.

(2) We know that $\lim_{x\to 1} f(x)$ exists.

(3) We also know that $\lim_{x\to 1} f(x)=2=f(1)$.

Since all three conditions are satisfied, $f(x)=x^2+2x-1$ is continuous at $x=1$.   #

Example 2.14   Show that

$$f(x)=\begin{cases}\dfrac{x^2+5x+6}{x+2}, & \text{if } x\neq-2,\\ 1, & \text{if } x=-2\end{cases}$$

is continuous at $x=-2$.

Solution   Again, we need to check all three conditions.

(1) $f(x)$ is defined at $x=-2$, namely, $f(-2)=1$.

(2) To check whether

$$\lim_{x\to-2}\frac{x^2+5x+6}{x+2}$$

exists, we factor the numerator, $x^2+5x+6=(x+3)(x+2)$. Hence, for $x\neq-2$,

$$\lim_{x\to-2}\frac{x^2+5x+6}{x+2}=\lim_{x\to-2}\frac{(x+3)(x+2)}{x+2}=\lim_{x\to-2}(x+3).$$

Note that we are able to cancel the term $x+2$ since $x\neq-2$. Now, $\lim_{x\to-2}(x+3)$ exists.

(3) Finally, $\lim_{x\to-2}(x+3)=1$, which is equal to $f(-2)$.

Since all three conditions are satisfied, $f(x)$ is continuous at $x=-2$.   #

Example 2.15   Given the function

$$f(x)=\begin{cases}\dfrac{x^2-16}{x-4}, & \text{if } x\neq4,\\ k, & \text{if } x=4,\end{cases}$$

find k such that the function is continuous at $x=4$.

Solution   For $f(x)$ to be continuous at 4, we must have $\lim_{x\to 4} f(x)=f(4)$. Note that $f(4)=k$. To find $\lim_{x\to 4} f(x)$, we note that for $x\neq4$,

$$\frac{x^2-16}{x-4}=x+4.$$

Thus

$$\lim_{x\to 4} f(x)=4+4=8.$$

We see that $k=8$.   #

Your Practice 2.11   Using the definition of continuity, discuss the continuity of each function at the indicated point.

(1) $f(x)=x+2$ at $x=2$;   (2) $g(x)=\dfrac{x^2-4}{x-2}$ at $x=2$.

Example 2.16   Discuss the continuity of

$$g(x) = \frac{x^2 + 5x + 6}{x + 2}, \quad x \neq -2$$

at $x = -2$.

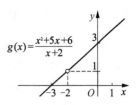

$$g(x) = \frac{x^2 + 5x + 6}{x + 2}$$

Figure 2. 17

Solution　$g(x)$ is not continuous at $x = -2$, since it is not even defined at $x = -2$ and therefore condition 1 does not hold. Figure 2. 17 shows the graph of $g(x)$.　#

Figure 2. 17 shows the graph of $g(x)$ has a "hole" at the discontinuous point $x = -2$. We can "fill" the hole to obtain a continuous function by simply assigning a "correct" value to $g(x)$ at $x = -2$, namely 1, as the function $f(x)$ in Example 2.14. In such cases where we can define a value so that $f(x)$ is continuous at that point, we can remove the discontinuity.

Formally, we say $f(x)$ has a **removable discontinuity** at $x = c$ if $\lim\limits_{x \to c} f(x)$ exists but is not equal to $f(c)$. Note that we do not require $f(c)$ to be defined in this case, that is, c need not belong to the domain of $f(x)$.

Example 2. 17　Show that $f(x) = \dfrac{|x|}{x}$, $x \neq 0$ is discontinuous at $x = 0$, and that the discontinuity at $x = 0$ cannot be removed.

Solution　Since $|x| = x$ for $x > 0$, and $|x| = -x$ for $x < 0$, we get

$$\lim_{x \to 0^+} f(x) = 1 \text{ and } \lim_{x \to 0^-} f(x) = -1.$$

The one-sided limits exist but they are not equal (which implies that $\lim\limits_{x \to 0} f(x)$ does not exist). This is enough to show that $f(x)$ is discontinuous at $x = 0$ (Figure 2. 18), as condition 2 does not hold. There is no way that we could assign a value to $f(0)$ so that the function would be continuous at $x = 0$.

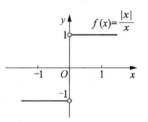

Figure 2. 18

This function does not exhibit even one-sided continuity because $f(x)$ is not defined at $x = 0$.　#

We say that $f(x)$ in Example 2. 17 has a **jump discontinuity** because the function jumps from one value to another.

Your Practice 2. 12　Show that

$$f(x) = \frac{|x - 2|}{x - 2}, \quad x \neq 2$$

is discontinuous at $x = 2$. Is this a removable or jump discontinuity?

Example 2. 18　Show that

$$f(x) = \frac{1}{x^2}, \quad x \neq 0$$

is discontinuous at $x = 0$, and that the discontinuity at $x = 0$ cannot be removed.

Solution　The graph of $f(x)$ is displayed in Figure 2. 19. $f(x) = \dfrac{1}{x^2}$ is discontinuous at $x = 0$ since $f(x)$ is not defined at $x = 0$ and hence condition 1 does not hold. We already

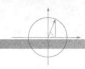

know $\lim\limits_{x\to 0}\dfrac{1}{x^2}=\infty$. Because ∞ is not a real number, we cannot assign a value to $f(0)$ so that $f(x)$ would be continuous at $x=0$. #

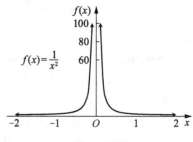

Figure 2. 19

We say that the function $f(x)$ in Example 2. 18 has an *infinite discontinuity* because the function goes off to infinity.

Example 2. 17 motivates the definition of one-sided continuity.

Definition 2. 6 (One-sided Continuity)

A function $f(x)$ is said to be continuous from the right at $x=c$ if

$$\lim_{x\to c^+} f(x)=f(c),$$

and continuous from the left at $x=c$ if

$$\lim_{x\to c^-} f(x)=f(c).$$

By this definition we can say the function $f(x)$ is continuous at $x=c$ if and only if

$$\lim_{x\to c^+} f(x)= \lim_{x\to c^-} f(x)=f(c).$$

Example 2. 19 Is the function

$$f(x)=\begin{cases} 2x+3, & \text{if } x<-2, \\ x-1, & \text{if } x\geqslant -2 \end{cases}$$

continuous at $x=-2$? Why or why not?

Solution To find out if $f(x)$ is continuous at -2, we must determine whether $\lim\limits_{x\to -2} f(x)=f(-2)$. Thus, we first note that $f(-2)=-2-1=-3$. To find $\lim\limits_{x\to -2} f(x)$, we look at left-hand and right-hand limits:

$$\lim_{x\to -2^-} f(x)=2\times(-2)+3=-1, \quad \lim_{x\to -2^+} f(x)=-2-1=-3.$$

Since $\lim\limits_{x\to -2^+} f(x)\neq \lim\limits_{x\to -2^-} f(x)$, we see that $\lim\limits_{x\to -2} f(x)$ does not exist. Thus $f(x)$ is not continuous at -2. #

One-sided limits allow us to extend the definition of continuity to closed intervals. Formally, a function is continuous on a closed interval if it is continuous in the interior of the interval and possesses the appropriate one-sided continuity at the end points of the interval.

2.3.2 Continuity Properties

The continuity of functions is preserved under the operations of addition, subtraction, multiplication and division (in the case that the function in the denominator is nonzero).

Theorem 2.5 (Operations of Continuous Functions)

If $f(x)$ and $g(x)$ are continuous at $x=c$ and k is a constant, then the following functions are also continuous at $x=c$:

(1) $f(x)\pm g(x)$;

(2) $kg(x)$;

(3) $f(x)g(x)$;

(4) $\dfrac{f(x)}{g(x)}$ (*provided* $g(c)\neq 0$).

Below we list some common functions known to be continuous on every interval inside their domains.

Theorem 2.6 (Common Types of Continuous Functions)

(1) *A constant function* $f(x)=k$, *where k is a constant, is continuous for all x.*

(2) *For n a positive integer,* $f(x)=x^n$ *is continuous for all x.*

(3) *A polynomial function is continuous for all x.*

(4) *A rational function is continuous for all x except those values that make a denominator* 0.

(5) *For n an odd positive integer greater than* 1, $\sqrt[n]{f(x)}$ *is continuous wherever* $f(x)$ *is continuous.*

(6) *For n an even positive integer,* $\sqrt[n]{f(x)}$ *is continuous wherever* $f(x)$ *is continuous and nonnegative.*

Example 2.20　Using Theorem 2.6 and the general properties of continuity, determine where each function is continuous.

(1) $f(x)=x^2+2x+1$;

(2) $f(x)=\dfrac{1}{(2x+1)(x-3)}$;

(3) $f(x)=\sqrt[3]{x^2+3x}$;

(4) $f(x)=\sqrt{x+1}$.

Solution

(1) Since f is a polynomial function, f is continuous for all x.

(2) Since f is a rational function, f is continuous for all x except $-\dfrac{1}{2}$ and 3 (values that make the denominator 0).

(3) Since $n=3$ is odd, the polynomial function $\sqrt[3]{x^2+3x}$ is continuous for all x.

(4) The polynomial function $f(x)=\sqrt{x+1}$ is continuous for all x and nonnegative for $x\geqslant -1$. Since $n=2$ is even, f is continuous for $x\geqslant -1$, or on the interval $[-1,+\infty)$.　　　　#

Your Practice 2.13　Using Theorem 2.6 and the general properties of continuity, determine where each function is continuous.

(1) $f(x)=x^3+4x+1$;

(2) $f(x)=\dfrac{x}{(x+1)(x-3)}$;

(3) $f(x) = \sqrt{x-2}$;   (4) $f(x) = \sqrt[3]{2x-1}$.

2.3.3 The Extreme Value Theorem

This subsection discusses some important properties of continuous functions on closed intervals.

Suppose that you look at the profile of the temperature in Jiangsu University for a whole year. You can easily convince yourself that there will be a time when you feel uncomfortably hot and another time when you feel uncomfortably cold. This intuitively represents the contents of the extreme value theorem: a continuous function over a closed, bounded interval has both an absolute maximum and an absolute minimum(Figure 2.20).

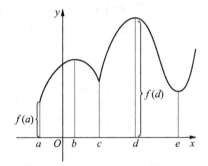

Figure 2. 20

To formalize this concept, we must introduce some terminology.

Definition 2.7

    Let f be a function defined over an interval I and let $c \in I$. We say f has an absolute maximum (or global maximum) at $x = c$ if $f(x) \leqslant f(c)$ for every x in I. The number $f(c)$ is called the maximum value of $f(x)$ on I. Similarly, $f(x)$ has an absolute minimum at c if $f(x) \geqslant f(c)$ for every x on I and the number $f(c)$ is called the minimum value of $f(x)$ on I.

If f has an absolute maximum on I at c or an absolute minimum on I at c, we say f has an absolute extremum on I at c.

Let us note two important issues regarding this definition. First, the term *absolute* here does not refer to absolute value. An absolute extremum may be positive, negative, or zero. Second, if a function f has an absolute extremum over an interval I at c, the absolute extremum is $f(c)$. The real number c is a point in the domain at which the absolute extremum occurs. For example, consider the function $f(x) = \dfrac{1}{x^2+1}$ over the interval $(-\infty, +\infty)$. Since

$$f(0) = 1 \geqslant \frac{1}{x^2+1} = f(x)$$

for all real numbers x, we say f has an absolute maximum over $(-\infty, +\infty)$ at $x = 0$. The absolute maximum is $f(0) = 1$ or occurs at $x = 0$.

A function may have both an absolute maximum and an absolute minimum, just one extremum, or neither. The following theorem gives conditions under which a function is guaranteed to possess extreme values.

Theorem 2.7 (Extreme Value Theorem)

    If f is continuous on a closed interval $[a, b]$, $-\infty < a < b < +\infty$, then f has an absolute maximum and an absolute minimum.

The proof of the extreme value theorem is beyond the scope of this text. Typically, it is proved in a course on real analysis. There are a couple of key points to note about the statement of this theorem. For the extreme value theorem to apply, the function must be continuous over a closed, bounded interval. If the interval is open or the function has even one point of discontinuity, the function may not have an absolute maximum or absolute minimum.

For example, consider the functions

$$f(x)=\begin{cases}x, & 0{\leqslant}x{\leqslant}1, \\ 3-x, & 1{<}x{\leqslant}3.\end{cases}$$

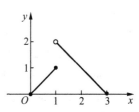

Note that $f(x)$ is defined on a closed interval, namely $[0, 3]$. However, $f(x)$ is discontinues at $x=1$, as can be seen in Figure 2.21. The graph of $f(x)$ shows that there is no value $c\in[0, 3]$ where $f(c)$ attains an absolute maximum. Though $\lim\limits_{x\to1^{+}}f(x)=2$,

Figure 2.21

the function $f(x)$ takes on value 1 at $x=1$. Hence, the function does not have an absolute maximum. It does, however, have absolute minima, namely at $x=0$ and $x=3$, where $f(x)$ takes on value 0.

Consider another example $f(x)=x$ for $0{<}x{<}1$. This function is continuous on its domain $(0, 1)$, but it is not defined on a closed interval. The function $f(x)$ attains neither an absolute maximum nor an absolute minimum. Though

$$\lim_{x\to0^{+}}f(x)=0\text{ and }\lim_{x\to1^{-}}f(x)=1$$

and $0{<}f(x){<}1$ for all $x\in(0, 1)$, there is no number c in the open interval $(0, 1)$ where $f(c)=0$ or $f(c)=1$.

2.3.4   The Intermediate Value Theorem

As you hike up a mountain, the temperature decreases with increasing elevation. Suppose the temperature at the bottom of the mountain is 70 ℉ and the temperature at the top of the mountain is 40 ℉. How do you know that at some time during your hike, you must have crossed a point where the temperature was exactly 50 ℉? Your answer will probably be something like: "To go from 70 ℉ and 40 ℉, I must have passed through 50 ℉, since 50 ℉ is between 40 ℉ and 70 ℉ and the temperature changed continuously as I hiked up the mountain."

Figure 2.22 shows the general case. If $f(x)$ is continuous and $f(a){<}L{<}f(b)$, then the graph of $f(x)$ must intersect the line $y=L$ at least once in the interval (a, b). This represents the content of the intermediate value theorem.

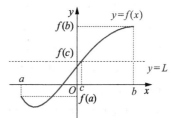

Figure 2.22

> **Theorem 2.8 (Intermediate Value Theorem)**
>
> *Suppose that $f(x)$ is continuous on the closed interval $[a, b]$. If L is any real number strictly between $f(a)$ and $f(b)$, then there exists at least one number c in the open interval (a, b) such that $f(c)=L$.*

You might wonder how the intermediate value theorem can be of any use. The theorem only gives us the existence of such a point c, it does not tell us how many such points there are or where they are located. One important application is that the theorem can be used to find approximate roots of equations, as shown in the following example. This method is called the ***method of interval bisection***. We will not pursue this method very far, because there are better methods to use once we have invoked this just to get going.

Example 2.21   Find a root of the equation $x^3 - x + 1 = 0$.

Solution   We probably do not know a formula to solve the cubic equation. The intermediate value theorem asserts: if a function f is continuous on an interval $[a, b]$ and if $f(a) < 0$ and $f(b) > 0$ (or vice versa), then there is some third point c with $a < c < b$ so that $f(c) = 0$. Now the function $f(x) = x^3 - x + 1$ is certainly continuous, so we can invoke the theorem as much as we would like. We start by finding a and b so that $f(a) < 0$ and $f(b) > 0$. For example,

$$f(-2) = -5 < 0 \text{ and } f(2) = 7 > 0.$$

So we know that there must be a number in the interval $(-2, 2)$ for which $f(c) = 0$. To locate this root with more precision, we take the midpoint of $(-2, 2)$, which is $\dfrac{-2+2}{2} = 0$, and evaluate the function at this midpoint, which is $f(0) = 1$. Thus we have

$$f(-2) < 0 \text{ and } f(0) > 0.$$

Using the intermediate value theorem again, we can conclude that there is a root in $(-2, 0)$. Since both $f(0) > 0$ and $f(2) > 0$, we cannot say anything at this point about whether or not there are roots in $(0, 2)$. Bisecting the new interval $(-2, 0)$ where we know there is a root, we compute $f(-1) = 1 > 0$. Thus, we know that there is a root in $(-2, -1)$ (and have no information about $(-1, 0)$). Repeating this procedure of bisecting and selecting a new (smaller) interval will eventually produce an interval that is small enough so that we can locate the root to any desired accuracy.   #

We give a final remark on continuous functions. Many functions in medical and pharmacy sciences are in fact discontinuous. For example, if we measure the size of a population over time, then this quantity takes on nonnegative integers only and therefore it does not change continuously. However, if the population size is large enough, increasing or decreasing the population size by one will changes the population size so slightly that it might be justified to approximate the population size by a continuous function. For example, if we measure the number of bacteria in a petri dish in millions, then the number 2.1 would correspond to 2100000 bacteria. An increase by one results in 2100001 bacteria, or if we measure the size in millions, in 2.100001, an increase of 10^{-6}.

2.3.5　Solving Inequalities Using Continuity Properties

One of the basic tools for analyzing graphs in calculus is a special line graph called a sign chart. We will make extensive use of this type of chart in later sections. In the discussion that follows, we use continuity properties to develop a simple and efficient procedure for constructing sign charts.

Suppose that a function $f(x)$ is continuous over the interval (1, 6) and $f(x)\neq 0$ for any x in (1, 6). Suppose also that $f(2)=5$, a positive number. Is it possible for $f(x)$ to be negative for any x in the interval (1, 6)? The answer is "No". If $f(5)=-3$, for example, as shown in Figure 2.23, then how would it be possible to join the points $(2, 5)$ to $(5, -3)$ with the graph of a continuous function without crossing the x-axis between 1 and 6 at least once? (Crossing the x-axis would violate our assumption that $f(x)\neq 0$ for any x in $(1,6)$)

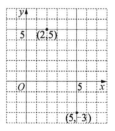

Figure 2.23

We conclude that $f(x)$ must be positive for all x in (1, 6). If $f(2)$ were negative, then, using the same type of reasoning, $f(x)$ would have to be negative over the entire interval (1, 6).

In general, if $f(x)$ is continuous and $f(x)\neq 0$ in the interval (a, b), then $f(x)$ cannot change sign in (a, b). This is the essence of Theorem 2.9.

Theorem 2.9 (Sign Properties on an Interval)

　　If $f(x)$ is continuous in (a, b) and $f(x)\neq 0$ for all x in (a, b), then either $f(x)>0$ for all x in (a, b) or $f(x)<0$ for all x in (a, b).

Theorem 2.9 provides the basis for an effective method of solving many types of inequalities. Example 2.22 illustrates the process.

Example 2.22　Solve $\dfrac{x+2}{x-1}>0$.

Solution　We start by using the left side of the inequality to form the function $f(x)=\dfrac{x+2}{x-1}$. The denominator is equal to 0 if $x=1$, and the numerator is equal to 0 if $x=-2$. So the rational function $f(x)$ is discontinuous at $x=1$ and $f(x)=0$ for $x=-2$. We plot $x=-2$ and $x=1$, which we call ***partition numbers***, on a real number line (Figure 2.24). (Note that the dot at 1 is open because the function is not defined at $x=1$)

The partition numbers 2 and 1 determine three open intervals: $(-\infty,-2)$, $(-2, 1)$, $(1,+\infty)$. The function $f(x)$ is continuous and nonzero on each of these intervals. From Theorem 2.9, we know that $f(x)$ does not change sign on any of these intervals. We can find the sign of $f(x)$ on each of the intervals by selecting a ***test number*** in each interval and evaluating $f(x)$ at that number. Since any number in each subinterval will do, we choose test numbers that are easy to evaluate: $-3,0$ and 2. Table 2.6 shows the results.

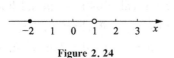

Figure 2.24

Table 2.6   Test Numbers

x	$f(x)$
-3	$\dfrac{1}{4}$
0	-2
2	4

The sign of $f(x)$ at each test number is the same as the sign of $f(x)$ over the interval containing that test number. Using this information, we construct a **sign chart** for $f(x)$ as shown in Figure 2.25. From the sign chart, we can easily write the solution of the given nonlinear inequality $\dfrac{x+2}{x-1} > 0$ is $x < -2$ or $x > 1$ (in inequality notation), or $(-\infty, -2) \cup (1, +\infty)$ (in interval notation).   #

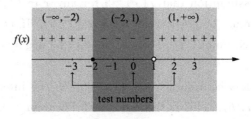

Figure 2.25

Your Practice 2.14   Solve $\dfrac{x^2-1}{x-3} < 0$.

Most of the inequalities we encounter will involve strict inequalities ($>$ or $<$). If it is necessary to solve inequalities of the form $\geq$ and $\leq$, we simply include the endpoint x of any interval if $f(x)$ is defined at x and $f(x)$ satisfies the given inequality. For example, from the sign chart Figure 2.25, the solution of the inequality $\dfrac{x+2}{x-1} \geq 0$ is

$$x \leq -2 \text{ or } x > 1, \qquad \text{(inequality notation)}$$
$$(-\infty, -2] \cup (1, +\infty). \qquad \text{(interval notation)}$$

Example 2.22 illustrates a general procedure for constructing sign charts.

Definition 2.8 (Partition Number)

A real number x is a partition number for a function $f(x)$ if $f(x)$ is discontinuous at x or $f(x) = 0$.

Suppose that p_1 and p_2 are consecutive partition numbers for $f(x)$, that is, there are no partition numbers in the open interval (p_1, p_2). Then $f(x)$ is continuous in (p_1, p_2) (since there are no points of discontinuity in that interval), so that $f(x)$ does not change sign in (p_1, p_2) (since $f(x) \neq 0$ for x in that interval). In other words, partition numbers determine open intervals on which $f(x)$ does not change sign. By using a test number from each interval, we can construct a sign chart for $f(x)$ on the real number line. It is then easy to solve the inequality $f(x) < 0$ or the inequality $f(x) > 0$.

We summarize the procedure for constructing sign charts in the following.

Procedure for Constructing Sign Charts

Given a function $f(x)$.

Step 1   Find all partition numbers of $f(x)$.

(1) Find all numbers x such that $f(x)$ is discontinuous at x. (Rational functions are discontinuous at values of x that make a denominator 0)

(2) Find all numbers x such that $f(x) = 0$. (For a rational function, this occurs where the numerator is 0 and the denominator is not 0)

Step 2   Plot the numbers found in Step 1 on a real number line, dividing the number line into intervals.

Step 3   Select a test number in each open interval determined in Step 2 and evaluate $f(x)$ at each test number to determine whether $f(x)$ is positive $(+)$ or negative $(-)$ in each interval.

Step 4   Construct a sign chart, using the real number line in Step 2. This will show the sign of $f(x)$ in each open interval.

There is an alternative to Step 3 in the procedure for constructing sign charts that may save time if the $f(x)$ is written in factored form. The key is to determine the sign of each factor in the numerator and denominator of $f(x)$. We will illustrate with Example 2.22. The partition numbers -2 and 1 divide the x-axis into three open intervals. If $x > 1$, then both the numerator and denominator are positive, so $f(x) > 0$. If $-2 < x < 1$, then the numerator is positive but the denominator is negative, so $f(x) < 0$. If $x < -2$, then both the numerator and denominator are negative, so $f(x) > 0$. Of course both approaches, the test number approach and the sign of factors approach, give the same sign chart.

Exercise 2.3

1.   Sketch a possible graph of a function that satisfies the given conditions at $x = 1$ and discuss the continuity of $f(x)$ at $x = 1$.

(1) $f(1) = 3$ and $\lim_{x \to 1} f(x) = 3$;

(2) $f(1) = -3$ and $\lim_{x \to 1} f(x) = 3$;

(3) $f(1) = 3$ and $\lim_{x \to 1} f(x) = -3$;

(4) $f(1) = -3$ and $\lim_{x \to 1} f(x) = -3$;

(5) $f(1) = -3$ and $\lim_{x \to 1^+} f(x) = 3$, and $\lim_{x \to 1^-} f(x) = -3$;

(6) $f(1) = 3$ and $\lim_{x \to 1^+} f(x) = 3$, and $\lim_{x \to 1^-} f(x) = -3$.

Questions $2 - 5$ are based on the function $f(x)$ shown in Figure 2.26. Use the graph to estimate the indicated function values and limits.

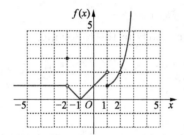

Figure 2.26

2. Find:

(1) $f(-2)$;

(2) $f(1)$;

(3) $\lim_{x \to 1^-} f(x)$;

(4) $\lim_{x \to 1^+} f(x)$;

(5) $\lim_{x \to 1} f(x)$;

(6) Is $f(x)$ continuous at $x=1$? Explain.

3. Find:

(1) $\lim_{x \to 2^-} f(x)$;

(2) $\lim_{x \to 2^+} f(x)$;

(3) $\lim_{x \to 2} f(x)$;

(4) $f(2)$;

(5) Is $f(x)$ continuous at $x=2$? Explain.

4. Find:

(1) $\lim_{x \to -2^-} f(x)$;

(2) $\lim_{x \to -2^+} f(x)$;

(3) $\lim_{x \to -2} f(x)$;

(4) $f(-2)$;

(5) Is $f(x)$ continuous at $x=-2$? Explain.

5. Find:

(1) $\lim_{x \to -1^-} f(x)$;

(2) $\lim_{x \to -1^+} f(x)$;

(3) $\lim_{x \to -1} f(x)$;

(4) $f(-1)$;

(5) Is $f(x)$ continuous at $x=-1$?

Explain.

Questions 6—8 are based on the function $f(x)$ shown in Figure 2.27. Use the graph to estimate the indicated function values and limits.

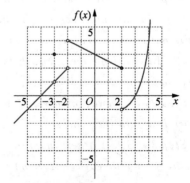

Figure 2.27

6. Find:

(1) $f(-3)$;

(2) $\lim_{x \to -3^-} f(x)$;

(3) $\lim_{x \to -3^+} f(x)$;

(4) $\lim_{x \to -3} f(x)$;

(5) Is $f(x)$ continuous at $x=-3$? Explain.

7. Find:

(1) $\lim_{x \to 2^-} f(x)$;

(2) $\lim_{x \to 2^+} f(x)$;

(3) $\lim_{x \to 2} f(x)$;

(4) $f(2)$;

(5) Is $f(x)$ continuous at $x=2$? Explain.

8. Find:

(1) $\lim_{x \to 4^-} f(x)$;

(2) $\lim_{x \to 4^+} f(x)$;

(3) $\lim_{x \to 4} f(x)$;

(4) $f(4)$;

(5) Is $f(x)$ continuous at $x=4$? Explain.

9. Use Theorem 2.4 to determine where each function is continuous.

(1) $f(x)=2x-4$;

(2) $f(x)=2-x$;

(3) $f(x)=\dfrac{x}{2x-1}$;

(4) $f(x)=\dfrac{2x}{2x-3}$;

(5) $f(x)=\dfrac{x-1}{x^2+2x-3}$;

(6) $f(x)=\dfrac{1-x^2}{x^2+1}$;

(7) $f(x)=\dfrac{x-1}{4x^2-9}$.

10. Find all partition numbers of the function.

(1) $f(x)=\dfrac{3x-1}{x-4}$;

(2) $f(x)=\dfrac{2x-4}{5x+1}$;

(3) $f(x)=\dfrac{1-x^2}{1+x^2}$;

(4) $f(x)=\dfrac{x^2-1}{x^2-9}$;

(5) $f(x)=\dfrac{x^2+4x-45}{x^2+6x}$;

(6) $f(x)=\dfrac{x^3+x}{x^2-x-42}$.

11. Use a sign chart to solve each inequality. Express answers in equality and interval notation.

(1) $x^2-x-12<0$;

(2) $x^2-2x-8<0$;

(3) $x^2+21>10x$;

(4) $x^2+7x>-10$;

(5) $x^3<3x$;

(6) $x^3-5x<0$;

(7) $\dfrac{x^2+x}{x^2-x}>0$;

(8) $\dfrac{x-4}{x^2+2x}<0$.

12. Use the graph of $f(x)$ in Figure 2.28 to determine where

(1) $f(x)>0$;

(2) $f(x)<0$.

Express answers in interval notation.

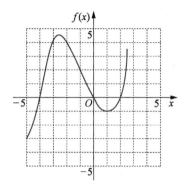

Figure 2.28

13. Graph each function in the following, locate all points of discontinuity, and discuss the behavior of $f(x)$ at these points.

(1) $f(x)=\begin{cases}2x+1, & \text{if } x<1,\\ x-1, & \text{if } x\geqslant1;\end{cases}$

(2) $f(x)=\begin{cases}x^2, & \text{if } x<1,\\ 2x, & \text{if } x\geqslant1;\end{cases}$

(3) $f(x)=\begin{cases}x^2, & \text{if } x<2,\\ 2x, & \text{if } x\geqslant2;\end{cases}$

(4) $f(x)=\begin{cases}-x, & \text{if } x<0,\\ 1, & \text{if } x=0,\\ x, & \text{if } x>0.\end{cases}$

14. Discuss the validity of each statement. If the statement is always true, explain why. If not, give a counter example.

(1) A polynomial function is continuous for all real numbers;

(2) A rational function is continuous for all but finitely many real numbers;

(3) If a function is continuous at $x=-1$ and $x=2$, then $f(x)$ is continuous at $x=0$;

(4) If a function that have no partition

numbers in the interval (a, b), then $f(x)$ is continuous in (a, b).

15. A medical laboratory raises its own rabbits. The number of rabbits $N(t)$ available at any time t depends on the number of births and deaths. When a birth or death occurs, the function N generally has a discontinuity, as shown in Figure 2. 29.

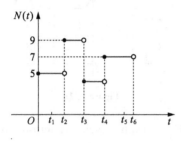

Figure 2. 29

(1) Where is the function N discontinuous?

(2) Find $\lim\limits_{t \to t_2} N(t)$ and $N(t_2)$;

(3) Find $\lim\limits_{t \to t_4} N(t)$ and $N(t_4)$.

16. Does each function satisfy the assumption of the Extreme Value Theorem? Then locate its absolute extremum if the answer is "Yes".

(1) $f(x) = 2x - 1$, $0 \leqslant x \leqslant 1$;

(2) $f(x) = \begin{cases} x, & 0 \leqslant x \leqslant 1, \\ 2 - x, & 1 < x \leqslant 2. \end{cases}$

17. Let $f(x) = x^2 - 1$, $0 \leqslant x \leqslant 2$. Show that $f(0) < 0 < f(2)$ and use the Intermediate Value Theorem to conclude that there exists a number $c \in (0, 2)$ so that $f(c) = 0$.

18. Invoke the Intermediate Value Theorem to find an interval of length 1 or less in which there is a root of $x^3 + x + 3 = 0$.

19. Invoke the Intermediate Value Theorem to find three different intervals of length 1 or less in each of which there is a root of $x^3 - 4x + 1 = 0$.

2.4　Limits at Infinity

Limits at infinity, which is opposed to infinite limits, determine the end behaviour of a function when its independent variable increases or decreases without bound.

Let us consider the behaviour of $f(x) = \dfrac{1}{x}$. As shown in Figure 2. 10, when x becomes very large and positive, the values of $f(x)$ approach zero. We say the limit as x approaches $+\infty$ of $f(x)$ is 0 and write

$$\lim_{x \to +\infty} \frac{1}{x} = 0.$$

Similarly, for $x < 0$, as the values $|x|$ get larger, the values of $f(x)$ approaches 0. We could represent this concept with notation as

$$\lim_{x \to -\infty} \frac{1}{x} = 0.$$

More generally, for any function $f(x)$, we say the limit as $x \to +\infty$ of $f(x)$ is L if $f(x)$ becomes arbitrarily close to L as long as x is sufficiently large. In that case, we write $\lim\limits_{x \to +\infty} \dfrac{1}{x} = L$. Similarly, we say the limit as $x \to -\infty$ of $f(x)$ is L if $f(x)$ becomes arbitrarily close to L as long as $x < 0$ and $|x|$ is sufficiently large. In that case, we write

$\lim\limits_{x \to -\infty} \dfrac{1}{x} = L$. We now give the definition of a function having a limit at infinity.

Definition 2.9 (Limits at Infinity)

    If the values of $f(x)$ become arbitrarily close to L as x becomes sufficiently large, then the function f has a limit at infinity and we write

$$\lim_{x \to +\infty} f(x) = L.$$

If the values of $f(x)$ becomes arbitrarily close to L for $x < 0$ as $|x|$ becomes sufficiently large, then the function f has a limit at negative infinity and we write

$$\lim_{x \to -\infty} f(x) = L.$$

Let us note that the limits laws given in Theorem 2.2 also hold if we replace $\lim\limits_{x \to c}$ with $\lim\limits_{x \to +\infty}$ or $\lim\limits_{x \to -\infty}$.

    The following two facts are very useful to find many limits at infinity.

Two Useful Limits at Infinity

    (1) *If r is a positive rational number, then*

$$\lim_{x \to +\infty} \frac{1}{x^r} = 0.$$

    (2) *If r is a positive rational number, and x^r is defined for $x < 0$, then*

$$\lim_{x \to -\infty} \frac{1}{x^r} = 0.$$

Let us think about the first part of this fact. Because r is positive, then x^r will stay in the denominator. As x increases, then x^r will also increase. So, we have one divided by an increasingly large number and the result will be increasingly small. Or, in the limit we will get zero.

    The second part is nearly identical except we need to worry about x^r being defined for negative x.

Infinity limits at infinity

Definition 2.10 (Infinity Limits at Infinity)

    Let $f(x)$ be a function defined in some interval $(a, +\infty)$. Then we say

$$\lim_{x \to +\infty} f(x) = +\infty$$

if the values of $f(x)$ can be made arbitrarily large by taking x sufficiently large.

    We give similar meaning to the statements

$$\lim_{x \to +\infty} f(x) = -\infty, \ \lim_{x \to -\infty} f(x) = -\infty, \ \lim_{x \to -\infty} f(x) = +\infty.$$

We have

$$\lim_{x \to -\infty} x^n = \infty, \ \lim_{x \to +\infty} x^{2n} = +\infty, \ \lim_{x \to -\infty} x^{2n+1} = -\infty$$

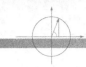

for all positive integers n.

Using this and power rule of limits in Theorem 2.2, we get that for all positive integers m, n:

$$\lim_{x \to +\infty} x^{\frac{n}{m}} = \infty, \quad \lim_{x \to -\infty} x^{\frac{2n}{2m+1}} = +\infty, \quad \lim_{x \to -\infty} x^{\frac{2n+1}{2m+1}} = -\infty.$$

We begin with the limit of rational functions.

Example 2.23 Find

$$\lim_{x \to +\infty} \frac{x}{x+1}.$$

Solution We set $f(x) = x$ and $g(x) = x+1$. Obviously, neither $\lim\limits_{x \to +\infty} f(x)$ nor $\lim\limits_{x \to +\infty} g(x)$ exists. Thus, the hypothesis of the limit laws does not hold, and we cannot use the quotient rule in Theorem 2.2. But we can divide both numerator and denominator by the largest power, that is, x, in the denominator. We find

$$\lim_{x \to +\infty} \frac{x}{x+1} = \lim_{x \to +\infty} \frac{1}{1 + \dfrac{1}{x}}.$$

Since

$$\lim_{x \to +\infty} \left(1 + \frac{1}{x}\right) = 1 + \lim_{x \to +\infty} \frac{1}{x} = 1 + 0 = 1,$$

which is nonzero, we can therefore apply the quotient rule after having done the algebraic manipulation, and find

$$\lim_{x \to +\infty} \frac{x}{x+1} = \lim_{x \to +\infty} \frac{1}{1 + \dfrac{1}{x}} = \frac{1}{1} = 1. \qquad \#$$

In Example 2.23, we computed the limit of a rational function as x tends to infinity. To find out how the limit of a rational function behaves as x tends to infinity, we will first compare the relative growth of functions of the form $y = x^n$. We find, for instance, that $x^4 > x^2$ for $x > 1$, since $\dfrac{x^4}{x^2} = x^2 \geqslant 1$ for $x \geqslant 1$. More generally, when $n \geqslant m$, we find

$$x^n \geqslant x^m \text{ for } x \geqslant 1.$$

To see why, note that $\dfrac{x^n}{x^m} = x^{n-m} \geqslant 1$, since $n - m \geqslant 0$. In fact, one can say quite a bit more: namely, if $n > m$, then x^n dominates x^m for large x, in the sense that

$$\lim_{x \to +\infty} \frac{x^n}{x^m} = \infty \text{ and } \lim_{x \to +\infty} \frac{x^n}{x^m} = 0.$$

This follows immediately if one simplifies the fractions. This property is important when we compute limits of rational functions as $x \to \infty$. We compare the following three examples.

Example 2.24 Find

$$\lim_{x \to +\infty} \frac{x^2 + 3x - 1}{x^3 - 2x + 1}.$$

Analyse To determine whether the numerator or the denominator grows faster, we look at the leading term of the polynomials in the numerator and the denominator (the leading term is the term with the largest exponent). The leading term tells us how quickly the function increases for large x.

Solution The leading term in the numerator is x^2, and the leading term in the denominator is x^3. As $x \to \infty$, the denominator grows much faster than the numerator. We therefore expect the limit to be equal to 0. We can show this by dividing both numerator and denominator by the largest power, namely x^3. We find

$$\lim_{x \to +\infty} \frac{x^2 + 3x - 1}{x^3 - 2x^2 + 1} = \lim_{x \to +\infty} \frac{\dfrac{1}{x} + \dfrac{3}{x^2} - \dfrac{1}{x^3}}{1 - \dfrac{2}{x} + \dfrac{1}{x^3}}.$$

Since

$$\lim_{x \to +\infty} \left(\frac{1}{x} + \frac{3}{x^2} - \frac{1}{x^3} \right) = 0,$$

and

$$\lim_{x \to +\infty} \left(1 - \frac{2}{x} + \frac{1}{x^3} \right) = 1,$$

which is nonzero, we can apply the quotient rule and find

$$\lim_{x \to +\infty} \frac{x^2 + 3x - 1}{x^3 - 2x^2 + 1} = \lim_{x \to +\infty} \frac{\dfrac{1}{x} + \dfrac{3}{x^2} - \dfrac{1}{x^3}}{1 - \dfrac{2}{x} + \dfrac{1}{x^3}} = \frac{\lim\limits_{x \to +\infty} \left(\dfrac{1}{x} + \dfrac{3}{x^2} - \dfrac{1}{x^3} \right)}{\lim\limits_{x \to +\infty} \left(1 - \dfrac{2}{x} + \dfrac{1}{x^3} \right)} = \frac{0}{1} = 0. \qquad \#$$

Example 2.25 Find

$$\lim_{x \to +\infty} \frac{x^3 + 4x - 1}{x^3 + x^2 + 2}.$$

Solution Both the leading terms in the numerator and the denominator are x^3. We divide the numerator and the denominator by x^3 and obtain

$$\lim_{x \to +\infty} \frac{x^3 + 4x - 1}{x^3 + x^2 + 2} = \lim_{x \to +\infty} \frac{1 + \dfrac{4}{x^2} - \dfrac{1}{x^3}}{1 + \dfrac{1}{x} + \dfrac{2}{x^3}} = \frac{\lim\limits_{x \to +\infty} \left(1 + \dfrac{4}{x^2} - \dfrac{1}{x^3} \right)}{\lim\limits_{x \to +\infty} \left(1 + \dfrac{1}{x} + \dfrac{2}{x^3} \right)} = \frac{1}{1} = 1. \qquad \#$$

Example 2.26 Find

$$\lim_{x \to +\infty} \frac{x^4 + 2x - 5}{x^2 + x + 2}.$$

Solution The leading term in the numerator is x^4, and the leading term in the denominator is x^2. As $x \to +\infty$, the numerator grows much faster than the denominator. We divide both the numerator and the denominator by x^2 and obtain

$$\lim_{x \to +\infty} \frac{x^4 + 2x - 5}{x^2 + x + 2} = \lim_{x \to +\infty} \frac{x^2 + \dfrac{2}{x} - \dfrac{5}{x^2}}{1 + \dfrac{1}{x} + \dfrac{2}{x^2}}.$$

As

$$\lim_{x \to +\infty} x^2 = +\infty, \quad \lim_{x \to +\infty} \left(\frac{2}{x} - \frac{5}{x^2} \right) = 0,$$

we have

$$\lim_{x \to +\infty} \left(x^2 + \frac{2}{x} - \frac{5}{x^2} \right) = +\infty.$$

By using the limits laws we get

$$\lim_{x \to +\infty} \frac{1}{1 + \frac{1}{x} + \frac{2}{x^2}} = \frac{1}{\lim_{x \to +\infty} \left(1 + \frac{1}{x} + \frac{2}{x^2} \right)} = \frac{1}{1} = 1 > 0.$$

Then using the facts of infinite limits we obtain

$$\lim_{x \to +\infty} \frac{x^4 + 2x - 5}{x^2 + x + 2} = \lim_{x \to +\infty} \left(x^2 + \frac{2}{x} - \frac{5}{x^2} \right) \frac{1}{1 + \frac{1}{x} + \frac{2}{x^2}} = +\infty. \qquad \#$$

Your Practice 2.15 Evaluate $\lim_{x \to +\infty} \frac{4x^2 + 3}{5 - 2x}$.

Let us summarize our findings.

Limits at Infinity for Rational Functions

If $f(x)$ is a rational function, we find that

$$\lim_{x \to \infty} \frac{a_m x^m + a_{m-1} x^{m-1} + \cdots + a_1 x + a_0}{b_n x^n + b_{n-1} x^{n-1} + \cdots + b_1 x + b_0} = \begin{cases} 0, & m < n, \\ \dfrac{a_m}{b_n}, & m = n, \\ \pm\infty, & m > n. \end{cases}$$

Example 2.27 Evaluate $\lim_{x \to +\infty} \frac{\sqrt{4x^2 + 3}}{2 - 5x}$.

Solution We write

$$\lim_{x \to +\infty} \frac{\sqrt{4x^2 + 3}}{2 - 5x} = \lim_{x \to +\infty} \frac{\sqrt{x^2 \left(4 + \frac{3}{x^2} \right)}}{2 - 5x} = \lim_{x \to +\infty} \frac{x}{2 - 5x} \sqrt{4 + \frac{3}{x^2}}.$$

Applying the limits results of rational functions, we have

$$\lim_{x \to +\infty} \frac{x}{2 - 5x} = \frac{1}{-5} = -\frac{1}{5}.$$

We also have

$$\lim_{x \to +\infty} \sqrt{4 + \frac{3}{x^2}} = \sqrt{\lim_{x \to +\infty} \left(4 + \frac{3}{x^2} \right)} = \sqrt{4 + 0} = 2.$$

Therefore,

$$\lim_{x \to +\infty} \frac{\sqrt{4x^2 + 3}}{2 - 5x} = -\frac{1}{5} \times 2 = -\frac{2}{5}.$$

Another way to solve this problem is to treat the square root function as a polynomial. As x is very large and positive, the values of $4x^2 + 3$ is approximately its leading term $4x^2$. Thus the leading term of the numerate can be said to be $\sqrt{4x^2} = 2x$. As the leading term of denominator is $-5x$, which is the same degree as the numerate, the limit required is the quotient of coefficients the two leading terms: $\frac{2}{-5} = -\frac{2}{5}$. $\qquad \#$

Your Practice 2.16　Compute:

(1) $\lim\limits_{x \to +\infty} \dfrac{1-x+x^2}{3x+x^2}$;

(2) $\lim\limits_{x \to +\infty} \dfrac{3x^2+4}{4x-1}$.

2.4.1　Horizontal Asymptotes

Figure 2.30 shows the graph of the rational function

$$f(x) = \frac{x^2+x+2}{x^2-1}.$$

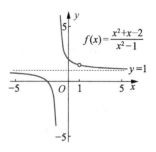

Note that function values get closer and closer to 1 as x is negative and $|x|$ is very large, meaning that

$$\lim_{x \to -\infty} f(x) = 1.$$

The line $y=1$ is called a horizontal asymptote.

Figure 2.30

Definition 2.11 (Horizontal Asymptote)

　The line $y=b$ is a horizontal asymptote if either or both of the following limit statements is true:

$$\lim_{x \to -\infty} f(x) = b \text{ and } \lim_{x \to +\infty} f(x) = b.$$

In Figure 2.31, we see two ways in which horizontal asymptotes can occur.

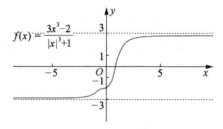

Figure 2.31

The graph of a rational function may or may not cross a horizontal asymptote. Horizontal asymptotes are found by determining the limit at infinity of a rational function. Thus, horizontal asymptotes occur when the degree of the numerator is less than or equal to that of the denominator (the degree of a polynomial in one variable is highest of that variable).

Example 2.28　Determine the horizontal asymptote of the function given by

$$f(x) = \frac{3x-4}{x}.$$

Solution　To find the horizontal asymptote, we consider

$$\lim_{x \to +\infty} f(x) = \lim_{x \to +\infty} \frac{3x-4}{x} = \frac{3}{1} = 1,$$

by applying the limits at infinity of rational functions.

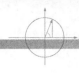

In a similar manner, it can be shown that

$$\lim_{x \to -\infty} f(x) = 3.$$

Therefore, the line $y = 3$ is a horizontal asymptote. #

Your Practice 2.17 Determine the horizontal asymptote of the function given by

$$f(x) = \frac{2x+5}{x}.$$

Example 2.29 Determine the horizontal asymptote of the function given by

$$f(x) = \frac{2x^2 + x + 1}{3x^2 - 2x + 4}.$$

Solution Note the degree of the numerator is the same as that of the denominator. We divide the numerator and the denominator by x^2 and find the limit as $|x|$ gets larger and larger:

$$f(x) = \frac{3x^2 + x + 1}{2x^2 - 2x + 4} = \frac{3 + \dfrac{1}{x} + \dfrac{1}{x^2}}{2 - \dfrac{2}{x} + \dfrac{4}{x^2}}.$$

As $|x|$ gets very large, the numerator approaches 3 and the denominator approaches 2. Therefore, the value of the function gets very close to $\frac{3}{2}$. Thus

$$\lim_{x \to -\infty} f(x) = \frac{3}{2} \text{ and } \lim_{x \to +\infty} f(x) = \frac{3}{2}.$$

We conclude that the line $y = \frac{3}{2}$ is a horizontal asymptote. #

We make the following conclusion from Examples 2.28 and 2.29.

Conclusion *For a rational function, when the degree of the numerator is the same as that of the denominator, the line $y = \frac{a}{b}$ is a horizontal asymptote, where a is the leading coefficient of the numerator and b is the leading coefficient of the denominator.*

Your Practice 2.18 Determine the horizontal asymptote of the function given by

$$f(x) = \frac{x^2 + 3x + 1}{2x^2 - 2x - 5}.$$

Example 2.30 Determine the horizontal asymptote of the function given by

$$f(x) = \frac{x+1}{x^2 - 2x + 3}.$$

Solution Since the degree of the numerator is less than that of the denominator, there is a horizontal asymptote. To identify that asymptote, we divide both the numerator and denominator by the highest power of x in the denominator, and find the limits as $|x| \to +\infty$:

$$f(x) = \frac{x+1}{x^2 - 2x + 3} = \frac{\dfrac{1}{x} + \dfrac{1}{x^2}}{1 - \dfrac{2}{x} + \dfrac{3}{x^2}}.$$

As x gets smaller and smaller negatively, $|x|$ gets larger and larger. Similarly, as x

gets larger and larger, $|x|$ become large. Thus, the numerator of $f(x)$ approaches 0 as its denominator approaches 1. Hence, the entire expression takes on values ever closer to 0. That is, we have

$$\lim_{x \to -\infty} \frac{x+1}{x^2-2x+3} = \lim_{x \to -\infty} \frac{\dfrac{1}{x}+\dfrac{1}{x^2}}{1-\dfrac{2}{x}+\dfrac{3}{x^2}} = \frac{0+0}{1-0+0} = 0.$$

$$\lim_{x \to +\infty} \frac{x+1}{x^2-2x+3} = \lim_{x \to +\infty} \frac{\dfrac{1}{x}+\dfrac{1}{x^2}}{1-\dfrac{2}{x}+\dfrac{3}{x^2}} = \frac{0+0}{1-0+0} = 0.$$

Therefore, the x-axis, or equivalently, the line $y=0$, is a horizontal asymptote.   ♯

Conclusion *Given a rational function, when the degree of the numerator is less than that of the denominator, the line $y=0$ is a horizontal asymptote.*

Your Practice 2.19 Determine the horizontal asymptote of the function given by

$$f(x) = \frac{x^2+1}{2x^3-x^2-5x}.$$

2.4.2 Exponential Functions

Cell division is an interesting phenomenon, and the speed with which new cells are created is astonishing. For example, when a certain cell divides, one divides into two, and two divides into four, etc. Therefore, the functional relationship between the number of new cells y obtained from the x division is $y=2^x$. The function above is the form of the exponential function, and the independent variable is a power. So let us consider such functions and many of their applications.

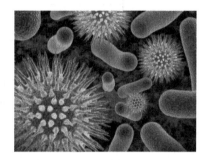

Figure 2.32

For $b>0$, the usual laws of exponents, such as

$$b^x b^y = b^{x+y}, \; b^x \div b^y = b^{x-y}, \; (b^x)^y = b^{xy}, \; b^{-x} = \frac{1}{b^x}$$

can be applied to real number exponents. Moreover, the function obtained $f(x)=b^x$, is continuous.

Definition 2.12 (Exponential Function)

An exponential function $f(x)$ is given by

$$f(x)=b^x$$

where x is any real number, $b>0$ and $b \neq 1$. The number b is called the base.

The following are examples of exponential functions:

$$f(x)=2^x, \; f(x)=\left(\frac{1}{2}\right)^x, \; f(x)=(0.3)^x.$$

Note that in contrast to power function like $y=x^2$ and $y=x^3$, an exponential function has the variable in the exponent, not as the base. For now, let us consider their graphs.

Example 2.31 Graph $y=2^x$.

Solution First we find some function values. Note that $y=2^x$ is always positive:

$$x=0, \qquad y=2^0=1;$$

$$x=\frac{1}{2}, \qquad y=2^{\frac{1}{2}}=\sqrt{2}\approx1.4;$$

$$x=1, \qquad y=2^1=2;$$

$$x=2, \qquad y=2^2=4;$$

$$x=3, \qquad y=2^3=8;$$

$$x=-1, \qquad y=2^{-1}=\frac{1}{2};$$

$$x=-2, \qquad y=2^{-2}=\frac{1}{2^2}=\frac{1}{4}.$$

We write these values in Table 2.7.

Table 2.7

x	0	$\frac{1}{2}$	1	2	3	-1	-2
$y=2^x$	1	1.4	2	4	8	$\frac{1}{2}$	$\frac{1}{4}$

Next we plot the points and connect them with a smooth curve, as shown in Figure 2.33. The graph is continuous, increasing without bound, and concave up. #

Your Practice 2.20 Graph $y=\left(\frac{1}{2}\right)^x$.

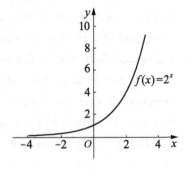

Figure 2.33

After we graph $y=\left(\frac{1}{2}\right)^x$, we can find that the graph

of $y=\left(\frac{1}{2}\right)^x$ is reflection of the graph of $f(x)=2^x$ across

the y-axis. Thus we expect the graphs of $y=\left(\frac{1}{2}\right)^x$ and

$f(x)=2$ to be symmetric with respect to the y-axis.

There is a very important exponential function that arises naturally in many places. This function is called **the natural exponential function**. We will give the definition of its base, the natural number e, using a special limit.

Consider the limit

$$\lim_{h\to0}\frac{b^h-1}{h}.$$

Note that the quotient rule of limits fails to be satisfied since the denominator tends to zero. Until now, we have not been able to calculate this limit.

However, we can look at some examples. Consider $b=2$ and $b=3$ (Tables 2.8 and 2.9):

Tables 2.8

h	$\dfrac{2^h-1}{h}$	h	$\dfrac{2^h-1}{h}$
-1	0.5	1	1
-0.1	0.6700	0.1	0.7177
-0.01	0.6910	0.01	0.6956
-0.001	0.6929	0.001	0.6934
-0.0001	0.6931	0.0001	0.6932
-0.00001	0.6932	0.00001	0.6932

Tables 2.9

h	$\dfrac{3^h-1}{h}$	h	$\dfrac{3^h-1}{h}$
-1	0.6667	1	2
-0.1	1.0404	0.1	1.1612
-0.01	1.0926	0.01	1.1047
-0.001	1.0980	0.001	1.0992
-0.0001	1.0986	0.0001	1.0987
-0.00001	1.0986	0.00001	1.0986

It turns out that

$$\lim_{h\to 0}\frac{2^h-1}{h}\approx 0.7 \text{ and } \lim_{h\to 0}\frac{3^h-1}{h}\approx 1.1.$$

Following this way, we will find that the limit varies directly with the base b: bigger b, bigger limit; smaller b, smaller limit. As we can already see, some of these limits will be less than 1 and some larger than 1. Somewhere between $b=2$ and $b=3$ the limit will be exactly 1. This happens when the base to be the natural number e:

$$b=e\approx 2.718281828459045\cdots$$

Figure 2.34 shows the graph of $f(x)=e^x$. There are in fact a variety of ways to define e. We will define the number e by this property in the next definition:

Definition 2.13 (The Natural Number e)

The number denoted by e, *called Euler's number*, *is defined to be the number satisfying the following relation*:

$$\lim_{h\to 0}\frac{e^h-1}{h}=1.$$

Rational function are not only function that involve limits as x tends to $+\infty$ (or $-\infty$). Many important applications in biology involve exponential functions. We will use the following result repeatedly and it is one of the important limits.

$$\boxed{\lim_{x\to +\infty} e^{-x}=0}$$

The graph of $f(x)=e^{-x}$ is given in Figure 2.35.

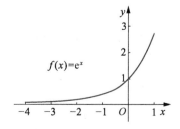

Figure 2.34

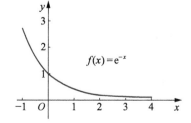

Figure 2.35

Example 2. 32 (*Logistic Growth*)   The logistic curve describes the density of a population over time, where the rate of growth depends on the population size. The per capita rate of growth decreases with increasing population size. If $N(t)$ denotes the size of the population at time t, then the logistic curve is given by

$$N(t)=\frac{K}{1+\left[\dfrac{K}{N(0)}-1\right]e^{-rt}} \quad \text{for } t \geqslant 0.$$

The parameters K and r are positive numbers that describe the population dynamics. The graph of $N(t)$ is shown in Figure 2. 36 with $K=100$, $N(0)=10$ and $r=1$.

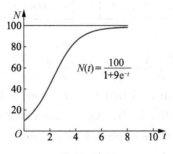

Figure 2. 36

We are interested in the long-term behavior of the population evolving according to the logistic growth curve. That is, we want to investigate what happens to $N(t)$ as $t \to \infty$. We find that

$$\lim_{t \to +\infty} \frac{K}{1+\left[\dfrac{K}{N(0)}-1\right]e^{-rt}}=K,$$

since

$$\lim_{t \to +\infty} e^{-rt}=0.$$

This value K which the population size approaches is called the **carrying capacity** of the population.

Exercise 2.4

1. Compute:

(1) $a^2 \cdot a^3$;

(2) $a^{\frac{1}{2}} \cdot a^{\frac{1}{3}}$;

(3) $a^3 \div a^2$;

(4) $a^4 \div a^5$;

(5) $(a^2)^3$;

(6) $(a^2)^{\frac{3}{2}}$;

(7) $(a^{-2})^{-3}$;

(8) $(a^2 \cdot a^3)^2$.

2. Graph the functions:

(1) $y=3^x$;

(2) $y=\left(\dfrac{1}{3}\right)^x$;

(3) $y=0.4^x$;

(4) $y=\left(\dfrac{3}{2}\right)^x$.

3. Solve equation $x^2 e^{-x} - 9e^{-x} = 0$ for x.

4. Solve equation $e^{3x-2} - e = 0$ for x.

5. Marine life depends on the microscopic plant life that exists in the photic zone, a zone that goes to a depth where only 1% of surface light remains. In some waters with a great deal of sediment, the photic zone may go down only 15 to 20 feet. In some murky harbors, the intensity of light d feet below the surface is given approximately by

$$I = I_0 e^{-0.23d}.$$

What percentage of the surface light will reach a depth of

(1) 10 feet;

(2) 20 feet?

6. Light intensity I relative to depth d (in feet) for one of the clearest bodies of water in the world, the Sargasso Sea in the West Indies, can be approximated by

$$I = I_0 e^{-0.00942d}$$

where I_0 is the intensity of light at the surface. What percentage of the surface light will reach a depth of

(1) 50 feet;

(2) 100 feet?

7. Evaluate the limits:

(1) $\lim\limits_{x\to+\infty} \dfrac{2x^2 - 2x + 5}{x^3 - 2x + 1}$;

(2) $\lim\limits_{x\to+\infty} \dfrac{x^2 + 3}{2x^3 - 2x + 2}$;

(3) $\lim\limits_{x\to+\infty} \dfrac{x^3 + 1}{x - 2}$;

(4) $\lim\limits_{x\to+\infty} \dfrac{2x - 1}{3x + 4}$;

(5) $\lim\limits_{x\to+\infty} \dfrac{3x^4 - x^3 + 1}{x^4 + 4}$;

(6) $\lim\limits_{x\to+\infty} \dfrac{5x^3 - 1}{4x^4 + 1}$.

8. Determine the horizontal asymptote of each function. If it does not exist, state that.

(1) $f(x) = \dfrac{6x + 2}{2x + 3}$;

(2) $f(x) = \dfrac{x^2 + 2}{6x^2 + 1}$;

(3) $f(x) = \dfrac{4x}{x^2 + 1}$;

(4) $f(x) = \dfrac{2x}{3x^3 + x^2}$;

(5) $f(x) = 5 - \dfrac{3}{x}$;

(6) $f(x) = 4 + \dfrac{2}{x}$.

9. Suppose the size of a population at time t is given by

$$N(t) = \dfrac{400t}{3 + t}, \quad t \geqslant 0.$$

Determine the size of the population as $t \to +\infty$. We call the limit **limiting population size**.

10. Suppose that the value V of the inventory at Fido's Pet Supply decreases, or depreciates, with time t, in months, where

$$V(t) = 50 - \dfrac{25t^2}{(t + 2)^2}.$$

(1) Find $V(0)$, $V(5)$, $V(10)$;

(2) Does there seem to be a value below which $V(t)$ will never fall? Explain.

11. Since 1970, the purchasing power of the dollar, as measured by consumer prices, can be modeled by the function

$$P(x) = \dfrac{2.632}{1 + 0.116x},$$

where x is the number of years since 1970. (Source: U. S. Bureau of Economic Analysis.)

(1) Find $P(10)$, $P(20)$, $P(40)$;

(2) When was the purchasing power

$0.50?

(3) Find $\lim\limits_{x \to +\infty} P(x)$.

12. After an injection, the amount of a medication A, in cubic centimeters (cc), in the bloodstream decreases with time t, in hours. Suppose that under certain conditions A is given by

$$A(t) = \frac{A_0}{t^2 + 1},$$

where A_0 is the initial amount of the medication. Assume that an intial amount of 100 cc is injected.

(1) Find $A(0)$, $A(1)$, $A(2)$, $A(4)$, $A(7)$.

(2) According to this function, does the medication ever completely leave the bloodstream? Explain your answer.

2.5　Precise Definition of Limits

In this section we are going to give the precise mathematical definition of the three kinds of limits in this chapter. We will discuss the precise definition of limits at finite points that have finite values, limits that are infinity and limits at infinity. The precise mathematical definition of continuity will also be given.

Quantifying Closeness

Before stating the formal epsilon-delta definition of a limit, we must introduce a few preliminary ideas.

Recall that the distance between two points a and b on a number line is given by $|a - b|$. Thus the statement $|f(x) - L| < \varepsilon$ may be interpreted as:

The distance between $f(x)$ and L is less than ε;

the statement $0 < |x - c| < \delta$ may be interpreted as:

$x \neq c$ and the distance between x and c is less than δ.

Look at the following equivalences for absolute value: The statement $|f(x) - L| < \varepsilon$ is equivalent to $L - \varepsilon < f(x) < L + \varepsilon$; the statement $0 < |x - c| < \delta$ is equivalent to $c - \delta < x < c + \delta$ and $x \neq c$.

With these clarifications, we can state the formal epsilon-delta definition of the limit.

Let us start this section with the definition of a limit at a finite point that has a finite value.

2.5.1　Limits at Finite Points that Have Finite Values

Definition 2.14

Let $f(x)$ be defined for all $x \neq c$ over an open interval containing c. Let L be a real number. Then

$$\lim_{x \to c} f(x) = L$$

if for every $\varepsilon > 0$, there exists a $\delta > 0$, such that if $0 < |x - c| < \delta$, then $|f(x) - L| < \varepsilon$.

It becomes easier to understand this definition if we break it down phrase by phrase. The statement itself involves something called a universal quantifier (for every $\varepsilon > 0$), an existential quantifier (there exists a $\delta > 0$), and, last, a conditional statement (if $0 < |x-c| < \delta$, then $|f(x)-L| < \varepsilon$). We can get a better handle on this definition by looking at the definition geometrically.

Starting from the universal quantifier, we pick any number $\varepsilon > 0$. We can get the graph (Figure 2.37) and sketch two horizontal lines at $L+\varepsilon$ and $L-\varepsilon$ to make a horizontal region, i. e. between $L-\varepsilon$ and $L+\varepsilon$. Then there is another number $\delta > 0$, which we will need to determine its existence, that will allow us to add in two vertical lines at $c-\delta$ and $c+\delta$. If we take any x in the vertical region bounded by the dashed lines, i. e. between

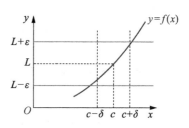

Figure 2.37

$c-\delta$ and $c+\delta$, then this x will be closer to c than either of $c-\delta$ and $c+\delta$, or
$$|x-c| < \delta.$$
If we now identify the point on the graph that our choice of x gives, then this point on the graph will lie in the intersection of the vertical and horizontal region. This means that this function value $f(x)$ will be closer to L than either of $L+\varepsilon$ and $L-\varepsilon$, or
$$|f(x)-L| < \varepsilon.$$
If we take any value of x in the vertical region then the graph for those values of x will lie in the horizontal region.

Notice that there are actually an infinite number of possible δ's that we can choose. What we need to do is to give the existence of δ.

Example 2.33　Use the precise definition of the limit to prove
$$\lim_{x \to c} x = c.$$

Proof　Let $\varepsilon > 0$ be any number. Now according to the definition of the limit, if this limit is to be true we will need to find some other number $\delta > 0$ so that the following statement will be true:
$$|x-c| < \varepsilon \quad \text{whenever} \quad 0 < |x-c| < \delta.$$
So, if we choose $\delta = \varepsilon$ we should get what we want.

We next need to verify that our choice of δ will give us what we want. Verification is in fact pretty much the same work as what we did to get our guess. First, let $\varepsilon > 0$ be any number and then choose $\delta = \varepsilon$. Now, assume that $0 < |x-c| < \delta$. By choosing x to satisfy this we will get
$$|x-c| < \varepsilon,$$
and according to our definition this means that,
$$\lim_{x \to c} x = c. \qquad\qquad \#$$

Next, give the precise definitions for the right-and-left-handed limits.

Definition 2.15 (One-side Limits)

For the right-hand limit we say that,

$$\lim_{x \to c^+} f(x) = L$$

if for every $\varepsilon > 0$, *there exists a* $\delta > 0$, *such that*

$$|f(x) - L| < \varepsilon \quad whenever \quad 0 < x - c < \delta.$$

For the left-hand limit we say that,

$$\lim_{x \to c^-} f(x) = L$$

if for every $\varepsilon > 0$, *there exists a* $\delta > 0$, *such that*

$$|f(x) - L| < \varepsilon \quad whenever \quad \delta < x - c < 0.$$

Example 2.34 Prove that $\lim\limits_{x \to 2^+} \sqrt{x-2} = 0$.

Proof Let $\varepsilon > 0$. We want to find a δ so that

$$|\sqrt{x-2} - 0| < \varepsilon \quad whenever \quad 0 < x - 2 < \delta.$$

We manipulate $|\sqrt{x-2} - 0| < \varepsilon$ to get $|x-2| < \varepsilon^2$ or, equivalently, $0 < x - 2 < \varepsilon^2$. It seems that we can take $\delta = \varepsilon^2$.

Let us verify this. Let $\varepsilon > 0$ be any number and chose $\delta = \varepsilon^2$. Assume $0 < x - 2 < \delta$. Thus, $0 < x - 2 < \varepsilon^2$. Hence, $0 < \sqrt{x-2} < \varepsilon$. Finally, $|\sqrt{x-2} - 0| < \varepsilon$. Therefore, $\lim\limits_{x \to 2^+} \sqrt{x-2} = 0$. #

2.5.2 Infinite Limits

Here are two definitions that we need to cover both possibilities, limits that are positive infinity and limits that are negative infinity.

Definition 2.16 (Infinity Limits)

If $f(x)$ *is defined on an interval that contains* $x = c$, *except possibly at* $x = c$, *then we say that,*

$$\lim_{x \to c} f(x) = +\infty$$

if for every number $M > 0$, *there is some number* $\delta > 0$, *such that*

$$f(x) > M \quad whenever \quad 0 < |x - c| < \delta.$$

We say that,

$$\lim_{x \to c} f(x) = -\infty$$

if for every number $M > 0$, *there is some number* $\delta > 0$, *such that*

$$f(x) < -M \quad whenever \quad 0 < |x - c| < \delta.$$

The definition of $\lim\limits_{x \to c} f(x) = +\infty$ tells us that no matter how large we choose M to be we can always find an interval around $x = c$, given by $0 < |x - c| < \delta$ for some number δ, so that as long as we stay within that interval the graph of the function will be above the line

$y=M$, as shown in Figure 2.38.

Also note that we do not need the function to actually exist at $x=c$ in order to hold the definition.

Note that we could also write down definitions for one-sided limits that are infinity if we wanted to.

Proving Limit Laws

We now demonstrate how to use the epsilon-delta definition of a limit to construct a rigorous proof of one of the limit laws. We first review the triangle inequality

$$|a+b| \leqslant |a| + |b|.$$

This key property of absolute value is used at a key point of the proof.

2.5.3　Definition of Limits at Infinity

We give a definition of limits at infinity and another for negative infinity.

Definition 2.17 (Limits at Infinity)

If $f(x)$ is defined on $x>K$ for some K, then we say that,

$$\lim_{x \to +\infty} f(x) = L$$

if for every number $\varepsilon>0$, there is some number $M>0$, such that

$$|f(x)-L|<\varepsilon \quad whenever \quad x>M.$$

If $f(x)$ is defined on $x<K$ for some K, then we say that,

$$\lim_{x \to -\infty} f(x) = L$$

if for every number $\varepsilon>0$, there is some number $M>0$, such that

$$|f(x)-L|<\varepsilon \quad whenever \quad x<-M.$$

Definition of $\lim_{x \to +\infty} f(x) = L$ tells us that no matter how close to L we want to get, mathematically this is given by $|f(x)-L|<\varepsilon$ for any chosen ε, we can determine another number M such that provided we take any x bigger than M, then the graph of the function for that x will be closer to L than either $L-\varepsilon$ and $L+\varepsilon$, or, in other words, the graph will be in the horizontal region bounded by the lines $y=L-\varepsilon$ and $y=L+\varepsilon$ (Figure 2.39).

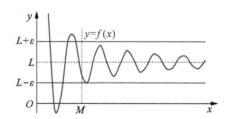

Figure 2.39

Exercise 2.5

In questions $1-4$, write the appro-　priate $\varepsilon-\delta$ definition for each of the given statements.

1. $\lim\limits_{x \to a} f(x) = M.$

2. $\lim\limits_{u \to b} g(u) = N.$

3. $\lim\limits_{t \to c} h(t) = P.$

4. $\lim\limits_{v \to s} g(v) = Q.$

In questions $5-11$, use the precise definition of limit to prove the given limits.

5. $\lim\limits_{x \to 1} 3x + 2 = 5.$

6. $\lim\limits_{x \to 1} \dfrac{x^2 - 1}{x - 1} = 2.$

7. $\lim\limits_{x \to 0} x^2 = 0.$

8. $\lim\limits_{x \to 4^+} \sqrt{x - 4} = 0.$

9. $\lim\limits_{x \to 3^-} \sqrt{3 - x} = 0.$

10. $\lim\limits_{x \to 0} \dfrac{1}{x^2} = +\infty.$

11. $\lim\limits_{x \to 1} -\dfrac{1}{(x - 1)^2} = -\infty.$

12. Use the precise definition of limits to prove

$$\lim\limits_{x \to c} [k f(x)] = k \lim\limits_{x \to c} f(x)$$

for any real constant k.

13. Use the precise definition of limits to prove

$$\lim\limits_{x \to c} [f(x) + g(x)] = \lim\limits_{x \to c} f(x) + \lim\limits_{x \to c} g(x)$$

provided both $\lim\limits_{x \to c} f(x)$ and $\lim\limits_{x \to c} g(x)$

exists.

Summary and Review

Important Terms, Symbols, and Concepts

- The limit of $f(x)$, as x approaches c, is equal to L means that $f(x)$ can be made arbitrarily close to L whenever x is sufficiently close to c (but not equal to c). We can denote this by $\lim\limits_{x \to c} f(x) = L$ or $f(x) \to L$ as $x \to c$.

- If $\lim\limits_{x \to c^-} f(x) = K$, we call K the left-hand limit which means that if $f(x)$ is close to K whenever x is close to, but to the left of, c on the real number line. If $\lim\limits_{x \to c^+} f(x) = L$, we call L the right-hand limit which means that if $f(x)$ is close to L whenever x is close to, but to the right of, c on the real number line.

  $x \to c^-$ is read "x approaches c from the left" and means $x \to c$ and $x < c$. $x \to c^+$ is read "x approaches c from the right" and means $x \to c$ and $x > c$.

- Let $f(x)$ be defined for all $x \neq c$ in an open interval containing c.

  1. If the values of $f(x)$ increase without bound as x (where $x \neq c$) approaches c, then we say that the limit as x approaches c is positive infinity and we write

  $$\lim\limits_{x \to c} f(x) = +\infty;$$

  2. If the values of $f(x)$ decrease without bound as x (where $x \neq c$) approaches c, then we say that the limit as x approaches c is negative infinity and we write

  $$\lim\limits_{x \to c} f(x) = -\infty.$$

- The vertical line $x = c$ is a vertical asymptote for the graph of $y = f(x)$ if

  $$f(x) \to +\infty \text{ or } f(x) \to -\infty \text{ as } x \to c^+ \text{ or } x \to c^-.$$

- A function $f(x)$ is said to be continuous at $x = c$ if $\lim\limits_{x \to c} f(x) = f(c)$.

  A function $f(x)$ is said to be continuous from the right at $x = c$ if $\lim\limits_{x \to c^+} f(x) = f(c)$

and continuous from the left at $x=c$ if $\lim\limits_{x \to c^-} f(x)=f(c)$.

- A function is continuous on a closed interval $[a, b]$ if it is continuous in the interior of the interval, is continuous from the right at $x=a$ and is continuous from the left at $x=b$.

- A real number x is a partition number for a function $f(x)$ if $f(x)$ is discontinuous at x or $f(x)=0$.

- An exponential function $f(x)$ is given by $f(x)=b^x$ where x is any real number, $b>0$ and $b \neq 1$. The number b is called the base.

- We call e the natural exponential base. $\lim\limits_{h \to 0} (1+h)^{\frac{1}{h}}=\mathrm{e} \approx 2.718281828459$.

- If the values of $f(x)$ become arbitrarily close to L as x becomes sufficiently large, then the function f has a limit at infinity and we write
$$\lim\limits_{x \to +\infty} f(x)=L.$$
If the values of $f(x)$ becomes arbitrarily close to L for $x<0$ as $|x|$ becomes sufficiently large, then the function f has a limit at negative infinity and we write
$$\lim\limits_{x \to -\infty} f(x)=L.$$

- The line $y=b$ is a horizontal asymptote if either or both of the following limit statements is true:
$$\lim\limits_{x \to -\infty} f(x)=b \text{ and } \lim\limits_{x \to +\infty} f(x)=b.$$

- Let f be a function defined over an interval I and let $c \in I$. We say f has an absolute maximum (or global maximum) at $x=c$ if $f(x) \leqslant f(c)$ for every x in I. The number $f(c)$ is called the maximum value of $f(x)$ on I. Similarly, $f(x)$ has an absolute minimum at c if $f(x) \geqslant f(c)$ for every x on I and the number $f(c)$ is called the minimum value of $f(x)$ on I.

Important Results

- Let $f(x)$ and $g(x)$ be two functions, and assume that
$$\lim\limits_{x \to c} f(x)=L, \qquad \lim\limits_{x \to c} g(x)=M$$
where L and M are real numbers (both limits exist). Then

    (1) $\lim\limits_{x \to c} k=k$　for any constant k;

    (2) $\lim\limits_{x \to c} x=c$;

    (3) $\lim\limits_{x \to c} kf(x)=k \lim\limits_{x \to c} f(x)=kL$　for any constant k;

    (4) $\lim\limits_{x \to c} [f(x) \pm g(x)]=\lim\limits_{x \to c} f(x) \pm \lim\limits_{x \to c} g(x)=L \pm M$;

    (5) $\lim\limits_{x \to c} [f(x) \cdot g(x)]=\lim\limits_{x \to c} f(x) \cdot \lim\limits_{x \to c} g(x)=LM$;

    (6) $\lim\limits_{x \to c} \dfrac{f(x)}{g(x)}=\dfrac{\lim\limits_{x \to c} f(x)}{\lim\limits_{x \to c} g(x)}=\dfrac{L}{M}$　if $M \neq 0$;

    (7) $\lim\limits_{x \to c} \sqrt[n]{f(x)}=\sqrt[n]{\lim\limits_{x \to c} f(x)}=\sqrt[n]{L}$,　$L>0$ for n even.

- For a (two-sided) limit to exist, the limit from the left and the limit from the right

must exist and be equal. That is,

$$\lim_{x \to c} f(x) = L \quad \text{if and only if} \quad \lim_{x \to c^-} f(x) = \lim_{x \to c^+} f(x) = L.$$

Extreme Value Theorem

If f is continuous on a closed interval $[a, b]$, $-\infty < a < b < +\infty$, then f has an absolute maximum and an absolute minimum.

Intermediate Value Theorem

Suppose that $f(x)$ is continuous on the closed interval $[a, b]$. If L is any real number strictly between $f(a)$ and $f(b)$, then there exists at least one number c on the open interval (a, b) such that $f(c) = L$.

Chapter 3 Derivatives

:: Introduction

Devised by Isaac Newton and G. W. Leibniz, differential calculus studies the rates at which quantities change. It concerns calculating derivatives and using them to solve problems involving nonconstant rates of change.

3.1 Definition of the Derivative

Suppose that you are on a freeway and you begin accelerating. Glancing at the speedometer, you see that at that instant your instantaneous rate of change is 55 m/h. These are two quite different concepts. The first you are probably familiar with. The second involves ideas of limits and calculus.

3.1.1 Instantaneous Rates of Change

To understand instantaneous rate of change, we first need to develop a solid understanding of average of change.

3.1.1.1 Average rates of change

Figure 3. 1 shows the total number of suits produced by Raggs, Ltd. , during one morning of work. Industrial psychologists have found curves like this typical of the production of factory workers.

Example 3. 1 Consider Figure 3. 1. What was the number of suits produced at Raggs, Ltd. , from 9 A. M. to 10 A. M. ?

Solution At 9 A. M. , 20 suits had been produced. At 10 A. M. , 55 suits had been produced. In the hour from 9 A. M. to 10 A. M. , the number of suits produced was

$$55-20=35 \text{ (suits).}$$

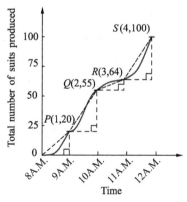

Figure 3. 1

Note that 35 is the slope of the line from Point P to Point Q.　　　　#

Example 3.2　Consider Figure 3.1. What was the average number of suits produced per hour from 9 A.M. to 11 A.M.?

Solution　We have

$$\frac{64-20}{11-9}=22 \text{ suits/h.}$$

Note that 22 is the slope of the line from Point P to Point R(Figure 3.2).　　　　#

Your Practice 3.1　Consider Figure 3.1. What was the average number of suits produced per hour from 9 A.M. to 12 A.M.?

Let us consider a function $y=f(x)$ and two inputs $x=a$ and $x=a+h$. The change in input or the change in x, is

$$(a+h)-a=h.$$

The change in output, or the change in y, is

$$f(a+h)-f(a).$$

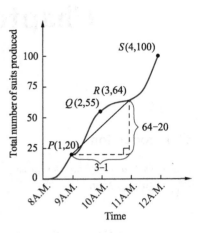

Figure 3.2

Definition 3.1 (Average Rate of Change)

Let $y=f(x)$. *The average rate of change of y with respect to x, as x changes from $x=a$ to $x=a+h$ is*

$$\frac{f(a+h)-f(a)}{(a+h)-a}=\frac{f(a+h)-f(a)}{h} \quad (h\neq 0). \tag{3.1}$$

Note that the numerator and denominator in Formula (3.1) are differences, so Formula (3.1) is a difference quotient.

Example 3.3　For $f(x)=x^2$, find the average rate of change as:

(1) x changes from 1 to 3;

(2) x changes from 1 to 2;

(3) x changes from 2 to 3.

Solution　(1) When $x=1$, and $h=3-1=2$, we plug them into Formula (3.1):

$$\frac{f(a+h)-f(a)}{h}=\frac{f(3)-f(1)}{2}.$$

Now $f(3)=3^2=9$, $f(1)=1^2=1$, and we have

$$\frac{f(3)-f(1)}{2}=\frac{9-1}{2}=4.$$

(2) When $x=1$, and $h=2-1=1$, from formula (3.1) we have

$$\frac{f(a+h)-f(a)}{h}=\frac{f(2)-f(1)}{1}.$$

Now $f(2)=2^2=4$, $f(1)=1^2=1$, and we get

$$\frac{f(2)-f(1)}{1}=\frac{4-1}{1}=3.$$

(3) When $x=2$, and $h=3-2=1$, Formula (3.1) becomes
$$\frac{f(a+h)-f(a)}{h}=\frac{f(3)-f(2)}{1}.$$

Now $f(2)=2^2=4$, $f(3)=3^2=9$, and we have
$$\frac{f(3)-f(2)}{1}=\frac{9-4}{1}=5.$$

Figure 3.3 shows the results.　　　　　　　　　　　　♯

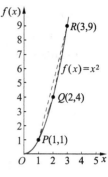

Figure 3.3

Example 3.4　The revenue (in dollars) from the sale of x plastic planter boxes is given by
$$f(x)=10x-0.02x^2, 0\leqslant x\leqslant 1000.$$

(1) What is the change in revenue if production is changed from 100 planters to 500 planters?

(2) What is the average rate of change in revenue for this change in production?

Solution　(1) The change in revenue is given by
$$\begin{aligned}
f(500)-f(100)&=10\times 500-0.02\times 500^2-(10\times 100-0.02\times 100^2)\\
&=0-800\\
&=-800.
\end{aligned}$$

Decreasing production from 100 planters to 500 planters will decrease revenue by \$800.

(2) To find the average rate of change in revenue, we divide the change in revenue by the change in production:
$$\frac{f(500)-f(100)}{500-100}=\frac{-800}{400}=-2.$$

The average of the change in revenue is -2 dollars per planter when production is increased from 100 to 500 planters.　　　　　　　　　　　♯

Your Practice 3.2　Refer to the revenue function in Example 3.4.

(1) What is the change in revenue if production is changed from 600 planters to 800 planters?

(2) What is the average rate of change in revenue for this change in production?

3.1.1.2　Instantaneous rates of change

Example 3.5　A small steel ball dropped from a tower will fall a distance of y feet in x seconds, as given approximately by the formula
$$y=16x^2.$$

Figure 3.4 shows the position of the ball on a coordinate line (positive direction down) at the end of 0, 1, 2 and 3 seconds.

(1) Find the average velocity from $x=1$ seconds to $x=3$ seconds.

(2) Find and simplify the average velocity from $x=1$ seconds to $x=1+h$ seconds, $h\neq 0$.

(3) Find the limit of the expression from part

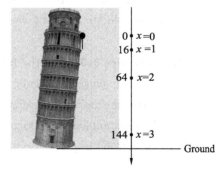

Figure 3.4

(2) as $h \to 0$ if that limit exists.

(4) Discuss possible interpretation of the limit from part (3).

Solution (1) Recall the formula $S = vt$, which can be written in the form of

$$v = \frac{S}{t} = \frac{Distance\ covered}{Elapsed\ time} = Average\ velocity.$$

So the average velocity of the steel ball from $x = 1$ seconds to $x = 3$ seconds is

$$Average\ velocity = \frac{Distance\ covered}{Elapsed\ time}$$

$$= \frac{f(3) - f(1)}{3 - 1}$$

$$= \frac{16 \times 3^2 - 16 \times 1^2}{2}$$

$$= 64\ (\text{feet per second}).$$

We see that if $y = f(x)$ is the position of the falling ball, then the average velocity is simply the average rate of change of $f(x)$ with respect to time x.

(2) Proceeding as in part (1), we have

$$Average\ velocity = \frac{Distance\ covered}{Elapsed\ time}$$

$$= \frac{f(1 + h) - f(1)}{(1 + h) - 1}$$

$$= \frac{16(1 + h)^2 - 16 \times 1^2}{h}$$

$$= \frac{16 + 32h + 16h^2 - 16}{h}$$

$$= 32 + 16h, h \neq 0.$$

Notice that if $h = 2$, the average velocity is 64 feet per second, which is the result in part (1).

(3) The limit of the average velocity expression from part (2) as $h \to 0$ is

$$\lim_{h \to 0} \frac{f(1 + h) - f(1)}{h} = \lim_{h \to 0} (32 + 16h) = 32\ (\text{feet per second}).$$

(4) The average velocity over smaller and smaller time intervals approaches 32 feet per second. This limit can be interpreted as the velocity of the ball at the instant that the ball has been falling for exactly 1 second. Therefore, 32 feet per second is referred to as the instantaneous velocity at $x = 1$ second, and we have solved one of the basic problems of calculus.   #

Your Practice 3.3   For the falling steel ball in Example 3.5.

(1) Find the average velocity from $x = 2$ seconds to $x = 3$ seconds.

(2) Find and simplify the average velocity from $x = 2$ seconds to $x = 2 + h$ seconds, $h \neq 0$.

(3) Find instantaneous velocity at $x = 2$ seconds.

The ideas in Example 3.5 can be applied to the average rate of change of any function.

Definition 3. 2 (Instantaneous Rate of Change)

For $y=f(x)$, *the instantaneous rate of change at $x=a$ is*

$$\lim_{h\to 0}\frac{f(a+h)-f(a)}{h}$$

if the limit exists.

The adjective instantaneous is often omitted with the understanding that the phrase rate of change and not the average rate of change. Similarly, velocity always refers to the instantaneous rate of change of distance with respect to time.

3.1.1.3　The derivative as an instantaneous rates of change

From Example 3. 5, it is not hard to see that it solved the problem through the following three steps (three-step method).

Three-step Method

Step 1　*When the independent variable x has a change quantity h, there is a change quantity Δy accordingly in the function $y=f(x)$:*

$$\Delta y=f(x+h)-f(x).$$

Step 2　*The difference quotient $\frac{f(x+h)-f(x)}{h}$ is the average rate of change of the function in the interval $(x, x+h)$.*

Step 3　*When the amount of change $h\to 0$, the limit of average rate of change*

$$\lim_{h\to 0}\frac{f(x+h)-f(x)}{h}$$

reflects the instantaneous rate of change of the function at x, which is called the derivative.

Therefore, the derivative of the function can be defined as:

Definition 3. 3 (Derivative)

For $y=f(x)$, *the derivative of $f(x)$ at x, denoted by $f'(x)$ or $\frac{dy}{dx}$, is defined as*

$$f'(x)=\lim_{h\to 0}\frac{f(x+h)-f(x)}{h}$$

if the limit exists. If $f'(x)$ exists for a given x, then $f(x)$ is said to be differentiable at the point x.

If $f'(x)$ exists for each x in the open interval (a, b), then $f(x)$ is said to be differentiable over (a, b).

So we know from Definition 3. 3 that instantaneous velocity is a derivative: $v=f'(t)$, where $f(t)$ is the position function.

3.1.1.4 Using the definition

To find derivatives, we can apply the three-step process in this section. In subsequent sections, we will develop rules for finding derivatives that do not involve limits. However, it is important that we master the limit process in order to fully comprehend and appreciate the various applications we will consider.

Example 3.6 (The Derivative of a Linear Function) Find $f'(x)$, the derivative of $f(x)$ at x, for $f(x)=kx+b$.

Solution We use the three-step process to find $f'(x)$.

Step 1 Find $f(x+h)-f(x)$.

$$f(x+h)-f(x)=k(x+h)+b-(kx+b)=kh.$$

Step 2 Find $\dfrac{f(x+h)-f(x)}{h}$.

$$\frac{f(x+h)-f(x)}{h}=\frac{kh}{h}=k.$$

Step 3 Find $f'(x)=\lim\limits_{h\to 0}\dfrac{f(x+h)-f(x)}{h}$.

$$f'(x)=\lim_{h\to 0}\frac{f(x+h)-f(x)}{h}=\lim_{h\to 0}k=k. \qquad\qquad \#$$

Example 3.7 Find $f'(x)$, the derivative of $f(x)$ at x, for $f(x)=2x-x^2$.

Solution To find $f'(x)$, we will use the three-step process.

Step 1 Find $f(x+h)-f(x)$.

$$\begin{aligned}
f(x+h)-f(x)&=2(x+h)-(x+h)^2-(2x-x^2)\\
&=2x+2h-x^2-2hx-h^2-2x+x^2\\
&=2h-2hx-h^2.
\end{aligned}$$

Step 2 Find $\dfrac{f(x+h)-f(x)}{h}$.

$$\begin{aligned}
\frac{f(x+h)-f(x)}{h}&=\frac{2h-2hx-h^2}{h}\\
&=2-2x-h,\ h\neq 0.
\end{aligned}$$

Step 3 Find $f'(x)=\lim\limits_{h\to 0}\dfrac{f(x+h)-f(x)}{h}$.

$$f'(x)=\lim_{h\to 0}\frac{f(x+h)-f(x)}{h}=\lim_{h\to 0}(2-2x-h)=2-2x. \qquad \#$$

Your Practice 3.4 Find $f'(x)$, the derivative of $f(x)$ at x, for $f(x)=x^2+4x$.

Example 3.8 Find $f'(x)$, the derivative of $f(x)$ at x, for $f(x)=\dfrac{1}{x}$.

Solution We use the three-step process to compute $f'(x)$.

Step 1 Find $f(x+h)-f(x)$.

$$\begin{aligned}
f(x+h)-f(x)&=\frac{1}{x+h}-\frac{1}{x}\\
&=\frac{x-(x+h)}{x(x+h)}
\end{aligned}$$

$$= \frac{-h}{x(x+h)}.$$

Step 2   Find $\frac{f(x+h)-f(x)}{h}$.

$$\frac{f(x+h)-f(x)}{h} = \frac{\dfrac{-h}{x(x+h)}}{h}$$

$$= \frac{-1}{x(x+h)}, \ h \neq 0.$$

Step 3   Find $f'(x) = \lim\limits_{h \to 0} \dfrac{f(x+h)-f(x)}{h}$

$$f'(x) = \lim \frac{f(x+h)-f(x)}{h} = \lim_{h \to 0} \frac{-1}{x(x+h)} = -\frac{1}{x^2}, \ x \neq 0. \qquad \#$$

Your Practice 3.5   Find $f'(x)$, the derivative of $f(x)$ at x, for $f(x) = \dfrac{1}{x+1}$.

3.1.2   Geometric Interpretation

So far, our interpretation of the difference quotient have been numerical in nature. Now we want to consider a geometric interpretation.

Tangent lines

A line through two points on the graph of a function is called a secant line. If $(a, f(a))$ and $(a+h, f(a+h))$ are two points on the graph of $y = f(x)$, then we can use the slope formula to find the slope of the secant line through these points (Figure 3.5):

$$\frac{y_2 - y_1}{x_2 - x_1} = \frac{f(a+h)-f(a)}{(a+h)-a}$$

$$= \frac{f(a+h)-f(a)}{h}.$$

The difference quotient can be interpreted as both the average rate of change and the slope of the secant line.

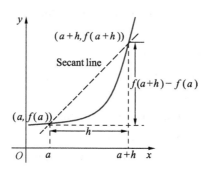

Figure 3.5

Example 3.9   Given $f(x) = x^2$.

(1) Find the slope of the secant line for $a = 1$, $h = 2$ and 1, respectively. Graph $y = f(x)$ and the two secant lines.

(2) Find and simplify the slope of the secant line for $a = 1$ and h any nonzero number.

(3) Find the limit of the expression in part (2).

(4) Discuss possible interpretations of the limit in part (3).

Solution

(1) For $a=1$ and $h=2$, the secant line goes through $(1,1)$ and $(3,9)$, and its slope is
$$\frac{f(1+2)-f(1)}{2}=\frac{3^2-1^2}{2}=4.$$

For $a=1$ and $h=1$, the secant line goes through $(1,1)$ and $(2,4)$, and its slope is
$$\frac{f(1+1)-f(1)}{1}=\frac{2^2-1^2}{1}=3.$$

The graph of $y=f(x)$ and the two secant lines are shown in Figure 3.6.

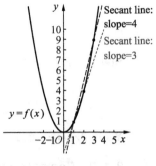

Figure 3.6

(2) For $a=1$ and h any nonzero number, the secant line goes through $(1, 1)$ and $(1+h, (1+h)^2)$, and its slope is
$$\frac{f(1+h)-f(1)}{h}=\frac{(1+h)^2-1^2}{h}$$
$$=\frac{2h+h^2}{h}$$
$$=2+h, h\neq0.$$

(3) The limit of the secant line slope from part (2) is
$$\lim_{h\to0}\frac{f(1+h)-f(1)}{h}=\lim_{h\to0}(2+h)=2.$$

(4) In part (3), we saw that the limit of the slope of the secant lines through the point $(1, f(1))$ with slope 2 (Figure 3.7), then this line is the limit of secant lines. The slope obtained from the limit of slopes of secant lines is called the slope of the graph at $x=1$. The line through the point $(1, f(1))$ with this slope is called the tangent line.

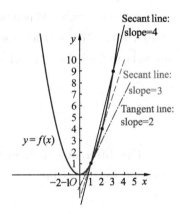

Figure 3.7

#

Your Practice 3.6   Given $f(x)=x^2$.

(1) Find the slope of the secant line for $a=2, h=2$ and 1, respectively. Graph $y=f(x)$ and the two secant lines.

(2) Find and simplify the slope of the secant line for $a=2$ and h any nonzero number.

(3) Find the limit of the expression in part (2).

(4) Find the slope of the graph and the slope of the tangent line at $a=2$.

The ideas introduced in the preceding example are summarized next:

Definition 3.4

Given $y=f(x)$, *the slope of the graph at the point* $(a, f(a))$ *is given by*
$$\lim_{h\to0}\frac{f(a+h)-f(a)}{h} \tag{3.2}$$

provided the limit exists. In this case, the tangent line to the graph is the line through $(a, f(a))$ *with the slope given by formula* (3.2).

We can give the equation of tangent line, since we know the slope and one point on the line. Using the point-slope form

$$y - y_0 = m(x - x_0)$$

where (x_0, y_0) is the point and m is the slope.

Definition 3.5 (Equation of the Tangent Line)

If the derivative of a given function f *exists at* $x = a$, *then* $f'(a)$ *is the slope of the tangent line at the point* $(a, f(a))$. *The equation of the tangent line is given by*

$$y - f(a) = f'(a)(x - a).$$

Using the geometric interpretation, it is easy to compute the equation of the tangent line.

Example 3.10   Given $y = x^2$, find the equation of the tangent line to the curve at $M(1, 1)$.

Solution   We know $f'(1) = 1$. We then find $(x_0, y_0) = (1, 1)$ and $m = 2$. So the equation of the line is given by (Figure 3.7)

$$y - 1 = 2(x - 1) \text{ or } y = 2x - 1. \qquad \sharp$$

Your Practice 3.7   Given $y = x^2$, find the equation of the tangent line to the curve at $M(2, 4)$.

3.1.3 Differentiability and Continuity

Using the geometric interpretation, it is easy to find situations in which $f'(a)$ does not exist.

Definition 3.6

The existence of a derivative at $x = a$ *depends on the existence of a limit at* $x = a$, *that is, on the existence of*

$$f'(a) = \lim_{h \to 0} \frac{f(a+h) - f(a)}{h}. \tag{3.3}$$

If the limit does not exist at $x = a$, *we say that the function* f *is non-differentiable at* $x = a$, *or* $f'(a)$ *does not exist.*

Example 3.11   Let

$$f(x) = |x| = \begin{cases} x, & \text{if } x \geqslant 0, \\ -x, & \text{if } x < 0. \end{cases}$$

Is $f(x)$ differentiable at $x = 0$?

Solution   A graph of $f(x)$ is shown in Figure 3.8. It should be clear from the graph there is no tangent line at $x = 0$. We can define the slope of the secant line when we approach 0 from the right and also from left; however, the slope converge to different values in the limit. The former is 1, the latter is -1, which are shown in the following calculation

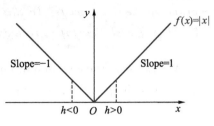

$$\lim_{h \to 0^+} \frac{f(0+h)-f(0)}{h} = \lim_{h \to 0^+} \frac{h-0}{h} = 1,$$

$$\lim_{h \to 0^-} \frac{f(0+h)-f(0)}{h} = \lim_{h \to 0^-} \frac{h-0}{h} = -1.$$

Figure 3.8

In the calculation, we used the fact that when $h \to 0^+$, $f(0+h) = |0+h| = |h| = h$ since $h > 0$, whereas when $h \to 0^-$, $f(0+h) = |0+h| = |h| = -h$ since $h < 0$. Since $1 \neq -1$, it follows that

$$\lim_{h \to 0} \frac{f(0+h)-f(0)}{h}$$

does not exist. Thus, $f'(0)$ does not exist. The function $f(x)$ is non-differentiable at $x = 0$.

Note that at all other points, the derivative in the above example exists. We can find the derivative by simply looking at the graph. We see that

$$f'(x) = \begin{cases} 1, & \text{if } x > 0, \\ -1, & \text{if } x < 0. \end{cases}$$

Note that we can consider $f'(x)$ itself as a function of x.   #

Your Practice 3.8   Let

$$f(x) = |x-1|.$$

Is $f(x)$ differentiable at $x = 1$?

We see in Example 3.11 that continuity alone is not enough for a function to be differentiable. The function $f(x) = |x|$ is continuous at all values of x but we see that it is not differentiable at $x = 0$. The example also shows that it is quite easy to draw the graph of a continuous function that is not differentiable at certain points: just put in "corners" at those points where we do not want the function to be differentiable (Figure 3.9).

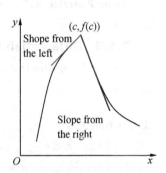

Figure 3.9

However, if a function is differentiable, it is also continuous. This means that continuity is a necessary but not a sufficient condition for differentiability. This result is important enough that we will formulate it as a theorem and prove it.

Theorem 3.1 (Differentiability and Continuity)

If $f(x)$ is differentiable at $x = a$, it is also continuous at $x = a$.

Proof   Since $f(x)$ is differentiable at $x = a$, we know that the limit

$$\lim_{x \to a} \frac{f(x)-f(a)}{x-a} \tag{3.4}$$

exists and is equal to $f'(a)$. To show that $f(x)$ is continuous at $x=a$, we must show that

$$\lim_{x\to a} f(x)=f(a) \text{ or } \lim_{x\to a}[f(x)-f(a)]=0.$$

First, note that $f(x)$ is defined at $x=a$. Now,

$$\lim_{x\to a}[f(x)-f(a)]=\lim_{x\to a}\frac{f(x)-f(a)}{x-a}(x-a).$$

Given that

$$\lim_{x\to a}\frac{f(x)-f(a)}{x-a}$$

exists and is equal to $f'(a)$ (Formula (3.4)), and that

$$\lim_{x\to a}(x-a)=0,$$

we can apply the product rule for limits and find

$$\lim_{x\to a}\frac{f(x)-f(a)}{x-a}(x-a)=\lim_{x\to a}\frac{f(x)-f(a)}{x-a}\lim_{x\to a}(x-a)$$

$$=f'(a)\cdot 0=0.$$

That is,

$$\lim_{x\to a}[f(x)-f(a)]=0,$$

hence, $f(x)$ is continuous at $x=a$.　　　　　　　　　　#

It follows from Theorem 3.1 that if a function $f(x)$ is not continuous at $x=a$ then $f(x)$ is not differentiable at $x=a$. The function $y=f(x)$ in Figure 3.10 is discontinuous at $x=a$, we can not draw a tangent line at $x=a$.

Finally, if a function has a vertical tangent at a point, it is not differentiable at that point. The following example shows the idea.

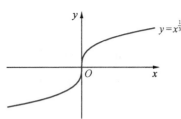

Figure 3.10

Example 3.12　Show that

$$f(x)=x^{\frac{1}{3}}$$

is not differentiable at $x=0$.

Solution　We see from the graph of $f(x)$ in Figure 3.11 that $f(x)$ is continuous at $x=0$. Using the formal definition, we find

$$f'(0)=\lim_{h\to 0}\frac{f(h)-f(0)}{h}$$

$$=\lim_{h\to 0}\frac{h^{\frac{1}{3}}-0}{h}$$

$$=\lim_{h\to 0}\frac{1}{h^{\frac{2}{3}}}=\infty$$

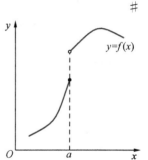

Figure 3.11

does not exist.

Since the limit does not exist, $f(x)$ is not differentiable at $x=0$. We see from the graph that the tangent line at $x=0$ is vertical.　　　　　　　#

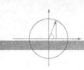

Exercise 3.1

1. For each function in the following, find a simplified form of the difference quotient and then complete Table 3.1.

Table 3.1

x	h	$\dfrac{f(x+h)-f(x)}{h}$
5	2	
5	1	
5	0.1	
5	0.01	

(1) $f(x)=2x^2$;

(2) $f(x)=5x^2$;

(3) $f(x)=-2x^2$;

(4) $f(x)=-5x^2$;

(5) $f(x)=x^2+x$;

(6) $f(x)=x^2-x$;

(7) $f(x)=x^2-3x+2$;

(8) $f(x)=x^2+4x-3$.

2. Find the indicated quantity for $y=5-x^2$ and interpret that quantity in terms of Figure 3.12.

(1) $\dfrac{f(2)-f(1)}{2-1}$;

(2) $\dfrac{f(1+h)-f(1)}{h}$;

(3) $\lim\limits_{h\to 0}\dfrac{f(1+h)-f(1)}{h}$;

(4) $\dfrac{f(-1)-f(-2)}{-1-(-2)}$;

(5) $\dfrac{f(-2+h)-f(-2)}{h}$;

(6) $\lim\limits_{h\to 0}\dfrac{f(-2+h)-f(-2)}{h}$.

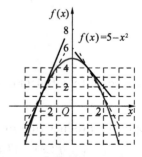

Figure 3.12

3. Find the indicates quantities for $f(x)=2x^2$.

(1) The slope of the secant line through the points $(1, f(1))$ and $(4, f(4))$.

(2) The slope of the graph at $(1, f(1))$.

4. Find the indicates quantities for $f(x)=3x^2$.

(1) The slope of the secant line through the points $(1, f(1))$ and $(2, f(2))$,

(2) The slope of the graph at $(1, f(1))$.

5. Suppose an object moves along the y-axis so that its location is $y=x^2-x$ at time x (y is in meters and x is in seconds). Find

(1) The average velocity (the average rate of change of y with respect to x) for x changing from 1 to 2 seconds;

(2) The average for x changing from 1 to $1+h$ seconds;

(3) The instantaneous velocity at $x=1$ second.

6. Suppose an object moves along the y-axis so that its location is $y=x^2+x$ at time x (y is in meters and x is in seconds). Find:

(1) The average velocity (the average

rate of change of y with respect to x) for x changing from 2 to 4 seconds;

(2) The average for x changing from 2 to $2+h$ seconds;

(3) The instantaneous velocity at $x=2$ second.

7. Refer to the function f in Figure 3.13. Use the graph to determine whether $f'(x)$ exists at each indicated value of x.

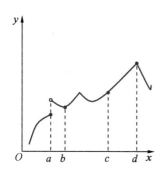

Figure 3.13

(1) $x=a$;

(2) $x=b$;

(3) $x=c$;

(4) $x=d$.

8. The amount of money, $A(t)$, in a saving account that pays 6% interest, compounded quarterly for t years, when an initial investment of \$2000 is made, is given by

$$A(t)=2000(1.015)^t.$$

(1) Find $A(2)$;

(2) Find $A(3)$;

(3) Find $A(3)-A(2)$;

(4) Find $\dfrac{A(3)-A(2)}{3-2}$, and interpret the result.

9. A person x inches tall has a pulse rate of y beats per minute, as given approximately by

$$y=590x^{-\frac{1}{2}}, 30\leqslant x\leqslant75.$$

What is the instantaneous rate of change of

pulse rate at the

(1) 35-inch level;

(2) 60-inch level?

10. Use the three-step process to find $f'(x)$ and then find $f'(1)$, $f'(2)$, and $f'(3)$.

(1) $f(x)=-2$;

(2) $f(x)=4$;

(3) $f(x)=3x-7$;

(4) $f(x)=-2x+6$;

(5) $f(x)=2x^2+3x$;

(6) $f(x)=x^3+x^2+x+1$;

(7) $f(x)=2\sqrt{x}$;

(8) $f(x)=\dfrac{1}{x+2}$.

11. Sketch the graph of $f(x)$ and determine where $f(x)$ is non-differentiable.

(1) $f(x)=\begin{cases}3, & \text{if } x\geqslant0, \\ 3x, & \text{if } x<0;\end{cases}$

(2) $f(x)=\begin{cases}2x, & \text{if } x\geqslant2, \\ 6-x, & \text{if } x<2;\end{cases}$

(3) $f(x)=\begin{cases}x^2+1, & \text{if } x\geqslant0, \\ 1, & \text{if } x<0;\end{cases}$

(4) $f(x)=\begin{cases}3-x^2, & \text{if } x\geqslant0, \\ 3, & \text{if } x<0.\end{cases}$

12. Determine whether $f(x)$ is differentiable at $x=0$ by considering

$$\lim_{h\to0}\frac{f(0+h)-f(0)}{h}.$$

(1) $f(x)=|x|$;

(2) $f(x)=|x|+1$;

(3) $f(x)=x^{\frac{1}{3}}$;

(4) $f(x)=\sqrt{1+x}$.

13. Discuss the validity of each statement. If the statement is always true, explain why. If not, give a counterexample.

(1) If $f(x)=C$ is a constant function, then $f'(x)=0$.

(2) If $f(x)=mx+b$ is a linear

function, then $f'(x) = m$.

(3) If a function f is differentiable in the interval (a, b), then f is continuous in the interval (a, b).

(4) If a function f is continuous in the interval (a, b), then f is differentiable in the interval (a, b).

(5) The function $f(x) = |x - 1|$ is differentiable.

(6) If the graph of f has a sharp corner at $x = a$, then f is not continuous at $x = a$.

14. The ozone level (in parts per billion) on a summer day in a metropolitan area is given by

$$P(t) = 80 + 6t - t^2.$$

(1) Use the three-step process to find $P'(t)$.

(2) Find $P(3)$ and $P'(3)$. Write a brief verbal interpretation of these results.

15. The body temperature (in degrees Fahrenheit) of a patient t hours after taking a fever-reducing drug is given by

$$F(t) = 98 + \frac{4}{t+1}.$$

(1) Use the three-step process to find $F'(t)$.

(2) Find $f(2)$ and $F'(2)$. Write a brief verbal interpretation of these results.

3.2　Basic Differentiation Properties

In Section 3.1, we defined the derivative of f at x as

$$f'(x) = \lim_{h \to 0} \frac{f(x+h) - f(x)}{h}$$

if the limit exists, and we used this definition and the three-step process to find the derivatives of several function. Now we want to develop some rules of differentiation. These rules will enable us to find the derivative of many functions without using the three-step process.

Before exploring these rules, we list some symbols that we often used to represent derivatives.

Derivative Symbols

If $y = f(x)$, then

$$f'(x),\ y',\ \frac{\mathrm{d}y}{\mathrm{d}x}$$

all represent the derivative of f at x.

Each of these derivative symbols has its particular advantage in certain situations. All of them will become familiar to you after a little experience.

3.2.1　Constant Function Rule

Example 3.13　Find $f'(x)$, the derivative of $f(x)$ at x, for $f(x) = C$.

Solution　We use the three-step process to find $f'(x)$.

Step 1　Find $f(x+h) - f(x)$.

$$f(x+h)-f(x)=C-C=0.$$

Step 2   Find $\dfrac{f(x+h)-f(x)}{h}$.

$$\frac{f(x+h)-f(x)}{h}=\frac{0}{h}.$$

Step 3   Find $f'(x)=\lim\limits_{h\to 0}\dfrac{f(x+h)-f(x)}{h}$.

$$f'(x)=\lim_{h\to 0}\frac{f(x+h)-f(x)}{h}=\lim_{h\to 0}0=0. \qquad\qquad \sharp$$

Theorem 3.2 (Constant Function Rule)

If $f(x)=C$, then

$$f'(x)=0.$$

Also, $y'=0$ and $\dfrac{\mathrm{d}y}{\mathrm{d}x}=0.$

Note   When we write $C'=0$ or $\dfrac{\mathrm{d}}{\mathrm{d}x}C=0$, we mean that $y'=\dfrac{\mathrm{d}y}{\mathrm{d}x}=0$ when $y=C$.

Your Practice 3.9

(1) If $f(x)=3$, find $f'(x)$;

(2) If $f(x)=-2$, find $f'(x)$;

(3) If $f(x)=\mathrm{e}$, find $f'(x)$;

(4) Find $\dfrac{\mathrm{d}}{\mathrm{d}x}4$.

3.2.2   The Power Rule

A function of the form $f(x)=x^{k}$, where k is a real number, is called a power function. The following elementary functions are examples of power functions:

$$r(x)=x^{3},\ s(x)=x^{\frac{1}{2}},\ t(x)=\sqrt[3]{x},\ u(x)=x^{-\frac{1}{3}}.$$

The definition of the derivative and the three-step process introduced in Section 3.1 can be used to find the derivative of many power functions. For example, it can be shown that

$$\text{If } f(x)=x^{2},\text{then } f'(x)=2x;$$
$$\text{If } f(x)=x^{3},\text{ then } f'(x)=3x^{3};$$
$$\text{If } f(x)=x^{4},\text{ then } f'(x)=4x^{4};$$
$$\text{If } f(x)=x^{5},\text{ then } f'(x)=5x^{5}.$$

Notice the pattern in these derivatives. In each case, the power in $f(x)$ becomes the coefficient in $f'(x)$ and the power in $f'(x)$ is 1 less than the power in $f(x)$. In general, for any positive integer n, if $f(x)=x^{n}$, then

$$f'(x)=nx^{n-1}. \qquad\qquad (3.5)$$

In fact, many more advanced techniques can be used to show that Equation (3.5) holds for any real number n. We will assume this general result for the remainder of the book.

Theorem 3.3 (Derivative of Power Functions)

If $f(x)=x^n$, where n is a real number, then
$$f'(x)=nx^{n-1}.$$

Also, $y'=nx^{n-1}$ and $\dfrac{\mathrm{d}y}{\mathrm{d}x}=nx^{n-1}$.

Example 3.14

(1) If $f(x)=x^6$, then $f'(x)=6x^{6-1}=6x^5$;

(2) If $f(x)=x^{20}$, then $f'(x)=20x^{20-1}=20x^{19}$;

(3) If $f(x)=x^{-3}$, then $f'(x)=-3x^{-3-1}=-3x^{-4}=-\dfrac{3}{x^4}$;

(4) $\dfrac{\mathrm{d}}{\mathrm{d}x}x^{\frac{3}{2}}=\dfrac{3}{2}x^{\frac{3}{2}-1}=\dfrac{3}{2}x^{\frac{1}{2}}$.   #

Your Practice 3.10 Find:

(1) $f'(x)$ for $f(x)=x^6$;

(2) y' for $y=x^{21}$;

(3) $\dfrac{\mathrm{d}y}{\mathrm{d}x}$ for $y=x^{-4}$;

(4) $\dfrac{\mathrm{d}}{\mathrm{d}x}x^{\frac{2}{3}}$.

3.2.3 Sum and Difference Rule

Since polynomials and rational functions are built from power functions of the form $y=x^n$, $n=0,1,2,\cdots$, by the basic operations of addition, subtraction, multiplication, and division, we need basic differentiation rules for such operations. We begin with the following rules.

Theorem 3.4 (Constant Multiple)

If $f(x)=ku(x)$, then
$$f'(x)=ku'(x)$$

Also,
$$y'=ku' \quad or \quad \frac{\mathrm{d}ku(x)}{\mathrm{d}x}=k\,\frac{\mathrm{d}u(x)}{\mathrm{d}x}.$$

Proof Using the three-step process, we have

Step 1 Find $f(x+h)-f(x)=ku(x+h)-ku(x)=k[u(x+h)-u(x)]$.

Step 2 $\dfrac{f(x+h)-f(x)}{h}=\dfrac{k[u(x+h)-u(x)]}{h}=k\left[\dfrac{u(x+h)-u(x)}{h}\right]$.

Step 3
$$f'(x)=\lim_{h\to 0}\frac{f(x+h)-f(x)}{h}$$
$$=\lim_{h\to 0}k\left[\frac{u(x+h)-u(x)}{h}\right]$$

$$=k \lim_{h \to 0} \left[\frac{u(x+h)-u(x)}{h} \right]$$

$$=ku'(x).$$ #

Example 3.15

(1) If $f(x)=3x^2$, then $f'(x)=3 \cdot 2x^{2-1}=6x$;

(2) If $f(x)=\dfrac{x^3}{3}$, then $f'(x)=\dfrac{1}{3} \cdot 3x^{3-1}=x^2$;

(3) If $f(x)=\dfrac{1}{2}x^{-3}$, then $f'(x)=\dfrac{1}{2} \cdot (-3)x^{-3-1}=-\dfrac{3}{2}x^{-4}=-\dfrac{3}{2x^4}$;

(4) $\dfrac{\mathrm{d}}{\mathrm{d}x}(3x^{\frac{2}{3}})=3 \cdot \dfrac{3}{2}x^{\frac{3}{2}-1}=\dfrac{9}{2}x^{\frac{1}{2}}$. #

Your Practice 3.11 Find:

(1) $f'(x)$ for $f(x)=4x^6$;

(2) y' for $y=3x^3$;

(3) $\dfrac{\mathrm{d}y}{\mathrm{d}x}$ for $y=4x^{-4}$;

(4) $\dfrac{\mathrm{d}}{\mathrm{d}x}(3x^{\frac{2}{3}})$.

Theorem 3.5 (Sum and Difference Rule)

If $f(x)=u(x) \pm v(x)$, then

$$f'(x)=u'(x) \pm v'(x).$$

Also,

$$y'=u' \pm v' \quad or \quad \frac{\mathrm{d}(u \pm v)}{\mathrm{d}x}=\frac{\mathrm{d}u}{\mathrm{d}x} \pm \frac{\mathrm{d}v}{\mathrm{d}x}.$$

Note This rule generalizes to the sum and difference of any given number of functions.

3.2.4 Derivative of Polynomials

With Theorem 3.2 to 3.5, we can compute the derivatives of all polynomials and a variety of other functions.

Example 3.16

(1) If $f(x)=3x^2+3x$, then

$$f'(x)=(3x^2)'+(3x)'=3(2x)+3(1)=6x+3.$$

(2) If $y=x^2+3x+1$, then

$$f'(x)=(x^2)'+(3x)'+1'=2x+3.$$

(3) If $y=\sqrt[3]{t}-2t$, then

$$\frac{\mathrm{d}y}{\mathrm{d}t}=\frac{\mathrm{d}}{\mathrm{d}t}t^{\frac{1}{3}}-\frac{\mathrm{d}}{\mathrm{d}t}2t=\frac{1}{3}t^{-\frac{2}{3}}-2=\frac{1}{3t^{\frac{2}{3}}}-2.$$

(4) $\dfrac{\mathrm{d}}{\mathrm{d}x}\left(\dfrac{5}{3x^2}-\dfrac{2}{x^4}+\dfrac{x^3}{9}\right)=\dfrac{\mathrm{d}}{\mathrm{d}x}\left(\dfrac{5}{3}x^{-2}\right)-\dfrac{\mathrm{d}}{\mathrm{d}x}(2x^{-4})+\dfrac{\mathrm{d}}{\mathrm{d}x}\left(\dfrac{1}{9}x^3\right)$

$$= \frac{5}{3}(-2)x^{-3} - 2(-4)x^{-5} + \frac{1}{9} \cdot 3x^2$$

$$= -\frac{10}{3x^3} + \frac{8}{x^5} + \frac{1}{3}x^2. \qquad \#$$

Your Practice 3.12 Find:

(1) $f'(x)$ for $f(x) = 4x^3 + x^2 - 5x$;

(2) y' for $y = 3x^3 - 2x$;

(3) $\dfrac{dy}{dt}$ for $y = 3t^{-3} - \sqrt[4]{t}$;

(4) $\dfrac{dy}{dx}$ for $y = -\dfrac{3}{4x} + \dfrac{4}{x^3} - \dfrac{x^4}{8}$.

Example 3.17 Find the derivative of

$$f(x) = \frac{1 - x^2}{x^4}.$$

Solution We know

$$f(x) = \frac{1 - x^2}{x^4}$$

$$= \frac{1}{x^4} - \frac{x^2}{x^4}$$

$$= x^{-4} - x^{-2}.$$

Note that we can apply those rules to find the derivative:

$$f'(x) = -4x^{-5} + 2x^{-3}. \qquad \#$$

Your Practice 3.13 Find the derivative of

$$f(x) = \frac{4x^2 - 2x + 1}{x}.$$

Example 3.18 An object moves along the y-axis (marked in feet) so that its position at time x (in seconds) is

$$f(x) = x^3 - 6x^2 + 9x.$$

(1) Find the instantaneous velocity function v.

(2) Find the velocity at $x = 2$ and $x = 5$ seconds.

(3) Find the time(s) when the velocity is 0.

Solution

(1) $v = f'(x) = (x^3)' - (6x^2)' + (9x)' = 3x^2 - 12x + 9$.

(2) $f'(2) = 3 \times 2^2 - 12 \times 2 + 9 = -3$(feet per second).

　　$f'(4) = 3 \times 4^2 - 12 \times 4 + 9 = 9$(feet per second).

(3) $v = f'(x) = 3x^2 - 12x + 9 = 0$, $3(x^2 - 4x + 3) = 0$, $3(x - 3)(x - 1) = 0$, $x = 1, 3$. $\#$

Your Practice 3.14 Repeat Example 3.18 for $f(x) = x^3 - 15x^2 + 72x$.

Exercise 3.2

1. Find the indicated derivatives.

(1) $f'(x)$ for $f(x)=7$;

(2) $\dfrac{\mathrm{d}}{\mathrm{d}x}3$;

(3) $\dfrac{\mathrm{d}y}{\mathrm{d}x}$ for $y=x^9$;

(4) $g'(x)$ for $g(x)=x^5$;

(5) $\dfrac{\mathrm{d}y}{\mathrm{d}x}$ for $y=x^{-5}$;

(6) $f'(x)$ for $f(x)=3x^{-2}$;

(7) $f'(x)$ for $f(x)=\dfrac{5}{x}$;

(8) y' for $y=0.4x^3$;

(9) $f'(x)$ for $f(x)=\dfrac{x}{25}$;

(10) $\dfrac{\mathrm{d}y}{\mathrm{d}x}$ for $y=\sqrt[5]{x}$.

2. Give the function f and g that satisfy $f'(2)=1$ and $g'(2)=3$. Find $h'(2)$ for the indicated function h.

(1) $h(x)=4f(x)$;

(2) $h(x)=5g(x)$;

(3) $h(x)=f(x)+g(x)$;

(4) $h(x)=2f(x)+3g(x)$;

(5) $h(x)=f(x)-g(x)+4$;

(6) $h(x)=3f(x)+4g(x)+5$.

3. Find the indicated derivatives.

(1) $\dfrac{\mathrm{d}y}{\mathrm{d}x}$ for $y=x^{-5}+3x+9$;

(2) $f'(x)$ for $f(x)=5x+3$;

(3) $f'(t)$ for $f(t)=t^3+4t^2-3t+1$;

(4) y' for $y=x^{-2}+x^{-3}$;

(5) $\dfrac{\mathrm{d}}{\mathrm{d}u}(8u^{\frac{2}{3}}+u^{\frac{1}{2}})$;

(6) $\dfrac{\mathrm{d}}{\mathrm{d}x}\left(\dfrac{3x^2}{2}-\dfrac{7}{5x^3}\right)$;

(7) y' for $y=\dfrac{1}{\sqrt[3]{x}}$;

(8) $h'(t)$ for $h(t)=\dfrac{1}{t}-\dfrac{3}{t^{\frac{3}{2}}}$;

(9) y' for $y=\dfrac{0.6}{\sqrt{x}}+0.5x^{-2}$;

(10) $\dfrac{\mathrm{d}}{\mathrm{d}x}(1.2x^{-2}-0.5x^{\frac{3}{2}})$.

4. Find:

(A) $f'(x)$;

(B) The slope of the graph of f at $x=2$ and $x=4$;

(C) The equation of the tangent at $x=2$ and $x=4$,

for the following functions:

(1) $f(x)=4x-x^2$;

(2) $f(x)=2x^2-3x$;

(3) $f(x)=3x^3-x^2$;

(4) $f(x)=x^4-x^3+2x^2+4$.

5. Find the indicated derivatives.

(1) $\dfrac{\mathrm{d}y}{\mathrm{d}x}$ for $y=(x-2)^2$;

(2) $f'(x)$ for $f(x)=(2x+3)^2$;

(3) y' for $y=\dfrac{x^2+3}{x^2}$;

(4) $\dfrac{\mathrm{d}}{\mathrm{d}x}\dfrac{4x+7}{x}$;

(5) y' for $y=\dfrac{3x-4}{12x^2}$;

(6) $\dfrac{\mathrm{d}y}{\mathrm{d}x}$ for $y=\dfrac{2x^4+x^3+x^2}{x^3}$.

6. A company's total sales (in millions of dollars) t months from now are given by

$$S(t)=0.02t^3+0.5t^2+2t+1.$$

(1) Find $S'(t)$;

(2) Find $S(3)$ and $S'(3)$ (to two decimal places), write a brief verbal interpretation of these results;

(3) Find $S(5)$ and $S(5)$ (to two decimal places), write a brief verbal interpretation of these results.

7. A marine manufacturer will sell $N(x)$ power boats after spending x thousand dollars on advertising, as given by

$$N(x) = 1000 - \frac{4200}{x}, \ 5 \leqslant x \leqslant 30.$$

(1) Find $N'(x)$;

(2) Find $N'(10)$ and $N'(20)$.

8. A coal-burning electrical generating plant emits sulfur dioxide into the surrounding air. The concentration $C(x)$, in parts per million, is given approximately by

$$C(x) = \frac{0.1}{x^2},$$

where x is the distance from the plant in miles. Find the instantaneous rate of change of concentration at

(1) $x = 1$ mile;

(2) $x = 2$ miles.

9. Animals or organisms living on other organisms (hosts) are called parasites. There is a kind of parasite that destroys spider eggs. Let the total number of spiders on a certain area be H, and the relative number of parasites be P, the function be

$$H(P) = M(1 - 2P^3),$$

find the derivative of $H(P)$.

10. Set the rule of some bacterial reproduction $p(t) = 30000 + 60t^2$, $p(t)$ is the number of bacteria at t. Find the reproduction rate of

(1) $t = 2$;

(2) $t = 0$;

(3) $t = 5$.

11. The body temperature (in degrees Fahrenheit) of a patient t hours after taking a fever-reducing drug is given by

$$F(t) = 0.12t^2 - 1.6t + 102,$$

find $F(4)$ and $F'(4)$.

3.3 Differentials

In this section, we introduce differentials. Differentials are often easier to compute than increments and can be used to approximate increments.

3.3.1 Differentials

In Section 3.1, we defined the derivative of f at x as the limit of the difference quotient

$$f'(x) = \lim_{h \to 0} \frac{f(x+h) - f(x)}{h}.$$

We consider various interpretations of this limit, including slope, velocity, and instantaneous rate of change. Increment notation enables us to interpret the numerator and denominator of the difference quotient separately.

Given $y = f(x) = x^2$, if x changes from 2 to 2.1, then y will change from $y = 2^2 = 4$ to $y = (2.1)^2 = 4.41$. The change in x is denoted by Δx (read as "delta x"). Similarly, the change in y is called increment in y and is denoted by Δy (Figure 3.14). In terms of the given example, we write

$$\Delta x = 2.1 - 2 = 0.1, \ \Delta y = f(2.1) - f(2) = 0.41.$$

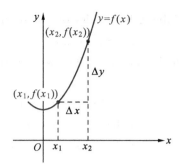

Figure 3.14

Definition 3.7 (Increments)

For $y=f(x)$, $\Delta x = x_2 - x_1$, so $x_2 = x_1 + \Delta x$ and

$$\Delta y = y_2 - y_1$$
$$= f(x_2) - f(x_1)$$
$$= f(x_1 + \Delta x) - f(x_1).$$

Δy represents the change in y corresponding to a change Δx in x. Δx can be either positive or negative.

Note Δy depends on the function $f(x)$, the input x_1, and the increment Δx.

Example 3.19   Given the function

$$y = x^3,$$

find $\dfrac{f(x_1 + \Delta x) - f(x_1)}{\Delta x}$ for $x_1 = 1$ and $\Delta x = 2$.

Solution

$$\frac{f(x_1 + \Delta x) - f(x_1)}{\Delta x} = \frac{f(1+2) - f(1)}{2}$$
$$= \frac{f(3) - f(1)}{2}$$
$$= \frac{27 - 1}{2} = 13. \qquad \#$$

Your Practice 3.15   Given the function

$$y = x^2 + 2,$$

find $\dfrac{f(x_1 + \Delta x) - f(x_1)}{\Delta x}$ for $x_1 = 1$ and $\Delta x = 2$.

Using Definition 3.7, we know that derivative is also defined by

$$f'(x) = \lim_{\Delta x \to 0} \frac{\Delta y}{\Delta x} \tag{3.6}$$

if the limit exists.

Assume that the limit in Equation (3.6) exists. Then, for small Δx, the difference quotient $\Delta y/\Delta x$ provides a good approximation for $f'(x)$. Also, $f'(x)$ provides a good approximation for $\Delta y/\Delta x$. We write

$$\frac{\Delta y}{\Delta x} \approx f'(x), \tag{3.7}$$

Δx is small, but $\Delta x \neq 0$. Multiplying both sides of Equation (3.7) by Δx gives us

$$\Delta y \approx f'(x)\Delta x, \qquad (3.8)$$

Δx is small, but $\Delta x \neq 0$. From Equation (3.8), we see that $f'(x)\Delta x$ provides a good approximation for Δy when Δx is small.

Because of the practical and theoretical importance of $f'(x)\Delta x$, we give it the special name **differential** and represent it with the special symbol $\mathrm{d}y$ or $\mathrm{d}f$:

$$\mathrm{d}y = f'(x)\Delta x \text{ or } \mathrm{d}f = f'(x)\Delta x.$$

For example,

$$\mathrm{d}(2x^3) = (2x^3)'\Delta x = 6x^2 \Delta x$$
$$\mathrm{d}(x) = (x)'\Delta x = 1 \cdot \Delta x = \Delta x.$$

In the second example, we usually drop the parentheses in $\mathrm{d}(x)$ and simply write

$$\mathrm{d}x = \Delta x.$$

In summary, we have the following definition:

Definition 3.8 (Differentials)

If $y = f(x)$ defines a differentiable function, then the differential $\mathrm{d}y$ or $\mathrm{d}f$, is defined as the product of $f'(x)$ and $\mathrm{d}x$, where $\mathrm{d}x = \Delta x$. Symbolically,

$$\mathrm{d}y = f'(x)\Delta x \text{ or } \mathrm{d}f = f'(x)\Delta x$$

where

$$\mathrm{d}x = \Delta x.$$

Note   The differential $\mathrm{d}y$ (or $\mathrm{d}f$) is actually a function involving two independent variables, x and $\mathrm{d}x$. A change in either one or both will affect $\mathrm{d}y$ (or $\mathrm{d}f$).

Example 3.20   Find $\mathrm{d}y$ for $f(x) = x^2 + 4x$. Evaluate $\mathrm{d}y$ for

(1) $x = 1$ and $\mathrm{d}x = 0.01$;

(2) $x = 2$ and $\mathrm{d}x = 0.1$;

(3) $x = 3$ and $\mathrm{d}x = 0.1$.

Solution $\mathrm{d}y = f'(x)\mathrm{d}x = (2x + 4)\mathrm{d}x.$

(1) When $x = 1$ and $\mathrm{d}x = 0.01$,

$$\mathrm{d}y = (2 \times 1 + 4) \times 0.01 = 0.06.$$

(2) When $x = 2$ and $\mathrm{d}x = 0.1$,

$$\mathrm{d}y = (2 \times 2 + 4) \times 0.1 = 0.8.$$

(3) When $x = 3$ and $\mathrm{d}x = 0.1$,

$$\mathrm{d}y = (2 \times 3 + 4) \times 0.01 = 0.1. \qquad \#$$

Your Practice 3.16   Find $\mathrm{d}y$ for $f(x) = x^2 + \sqrt{x}$. Evaluate $\mathrm{d}y$ for

(1) $x = 1$ and $\mathrm{d}x = 0.1$;

(2) $x = 4$ and $\mathrm{d}x = 0.01$;

(3) $x = 9$ and $\mathrm{d}x = 0.12$.

We now have two interpretation of the symbol $\dfrac{\mathrm{d}y}{\mathrm{d}x}$. Referring to the function $f(x) =$

x^2+4x in Example 3.20 with $x=2$ and $dx=0.01$, we have

$$\frac{dy}{dx}=f'(1)=6 \qquad \text{(derivative)}$$

and

$$\frac{dy}{dx}=\frac{0.06}{0.01}=6. \qquad \text{(ratio of differentials)}$$

3.3.2 Linear Approximation

Earlier, we noted that for small Δx,

$$\frac{\Delta y}{\Delta x}\approx f'(x) \text{ and } \Delta y\approx f'(x)\Delta x.$$

Also since

$$dy=f'(x)dx,$$

it follows that

$$\Delta y\approx dy$$

and dy can be used to approximate Δy.

To interpret this result geometrically, we need to recall a basic property of the slope. The vertical change in a line is equal to the product of the slope and the horizontal change (Figure 3.15). Now consider the line tangent to the graph of $y=f(x)$, as shown in Figure 3.16. Since $f'(x)$ is the slope of the tangent line and dx is the horizontal change in the tangent line, it follows that the vertical change in tangent line is given by $dy=f'(x)dx$, as indicated in Figure 3.15.

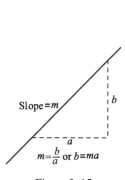

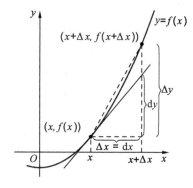

Figure 3.15   Figure 3.16

Example 3.21 Given $f(x)=x^2-3x$.

(1) Find Δy and dy when $x=2$;

(2) Compare Δy and dy from part (1) for $\Delta x=0.1,\ 0.2,\ 0.3$.

Solution (1)
$$\Delta y = f(2+\Delta x)-f(2)$$
$$=(2+\Delta x)^2-3(2+\Delta x)-(2^2-3\times 2)$$
$$=\Delta x^2+\Delta x.$$

Since $f'(x)=2x-3$, $f'(2)=1$, and $dx=\Delta x$, $dy=f'(2)dx=\Delta x$.

(2) Table 3.2 compares the values of Δy and dy for the indicated values of Δx.

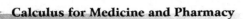

Table 3.2

Δx	Δy	dy
0.1	0.11	0.1
0.2	0.24	0.2
0.3	0.39	0.3

#

Your Practice 3.17 Repeat Example 3.21 for $x=3$ and $\Delta x=dx=-0.1,-0.2,-0.3$.

Example 3.22 There are spheres with a diameter of 10 cm, copper plating outside, copper thickness of 0.005 cm, to find the approximate volume of copper used.

Solution A sphere with a radius of R is

$$V=\frac{4}{3}\pi R^3 ,$$

then $dV=4\pi R^2 \cdot \Delta R$.

The known condition $R=5$ cm, $\Delta R=0.005$ cm$=\dfrac{1}{200}$ cm is substituted

$$dV=4\pi \cdot 5^2 \cdot \frac{1}{200}=\frac{\pi}{2}\approx 1.57.$$

And so the volume of copper is about 1.57 cm^3.   #

Example 3.23 After the patient takes the medicine, the function $c(t)=c_0(1-e^t)$ stands for the relationship of the blood drug concentration and time of the drug excreted through the kidney, where k is a constant and the constant c_0 is the initial concentration of the blood drug. After $\Delta t=0.1$ seconds, what is the increase in drug blood concentration?

Solution We know that $\Delta y\approx dy=f'(x)\Delta x$, since

$$c'(t)=c_0(1-e^t)'=-c_0 e^t.$$

The increase in drug concentration in blood is:

$$\Delta c \approx dc(t)=c'(t)dt$$
$$=c'(t)\Delta t=-c_0 e^t \cdot 0.1$$
$$=-\frac{c_0 e^t}{10}.$$ #

Exercise 3.3

1. Let $y=x^2$ and find the given values without using a calculator.

    (1) $f(0)$, $f(0.1)$;

    (2) $f(1)$, $f(1.1)$;

    (3) $f(10)$, $f(10.1)$;

    (4) $f(2.9)$, $f(3)$.

2. Find the indicated quantities for $y=2x^2$.

    (1) $\dfrac{\Delta y}{\Delta x}$, given $x_1=1$ and $x_2=3$;

    (2) $\dfrac{\Delta y}{\Delta x}$, given $x_1=2$ and $x_2=4$;

(3) $\dfrac{f(x_1+\Delta x)-f(x_1)}{\Delta x}$, given $x_1=1$

and $\Delta x=2$;

(4) $\dfrac{f(x_1+\Delta x)-f(x_1)}{\Delta x}$, given $x_1=2$

and $\Delta x=1$;

(5) $\dfrac{\Delta y}{\Delta x}$, given $x_1=2$ and $x_2=5$;

(6) $\dfrac{\Delta y}{\Delta x}$, given $x_1=3$ and $x_2=4$.

3. Find $\mathrm{d}y$ for each function.

(1) $y=x^2+12x+15$;

(2) $y=10x-\dfrac{x^2}{20}$;

(3) $y=x^2(1+x)$;

(4) $y=x^2(x+1)$;

(5) $y=x^2(x^2+x)$;

(6) $y=x^3(6-x)$.

4. Find the indicated quantities for $y=3x^2$.

(1) $\dfrac{f(1+\Delta x)-f(1)}{\Delta x}$;

(2) What does the quantity in part (1) approach as Δx approaches 0?

(3) $\dfrac{f(2+\Delta x)-f(2)}{\Delta x}$;

(4) What does the quantity in part (3) approach as Δx approaches 0?

5. Find $\mathrm{d}y$ for each function.

(1) $y=\dfrac{25}{\sqrt{x}}$;

(2) $y=\dfrac{x+1}{x}$;

(3) $y=\dfrac{(x+1)^2}{x^2}$;

(4) $y=(3x+5)^2$.

6. Evaluate $\mathrm{d}y$ and Δy for each function for the indicated values.

(1) $y=x^2-3x+2$, $x=5$, $\mathrm{d}x=\Delta x=0.2$;

(2) $y=x^3+2x+1$, $x=2$, $\mathrm{d}x=\Delta x=0.1$;

(3) $y=75\left(1-\dfrac{2}{x}\right)$, $x=5$, $\mathrm{d}x=\Delta x=-0.2$

(4) $y=100\left(x-\dfrac{2}{x^2}\right)$, $x=2$, $\mathrm{d}x=\Delta x=-0.1$.

7. Find $\mathrm{d}y$ and Δy for each function for the indicated values and compare the values of Δy and $\mathrm{d}y$.

(1) $y=x^2+2x+4$, $x=-0.5$, $\Delta x=\mathrm{d}x=0.1,\ 0.2,\ 0.3$;

(2) $y=x^2+2x+4$, $x=-2$, $\Delta x=\mathrm{d}x=0.1,\ 0.2,\ 0.3$;

(3) $y=x^3+2x^2$, $x=1$, $\Delta x=\mathrm{d}x=0.05,\ 0.1,\ 0.15$;

(4) $y=x^3+2x^2$, $x=2$, $\Delta x=\mathrm{d}x=0.05,\ 0.1,\ 0.15$.

8. A cube with 10-inch sides is covered with a coat of fiberglass 0.1 inch thick. Use differentials to estimate the volume of fiberglass shell.

9. A sphere with a radius of 5 cm is coated with 0.2 cm thick. Use differentials to estimate the volume of the ice.

10. Discuss the validity of each statement. If the statement is always true, explain why. If not, give a counter-example.

(1) If the graph of $y=f(x)$ is a line, then the functions Δy and $\mathrm{d}y$ (of the independent variable $\Delta x=\mathrm{d}x$) for $f(x)$ at $x=2$ are identical.

(2) If the graph of $y=f(x)$ is a parabola, then the functions Δy and $\mathrm{d}y$ (of the independent variable $\Delta x=\mathrm{d}x$) for $f(x)$ at $x=1$ are identical.

(3) Suppose that $y=f(x)$ defines a differentiable function whose domain is the set of all real numbers. If every differential

dy at $x=2$ is equal to 0, then $f(x)$ is a constant function.

(4) Suppose that $y=f(x)$ defines a function whose domain is the set of all real numbers. If every differential dy at $x=2$ is equal to 0, then $f(x)$ is a constant function.

11. Find dy if $y=(1-2x)\sqrt{x}$.

12. Find dy if $y=(2x-1)\sqrt[3]{x}$.

13. Find dy and Δy for $y=32\sqrt{x}$, $x=4$ and $\Delta x=dx=0.2$.

14. Find dy and Δy for $y=\dfrac{12}{\sqrt{x}}$, $x=16$ and $\Delta x=dx=1$.

15. One after x milligrams of a particular drug are given to a person, the change in body temperature T (in degrees Fahrenheit) is given by

$$T=x^2\left(1-\frac{x}{5}\right),\ 0\leqslant x\leqslant 5.$$

Approximate the changes in body temperature produced by the following changes in drug dosages

(1) from 1 to 1.1 milligrams;

(2) from 2 to 2.1 milligrams;

(3) from 3 to 3.1 milligrams.

16. A drug are given to a person to dilate her arteries. If the radius of an artery is increased from 2 to 2.1 millimeters, approximately how much is the cross-sectional area increased? (Assume that the cross section of the artery is circular; that is, $A=\pi r^2$)

17. The average pulse rate y (in beats per minute) of a healthy person x inches tall is given approximately by

$$y=\frac{590}{\sqrt{x}},\ 30\leqslant x\leqslant 75.$$

Approximate how will the pulse rate

change for a change in height

(1) from 32 to 33 inches?

(2) from 63 to 64 inches?

18. A company manufactures and sells x bicycles per a month. If the cost and the revenue equations are

$$C(x)=720+20x,\ x\in \mathbf{R},$$

$$R(x)=20x-\frac{x^2}{3},\ 0\leqslant x\leqslant 300.$$

What will the approximate changes in revenue and profit be if production is in-creased

(1) from 150 to 200?

(2) from 200 to 300?

19. A particular person learning to type has an achievement record given approximately by

$$N=60\left(1-\frac{2}{t}\right),\ 3\leqslant t\leqslant 15,$$

where N is the number of words per minute typed after t weeks of practice. What is the approximate improvement from 4 to 5 weeks of practice?

20. The median weight of a boy whose age is between 0 to 36 months can be approximated by the function

$$w(t)=9+2t-0.06t^2+0.0008t^3,$$

where t is measured in months and w is measured in pounds (Figure 3.17).

Approximate the change of weight for a boy from 1 to 3 months old.

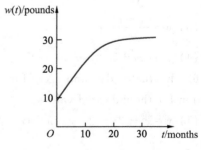

Figure 3.17

Summary and Review

Important Terms, Symbols, and Concepts

- The average rate of change of y with respect to x, as x changes from $x=a$ to $x=a+h$ is $\dfrac{f(a+h)-f(a)}{(a+h)-a}=\dfrac{f(a+h)-f(a)}{h}$, $h \neq 0$.

- For $y=f(x)$, the instantaneous rate of change at $x=a$ is

$$\lim_{h \to 0} \frac{f(a+h)-f(a)}{h}$$

if the limit exists.

- The derivative of $f(x)$ at x is defined by

$$f'(x)=\lim_{h \to 0} \frac{f(x+h)-f(x)}{h}$$

if the limit exists.

If the limit exists, we say that the function f is differentiable at x.

If $f(x)$ is differentiable at each x in an open interval (a, b), then $f(x)$ is said to be differentiable over (a, b).

- A line through two points on the graph of a function is called a secant line.

- The limit of secant lines is called the tangent line.

- If the derivative of a given function f exists at $x=a$, then $f'(a)$ is the slope of the tangent line at the point $(a, f(a))$. The equation of the tangent line is given by

$$y-f(a)=f'(a)(x-a).$$

- To find $f'(x)$, we use the three-step process.

Step 1: Find $f(x+h)-f(x)$.

Step 2: Find $\dfrac{f(x+h)-f(x)}{h}$.

Step 3: Find $f'(x)=\lim\limits_{h \to 0} \dfrac{f(x+h)-f(x)}{h}$.

- For $y=f(x)$, let $\Delta x=x_2-x_1$, then $\Delta y=f(x_2)-f(x_1)=f(x_1+\Delta x)-f(x_1)$ represents the change in y corresponding to a change Δx in x.

- If $y=f(x)$ defines a differentiable function, then the differential $\mathrm{d}y$ or $\mathrm{d}f$, is defined as the product of $f'(x)$ and $\mathrm{d}x$, where $\mathrm{d}x=\Delta x$. Symbolically,

$$\mathrm{d}y=f'(x)\Delta x \text{ or } \mathrm{d}f=f'(x)\Delta x$$

where

$$\mathrm{d}x=\Delta x.$$

Important Formula

Differentiation Formulas

$$\frac{\mathrm{d}}{\mathrm{d}x}k=0, \ \frac{\mathrm{d}}{\mathrm{d}x}x^n=nx^{n-1},$$

$$[cf(x)]'=cf'(x), \ [f(x) \pm g(x)]'=f'(x) \pm g'(x).$$

Chapter 4　Additional Derivative Topics

⋮ Introduction

4.1　Derivatives of Products and Quotients

This section discusses how to differentiate new functions formed from old functions by multiplication or division.

4.1.1　Derivatives of Products

We have found that the derivative of a sum is the sum of the derivatives. By analogy, one might be tempted to guess that the derivative of a product is the product of the derivatives. However, this guess is wrong by looking at a particular case.

Your Practice 4.1　Let $u(x)=x^3$, $v(x)=x^2$, $f(x)=u(x)v(x)=x^5$, which of the following is $f'(x)$?

(A) $u'(x)v'(x)$　　　　　　　　　(B) $u(x)v'(x)$

(C) $u'(x)v(x)$　　　　　　　　　(D) $u'(x)v(x)+u(x)v'(x)$

Comparing those expressions, we see that the derivative of a product is not the product of the derivatives. To see this, note that $f'(x)=(x^5)'=5x^4$, $u'(x)v'(x)=3x^2 \cdot 2x=6x^3$, $u(x)v'(x)=x^3 \cdot 2x=2x^4$, $u'(x)v(x)=3x^2 \cdot x^2=3x^4$, $u'(x)v(x)+u(x)v'(x)=5x^4$.

This practice shows that, in general, the derivative of a product is not the product of the derivatives. How can we discover the correct formula for general function of product form?

We start by assuming that both $u(x)$ and $v(x)$ are positive differentiable functions. Then the product $u(x)v(x)$ can be considered as an area of a rectangle (Figure 4.1). If x changes by an amount Δx, then the corresponding changes in u and v are

$$\Delta u=u(x+\Delta x)-u(x),$$

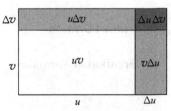

Figure 4.1

$$\Delta v = v(x + \Delta x) - v(x),$$

and the new value of the product $(u + \Delta u)(v + \Delta v)$, can be viewed as the area of the large rectangle in Figure 4. 1 (given that Δu and Δv happen to be positive).

The change in the area of the rectangle is the sum of the three shaded areas, then

$$\Delta(uv) = (u + \Delta u)(v + \Delta v) - uv$$
$$= u\Delta v + v\Delta u + \Delta u \Delta v. \tag{4.1}$$

Dividing the change by Δx, we get

$$\frac{\Delta(uv)}{\Delta x} = u\frac{\Delta v}{\Delta x} + v\frac{\Delta u}{\Delta x} + \Delta u\frac{\Delta v}{\Delta x}.$$

If we now let $\Delta x \to 0$, we get the derivative of uv:

$$\frac{d}{dx}(uv) = \lim_{\Delta x \to 0}\frac{\Delta(uv)}{\Delta x} \qquad (Recall \ that \ \frac{dy}{dx} = \lim_{\Delta x \to 0}\frac{\Delta y}{\Delta x})$$

$$= \lim_{\Delta x \to 0}\left(u\frac{\Delta v}{\Delta x} + v\frac{\Delta u}{\Delta x} + \Delta u\frac{\Delta v}{\Delta x}\right)$$

$$= u\lim_{\Delta x \to 0}\frac{\Delta v}{\Delta x} + v\lim_{\Delta x \to 0}\frac{\Delta u}{\Delta x} + (\lim_{\Delta x \to 0}\Delta u)\left(\lim_{\Delta x \to 0}\frac{\Delta v}{\Delta x}\right)$$

$$= u\frac{dv}{dx} + v\frac{du}{dx} + 0 \cdot \frac{dv}{dx}.$$

Notice that $\Delta u \to 0$ as $\Delta x \to 0$ since $u(x)$ is differentiable and therefore continuous. Thus

$$\frac{d}{dx}(uv) = \frac{du}{dx}v + u\frac{dv}{dx}. \tag{4.2}$$

We notice that Equation (4. 1) is always true despite the geometric interpretation that all the quantities are positive. The algebra is valid whether u, v, Δu, and Δv are positive or negative. So we have proved Equation (4. 2), known as **the Product Rule**, for all differentiable functions u and v.

The Product Rule

   Given $y = u(x)v(x)$. If $u'(x)$ and $v'(x)$ exist, then
$$(u(x)v(x))' = u'(x)v(x) + u(x)v'(x).$$
Also

$$(uv)' = u'v + uv', \quad \frac{dy}{dx} = \frac{du}{dx}v + u\frac{dv}{dx}.$$

The Product Rule says that the derivative of a product of two functions is the derivative of the first function times the second function plus the first function times the derivative of the second function.

Example 4. 1   Use two different methods to find $f'(x)$ for $f(x) = 3x^2(4x^3 - 2)$.

Solution   (**Method 1**) Use the Product Rule. We write $u = 3x^2$ and $v = 4x^3 - 2$. Both u and v are differentiable since they are polynomials. We have

$$u' = 6x, \ v' = 12x^2.$$

Then

$$f'(x) = u'v + uv'$$
$$= 6x(4x^3 - 2) + 3x^2(12x^2)$$
$$= 24x^4 - 12x + 36x^4$$
$$= 60x^4 - 12x.$$

(**Method 2**) Multiply first, then take derivatives:

$$f(x) = 12x^5 - 6x^2,$$
$$f'(x) = 60x^4 - 12x.$$ #

Your Practice 4.2 Use two different methods to find $f'(x)$ for $f(x) = 2x^3(3x^2 - 2x - 1)$.

At this point, all the product we encounter can be differentiated by either of the methods described in the above example. It is sometimes easier to simplify a product of functions than to use the Product Rule. In the next and later sections, we will see that the Product Rules is the only possible method in certain situations. Unless stated otherwise, we should use the Product Rule to differentiate all products in this section to gain experience with the use of this importance rule.

Example 4. 2 If $f(x) = \sqrt{x}\,g(x)$, where $g(x)$ is differentiable, $g(4) = 2$ and $g'(4) = 3$, find $f'(4)$.

Solution Applying the Product Rule, we get

$$f'(x) = [\sqrt{x}\,g(x)]' = (\sqrt{x})'g(x) + \sqrt{x}\,g'(x)$$
$$= \frac{1}{2\sqrt{x}}g(x) + \sqrt{x}\,g'(x).$$

Therefore, $f'(4) = \frac{1}{2\sqrt{4}}g(4) + 4g'(4) = \frac{1}{2\times 2}\times 2 + 2\times 3 = 6.5.$ #

Your Practice 4.3 If $f(x) = x^3 g(x)$, where $g(x)$ is differentiable, $g(2) = 4$ and $g'(2) = -3$, find $f'(2)$.

4.1.2 Derivatives of Quotients

Your Practice 4.4 Let $u(x) = x^5$, $v(x) = x^3$, $f(x) = \dfrac{u(x)}{v(x)} = \dfrac{x^5}{x^3} = x^2$, which of the following formulas is $f'(x)$?

(A) $\dfrac{u'(x)}{v'(x)}$;   (B) $\dfrac{u'(x)v(x)}{[v(x)]^2}$;   (C) $\dfrac{u(x)v'(x)}{[v(x)]^2}$;

(D) $\dfrac{u'(x)v(x)}{[v(x)]^2} - \dfrac{u(x)v'(x)}{[v(x)]^2} = \dfrac{u'(x)v(x) - u(x)v'(x)}{[v(x)]^2}.$

The expressions in Practice 4. 4 show that the derivative of a quotient leads to a more complicated quotient than you might expect.

We find a rule for differentiating the quotient of two differentiable functions by using the Product Rule. We write the function $u(x)$ by a product

$$u = \frac{u}{v} \cdot v$$

then apply the Product Rule to obtain

$$u' = \left(\frac{u}{v}\right)' \cdot v + \left(\frac{u}{v}\right) \cdot v'.$$

Solving the last equation with the unknown

$$\left(\frac{u}{v}\right)' = \frac{u' - \left(\frac{u}{v}\right) \cdot v'}{v} = \frac{u'v - uv'}{v^2}.$$

The Quotient Rule

If $y = \dfrac{u(x)}{v(x)}$, $v(x) \neq 0$, *both* $u'(x)$ *and* $v'(x)$ *exist, then*

$$\left[\frac{u(x)}{v(x)}\right]' = \frac{u'(x)v(x) - u(x)v'(x)}{[v(x)]^2}.$$

Also

$$\left(\frac{u}{v}\right)' = \frac{u'v - uv'}{v^2}, \quad \frac{dy}{dx} = \frac{\dfrac{du}{dx}v - u\dfrac{dv}{dx}}{v^2}.$$

In other words, the Quotient Rule says that the derivative of the quotient of two functions is the bottom function times the derivative of the top function minus the top function times the derivative of the bottom function, all over the bottom function squared.

Carefully note the exact form of the product and the quotient rules. In the product rule, we add $u'v$ and uv', whereas in the quotient rule, we subtract uv' from $u'v$.

Example 4.3　Find $f'(x)$ if $f(x) = \dfrac{2x-1}{4x^2+3}$. (This function is defined for all $x \in \mathbf{R}$ because $4x^2 + 3 \neq 0$)

Solution　We set $u = 2x - 1$ and $v = 4x^2 + 3$. Both u and v are differentiable since they are polynomials. We find

$$u' = 2, \; v' = 8x.$$

Using the quotient rule, we can calculate $f'(x)$.

$$f'(x) = \frac{u'v - uv'}{v^2}$$

$$= \frac{2 \cdot (4x^2+3) - (2x-1) \cdot 8x}{(4x^2+3)^2}$$

$$= \frac{8x^2 + 6 - 16x^2 + 8x}{(4x^2+3)^2}$$

$$= \frac{-8x^2 + 8x + 6}{(4x^2+3)^2}. \qquad \#$$

Your Practice 4.5　Find the derivatives of $f(x) = \dfrac{3x+7}{5x^2+8}$.

Example 4.4　The Monod growth function is named after French biologist Sir Jacques Monod. This function describes the rate of microbial growth as a function of nutrient density. It is given as

$$f(R) = c\,\frac{R}{s+R}, \; R \geqslant 0 \qquad (4.3)$$

where $c>0$ is the maximum growth rate and $s>0$ is semi-saturation constant. Find the derivative $f'(R)$.

Solution Since c and s are constant, $f(R)$ is defined for all $R\geqslant0$. We denote $u=cR$ and $v=s+R$, and obtain

$$u'=c,\ v'=1.$$

So

$$\frac{\mathrm{d}f(R)}{\mathrm{d}R}=\frac{u'v-uv'}{v^2}$$

$$=\frac{c(s+R)-cR\cdot1}{(s+R)^2}$$

$$=\frac{cs}{(s+R)^2}.\qquad\#$$

Example 4.5 Assume that $f(x)$ is differentiable. Find the derivative of $y=\dfrac{f(x)+2}{x^4+1}$.

Solution We set

$$u=f(x)+2, v=x^4+1,$$
$$u'=f'(x), v'=4x^3,$$

and use the Quotient Rule. We get that

$$y'=\frac{f'(x)(x^4+1)-[f(x)+2]\cdot4x^3}{(x^4+1)^2}$$

$$=\frac{f'(x)x^4+4(f(x)+2)x^3+f'(x)}{(x^4+1)^2}.\qquad\#$$

Your Practice 4.6 Suppose that $f(x)$ is differentiable. Find an expression for the derivative of $y=\dfrac{f(x)}{x^2}$.

Exercise 4.1

1. Find $f'(x)$.

(1) $f(x)=(4-2x^3)(x^2-2)$;

(2) $f(x)=(2x^2-3x)^2$;

(3) $f(x)=\sqrt{x}(2x^4-5x+2)$;

(4) $f(x)=(x^3-3+2)\left(\sqrt{x}+\dfrac{1}{\sqrt{x}}\right)$;

(5) $f(x)=\dfrac{3x^4-5}{2x+1}$;

(6) $f(x)=\dfrac{x^3-3x+1}{x+1}$;

(7) $f(x)=\dfrac{x^2-5}{x^3+1}$;

(8) $f(x)=\dfrac{3}{2x+1}-\dfrac{4}{\sqrt{x}}+\dfrac{2}{x^2}$.

2. Find $h'(x)$, where $f(x)$ is an unspecified differentiable function.

(1) $h(x)=x^3f(x)$;

(2) $h(x)=x^2[f(x)]^2$;

(3) $h(x)=[f(x)]^2-\dfrac{x}{f(x)}$;

(4) $h(x)=\dfrac{x^3+5f(x)}{f(x)}$;

(5) $h(x)=\dfrac{f(x)}{f(x)+x^2}$.

3. Find $f'(x)$ and find the equation of the line tangent to the graph of f at $x=2$.

(1) $f(x)=(7-3x)(1+2x)$;

(2) $f(x)=\dfrac{x-8}{3x-4}$.

4. One hour after x milligrams of a particular drug are given to a person, the change in body temperature T in degrees Fahrenheit is given approximately by

$$T(x)=x^2\left(1-\dfrac{x}{9}\right),\ 0\leqslant x\leqslant 7.$$

The rate $T'(x)$ at which T changes with respect to the size of the dosage, x, is called the sensitivity of the body to the dosage.

(1) Find $T'(x)$;

(2) Find $T'(1)$, $T'(3)$ and $T'(6)$, and interpret the results.

5. A drug is injected into a patient's bloodstream through her right arm. The drug concentration (in milligrams per cubic centimeter) in the bloodstream of the left arm t hours after the injection is given by

$$C(t)=\dfrac{0.14t}{t^2+1}.$$

(1) Find $C'(t)$;

(2) Find $C'(0.5)$ and $C'(3)$, and interpret the results.

6. Suppose that $f(1)=4$, $g(1)=-2$, $f'(1)=1$, $g'(1)=2$. Find:

(1) $(fg)'(1)$;

(2) $\left(\dfrac{f}{g}\right)'(1)$;

(3) $\left(\dfrac{g}{f}\right)'(1)$;

(4) $\left(\dfrac{1}{f+g}\right)'(1)$.

7. Suppose that $f(1)=4$, $g(1)=-3$, $f'(1)=1$, $g'(1)=-2$. Find $h'(1)$.

(1) $h(x)=5f(x)-4g(x)$;

(2) $h(x)=f(x)g(x)$;

(3) $h(x)=\dfrac{f(x)}{g(x)}$;

(4) $h(x)=\dfrac{g(x)}{f(x)-2}$.

8. If f and g are the functions whose graphs are shown in Figure 4.2, let $u(x)=f(x)g(x)$ and $v(x)=\dfrac{f(x)}{g(x)}$.

(1) Find $u'(1)$;

(2) Find $v'(5)$.

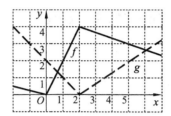

Figure 4.2

9. If F and G are the functions whose graphs are shown in Figure 4.3, let $u(x)=F(x)G(x)$ and $v(x)=\dfrac{F(x)}{G(x)}$.

(1) Find $u'(2)$;

(2) Find $v'(7)$.

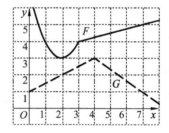

Figure 4.3

10. (1) Use the Product Rule twice to prove that if u, v, and w are differentiable, then $(uvw)'=u'vw+uv'w+uvw'$;

(2) Taking $u=v=w$ in part (1), show that

$$\dfrac{\mathrm{d}}{\mathrm{d}x}[u(x)]^3=3[u(x)]^2\,u'(x);$$

(3) Use part (2) to differentiate $y=(3x^2-4x+5)^3$.

11. (1) Use the Quotient Rule to prove **the Reciprocal Rule**

$$\dfrac{\mathrm{d}}{\mathrm{d}x}\left[\dfrac{1}{v(x)}\right]=-\dfrac{v'(x)}{[v(x)]^2};$$

(2) Use the Reciprocal Rule to differentiate the function $y=\dfrac{1}{x^2+4}$;

(3) Use the Reciprocal Rule to verify that the Power Rule is valid for negative integers, that is,

$$\frac{\mathrm{d}}{\mathrm{d}x}(x^{-n})=-nx^{-n-1}$$

for all positive integers n.

4.2 The Chain Rule

Suppose you are asked to differentiate the function

$$F(x)=\sqrt{x^4+1}.$$

The differentiation formulas you learned in the previous sections of this book do not enable you to calculate.

We try to write $F(x)$ in a familiar form. If we let $y=f(u)=\sqrt{u}$ and let $u=g(x)=x^4+1$, then we can write $y=F(x)=f[g(x)]=\sqrt{x^4+1}$. We call $f[g(x)]$ the **composition** of f and g. We know how to differentiate both f and g, so it would be useful to have a rule that tells us how to find the derivative of $f[g(x)]$ in terms of the derivatives of f and g. It turns out that the derivative of the composite function is the product of the derivative of f and g.

4.2.1 Composite Functions

We will now discuss the case of composite functions. Suppose that $y=f(u)$ and let $u=g(x)$. We can express f as a function of x by substituting $g(x)$ for u, that is, $y=f[g(x)]$. Functions that are defined in such a way are called composite functions.

> **Definition 4.1**
>
> Given two functions, the composite function $f\circ g$ (also called the composition of f and g) is defined by
>
> $$(f\circ g)(x)=f[g(x)]$$
>
> for each x in the domain of g for which $g(x)$ is in the domain of f.

The composition of functions is illustrated in Figure 4.4. To compute $f[g(x)]$, we start from the most inner part. Given the input x, we first compute $g(x)$ to be the output of the function $g(x)$. Then the quantity $g(x)$ is used as the input of f. Finally we get the output $f[g(x)]$ with respect to that x. This figure well explains the phrase "for each x in the domain of g for which $g(x)$ is in the domain of f". In order to compute $f(u)$, u needs to be in the domain of f. But since $u=g(x)$, we really require that $g(x)$ is in the domain of f for values of x we use to find $g(x)$. We usually call $g(x)$ the inner function and $f(u)$ the outer function.

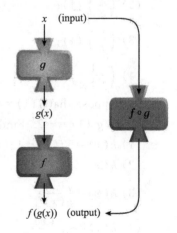

Figure 4.4

Example 4.6 Let $f(x) = \sqrt{x}$, $x \geqslant 0$ and $g(x) = x^2 + 3$. Calculate $f[g(x)]$ and $g[f(x)]$.

Solution Since $f(x) = \sqrt{x}$, we have $f[g(x)] = \sqrt{g(x)} = \sqrt{x^2 + 3}$ for $x \in \mathbf{R}$.

Since $g(x) = x^2 + 3$, we have $g[f(x)] = [f(x)]^2 + 3 = (\sqrt{x})^2 + 3 = x + 3$ for $x \geqslant 0$. #

You can see from the above example that, in general, $(f \circ g)$ is different from $(g \circ f)$. The order in the composition is important. Remember, the notation $(f \circ g)$ means that you apply the function g first and then f. In this example, $(f \circ g)$ is the function that first squares and adds 3 and then takes the square root; $(g \circ f)$ is the function that first takes the square root then squares and adds 3. In addition, you should pay attention to the domains of composite functions. The domain of $(g \circ f)$ in the last example is only the right half line $\{x \mid x \geqslant 0\}$ as f is defined for $x \geqslant 0$; the range of f is $\{u \mid u \geqslant 0\}$ and g is defined for all values in the range of f.

Your Practice 4.7 Given $f(x) = x^2 + x$, $g(x) = x^3 - x$, find $f[g(x)]$ and $g[f(x)]$.

We have used composition to make complicated functions from simpler ones. But in calculus it is often useful to decompose a complicated function into simpler ones, as in the following example.

Example 4.7 Write the function $m(x) = e^{x^2 + 4}$ as the composition of two functions g and f.

Solution Since $m(x) = e^{x^2 + 4}$, the formula for $m(x)$ says: first add 4 to the square of the input, then take the natural exponent of the result square. So we let

$$g(x) = x^2 + 4, \quad f(u) = e^u.$$

Then

$$(f \circ g)(x) = f[g(x)] = f(x^2 + 4) = e^{x^2 + 4} = m(x). \qquad \#$$

Your Practice 4.8 Write $k(x) = (2x^3 + 3)^2$ as the composition of two functions g and f.

The following result is useful in determining whether a composition of function is continuous.

Theorem 4.1 (Continuity of Composition Function)

   If $g(x)$ is continuous at $x = c$ with $g(c) = L$, and $f(x)$ is continuous at $x = L$, then the composite function $f[g(x)]$ is continues at c, that is,

$$\lim_{x \to c} (f \circ g)(x) = \lim_{x \to c} f[g(x)] = f[\lim_{x \to c} g(x)] = f[g(c)] = f(L).$$

To explain this theorem, we recall what it means to compute $(f \circ g)(c) = f[g(c)]$. When we compute $f[g(c)]$, we take the value c, compute $g(c)$, then take the result $g(c)$ and plug it into the function f to obtain $f[g(c)]$. If at each step the functions are continuous, the resulting function will be continuous.

Example 4.8 Determine the continuity of each function.

(1) $f(x) = e^{\frac{\pi}{x}}$; (2) $f(x) = e^{x^2}$; (3) $f(x) = \dfrac{1}{\sqrt{x+1}}$.

Solution　(1) We set $g(x) = \dfrac{\pi}{x}$ and $h(x) = e^x$. $g(x)$ is continuous for all $x \neq 0$. The range of $g(x)$ is $\mathbf{R}/0$, that is, the set of real numbers without 0. $h(x)$ is continuous for all x in the range of $g(x)$. Hence, $f(x)$ is continuous for all $x \neq 0$. Since $f(x)$ is not defined on $x = 0$, it is discontinuous at $x = 0$.

(2) Let $g(x) = x^2$ and $h(x) = e^x$. Then $f(x) = (h \circ g)(x)$. Since $g(x)$ is a polynomial, it is continuous for all $x \in \mathbf{R}$, and the range of $g(x)$ is $[0, +\infty)$, $h(x)$ is continuous for all values in the range of $g(x)$. Therefore, it follows that $f(x)$ is continuous for all $x \in \mathbf{R}$.

(3) We set $g(x) = \dfrac{1}{x+1}$ and $h(x) = x^{\frac{1}{2}}$. Then $f(x) = (h \circ g)(x)$ and $g(x)$ are both continuous for all $x \in \mathbf{R}/-1$. Since $h(x) = x^{\frac{1}{2}} = \sqrt{x}$, the range of $g(x)$ is $[0, +\infty)$, $h(x)$ is continuous for all $x \in [0, +\infty)$. So $f(x)$ is continuous for $x \in (-1, +\infty)$.　　＃

4.2.2　Proof of the Chain Rule

In many practical situations, you find that the rate at which one quantity is changing can be expressed as the product of other rates. For example, suppose the length of a metal bar is increasing at the rate of 2 mm for every degree increase in temperature and that temperature is increasing at the rate of 4 degree per hour. Then, to find out how much the metal bar is being expanded each hour, you would multiply the rates:

$$2 \text{ mm/degree} \times 4 \text{ degree/hour} = 8 \text{ mm/hour}.$$

Or, suppose the length be a function of temperature $L = f(p)$, and the function of time $p = g(t)$. Then the composition function $L = f(p) = f[g(t)]$ gives length as a function of time and

$$\frac{\mathrm{d}L}{\mathrm{d}p} = \left(\begin{array}{c}\text{the rate of change of length} \\ \text{with respect to temperature}\end{array}\right) \quad (\text{mm/degree}),$$

$$\frac{\mathrm{d}L}{\mathrm{d}p} = \left(\begin{array}{c}\text{the rate of change of temperature} \\ \text{with respect to time}\end{array}\right) \quad (\text{degree/hour}).$$

The product of these two rates is the rate of change of length with respect to time, that is,

$$\frac{\mathrm{d}L}{\mathrm{d}t} = \frac{\mathrm{d}L}{\mathrm{d}p} \cdot \frac{\mathrm{d}p}{\mathrm{d}t} \quad (\text{mm/hour}).$$

This formula is a special case of an important result in calculus called *the Chain Rule*.

The Chain Rule

Suppose $y = f(u)$ is a differentiable function of u, and $u = g(x)$ is a differentiable function of x. Then y is a composite function of x and

$$\frac{\mathrm{d}y}{\mathrm{d}x} = \frac{\mathrm{d}y}{\mathrm{d}u}\frac{\mathrm{d}u}{\mathrm{d}x}.$$

That is, the derivative of y with respect to x is the derivative of y with respect to u times the derivative of u with respect to x.

We will set the relationship between the increment of a function and its derivative. By definition we have

$$u'(x) = \lim_{\Delta x \to 0} \frac{u(x + \Delta x) - u(x)}{\Delta x},$$

rewrite which to get

$$\lim_{\Delta x \to 0} \left[\frac{u(x + \Delta x) - u(x)}{\Delta x} - u'(x) \right] = \lim_{\Delta x \to 0} \frac{u(x + \Delta x) - u(x)}{\Delta x} - \lim_{\Delta x \to 0} u'(x) = u'(x) - u'(x) = 0.$$

Now, define

$$\varepsilon(\Delta x) = \begin{cases} \dfrac{u(x + \Delta x) - u(x)}{\Delta x} - u'(x), & \text{if } \Delta x \neq 0, \\ 0, & \text{if } \Delta x \neq 0, \end{cases}$$

and notice that

$$\lim_{\Delta x \to 0} \varepsilon(\Delta x) = 0 = \varepsilon(0).$$

Therefore, $\varepsilon(\Delta x)$ is continuous at $\Delta x = 0$.

Now we have

$$u(x + \Delta x) = u(x) + \Delta x [\varepsilon(\Delta x) + u'(x)] \tag{4.4}$$

which is valid either for $\Delta x \neq 0$ or $\Delta x = 0$.

Thus, for a differentiable function f, we can write

$$\Delta u = u'(x) \Delta x + \varepsilon \cdot \Delta x \text{ where } \varepsilon \to 0 \text{ as } \Delta x \to 0 \tag{4.5}$$

and ε is a continuous function of Δx. This property of differentiable functions enables us to prove the Chain Rule.

Proof We would like to express the derivative $\dfrac{\mathrm{d}y}{\mathrm{d}x}$ in terms of the derivatives of f and g. Suppose $u = g(x)$ is differentiable at a and $y = f(u)$ is differentiable at $b = g(a)$.

Let Δx be an increment in x, Δu and Δy the corresponding increments in u and y. Then, by Equation (4.5) we have

$$\Delta u = g'(a) \Delta x + \varepsilon_1 \Delta x = [g'(a) + \varepsilon_1] \Delta x \tag{4.6}$$

where $\varepsilon_1 \to 0$ as $\Delta x \to 0$. By analogue,

$$\Delta y = f'(b) \Delta u + \varepsilon_2 \Delta u = [f'(b) + \varepsilon_2] \Delta u \tag{4.7}$$

where $\varepsilon_2 \to 0$ as $\Delta u \to 0$. Plugging Equation (4.6) into Equation (4.7) gives

$$\Delta y = [f'(b) + \varepsilon_2][g'(a) + \varepsilon_1] \Delta x. \tag{4.8}$$

So

$$\frac{\Delta y}{\Delta x} = [f'(b) + \varepsilon_2][g'(a) + \varepsilon_1].$$

As $\Delta x \to 0$, we have $\Delta u \to 0$ from Equation (4.6). Therefore both $\varepsilon_1 \to 0$ and $\varepsilon_2 \to 0$ as $\Delta x \to 0$. So

$$\frac{\mathrm{d}y}{\mathrm{d}x} = \lim_{\Delta x \to 0} \frac{\Delta y}{\Delta x} = \lim_{\Delta x \to 0} [f'(b) + \varepsilon_2][g'(a) + \varepsilon_1]$$

$$= f'(b) g'(a) = f'[g(a)] g'(a).$$

This is exactly what we need to prove and so we are done. #

Notice that one way to remember the Chain Rule is to pretend that the derivatives $\dfrac{\mathrm{d}y}{\mathrm{d}u}$

and $\dfrac{du}{dx}$ are quotients and to cancel du.

Example 4.9   Find $\dfrac{dF}{dx}$ if $F(x)=\sqrt{x^2+1}$.

Solution   write $F(x)=f[g(x)]$ where $y=f(u)=\sqrt{u}$ and $u=g(x)=x^2+1$. Since

$$\frac{dy}{du}=\frac{1}{2\sqrt{u}} \text{ and } \frac{du}{dx}=2x,$$

it follows that

$$\frac{dF}{dx}=\frac{dy}{dx}=\frac{dy}{du}\frac{du}{dx}$$

$$=\frac{1}{2\sqrt{u}}\cdot 2x.$$

Notice that this derivative is expressed in terms of the variables x and u. Since you are thinking of y as a function of x, you may want to express in terms of x alone. To do this, substitute x^2+1 for u in the expression for $\dfrac{dy}{dx}$ and simplify the answer as follows:

$$\frac{dF}{dx}=\frac{1}{2\sqrt{x^2+1}}\cdot 2x=\frac{x}{\sqrt{x^2+1}}. \qquad\qquad \#$$

Your Practice 4.9   Find $\dfrac{dy}{dx}$ if $y=(x^3+4x+1)^5$.

Recall that the composite function $f[g(x)]$ is the function formed from functions $f(u)$ and $g(x)$ by substituting $f(u)$ for u in the formula for $g(x)$. The Chain Rule is actually a rule for differentiating composite functions and can be rewritten using functional notation as follows:

> **The Chain Rule in Functional Notation**
>
> *If $y=f(u)$, $u=g(x)$ are differential functions and $f(x)=f[g(x)]$, then*
> $$F'(x)=\{f[g(x)]\}'=f'[g(x)]\cdot g'(x). \qquad (4.9)$$

The next example illustrates the use of this form of the Chain Rule.

Example 4.10   Find $f'(x)$ if $f(x)=\sqrt[3]{x^2-3x+1}$.

Solution   The form of the function is

$$f(x)=(\odot)^{\frac{1}{3}}$$

where the circle contains the expression x^2-3x+1, then

$$(\odot)'=(x^2-3x+1)'=2x-3.$$

According to the Chain Rule, the derivative of the composite function $f(x)$ is

$$f'(x)=\frac{1}{3}(\odot)^{-\frac{2}{3}}\cdot(\odot)'$$

$$=\frac{1}{3}(\odot)^{-\frac{2}{3}}\cdot(2x-3)$$

$$=\frac{1}{3}(x^2-3x+1)^{-\frac{2}{3}}\cdot(2x-3)$$

$$= \frac{2x-3}{3 \sqrt[3]{(x^2-3x+1)^2}}.$$ #

Your Practice 4.10　Find $F'(x)$ if $f(x)=\sqrt{x^2+1}$.

4.2.3　The General Power Rule

We have learned the rule

$$\frac{\mathrm{d}}{\mathrm{d}x}x^n=nx^{n-1}$$

for differentiating power functions. We will now turn to functions of form $[g(x)]^n$.

To derive the derivative $\frac{\mathrm{d}}{\mathrm{d}x}[g(x)]^n$, think of $[g(x)]^n$ as the composite function

$$[g(x)]^n=f[g(x)] \text{ where } f(u)=u^n,\ u=g(x).$$

Then

$$f'(u)=nu^{n-1} \text{ and } g'(x)=\frac{\mathrm{d}u}{\mathrm{d}x},$$

by the Chain Rule,

$$\frac{\mathrm{d}}{\mathrm{d}x}[g(x)]^n=\frac{\mathrm{d}}{\mathrm{d}x}f[g(x)]=f'[g(x)]g'(x)=nu^{n-1}\frac{\mathrm{d}u}{\mathrm{d}x}=n[g(x)]^{n-1}\frac{\mathrm{d}u}{\mathrm{d}x}.$$

Thus, by combining this rule with the Chain Rule, you have obtained the General Power Rule as follows:

The General Power Rule

If $u=g(x)$ is differentiable and n is a real number, then

$$\frac{\mathrm{d}}{\mathrm{d}x}[g(x)]^n=n[g(x)]^{n-1}\cdot\frac{\mathrm{d}g(x)}{\mathrm{d}x}.$$

In short,

$$\frac{\mathrm{d}}{\mathrm{d}x}u^n=nu^{n-1}\cdot\frac{\mathrm{d}u}{\mathrm{d}x}.$$

Example 4.11　Differentiate $y=(5x^3+1)^4$.

Solution　The function is a General Power $(\odot)^n$ where $\odot=5x^3+1$, $n=4$ and $(\odot)'=15x^2$. Applying the General Power Rule, we obtain

$$y'=\frac{\mathrm{d}y}{\mathrm{d}x}=n(\odot)^{n-1}\cdot(\odot)'$$
$$=4(5x^3+1)^3\cdot(15x^2)$$
$$=60x^2(5x^3+1)^3$$ #

Your Practice 4.11　Another way to do Example 4.11 is to expand the function and rewrite it as a polynomial and then differentiate this polynomial term by term. Do this way and compare your result with the example.

Your Practice 4.12　Find y' if $y=(4x^2-7)^3$.

Example 4.12　Differentiate $y=\dfrac{1}{\sqrt{x^2+x+1}}$.

Solution Do not use the Quotient Rule in this case! It is much easier to rewrite the function as

$$y=(x^2+x+1)^{-1/2}$$

and apply the General Power Rule to get

$$y'=-\frac{1}{2}(x^2+x+1)^{-1/2-1} \cdot \frac{d}{dx}(x^2+x+1)=-\frac{1}{2}(x^2+x+1)^{-3/2} \cdot (2x+1)$$

$$=-\frac{2x+1}{2(x^2+x+1)^{3/2}}.$$

#

Example 4.13 Suppose $f(x)$ is differentiable. Find $\dfrac{d}{dx}\dfrac{1}{\sqrt{f(x)}}$.

Solution The given function is similar as that in the previous example except that the inner function is not specified. We set

$$h(x)=\frac{1}{\sqrt{f(x)}}=[f(x)]^{-1/2}.$$

Now, apply the General Power Rule to get

$$\frac{d}{dx}h(x)=-\frac{1}{2}[f(x)]^{-1/2-1} \cdot f'(x)=-\frac{f'(x)}{2[f(x)]^{3/2}}.$$

#

Your Practice 4.13 Find y' if $y=\dfrac{1}{(2-x^4)^3}$.

The Chain Rule is usually used in combination with the other rules we learned in previous sections. The next example involves the Product Rule.

Example 4.14 Differentiate the function $f(x)=(x^2-1)(3x+5)^5$ and simplify your answer.

Solution We first use the Product Rule to obtain

$$f'(x)=(x^2-1)' \cdot (3x+5)^5+(x^2-1) \cdot [(3x+5)^5]'.$$

The term $(x^2-1)'=2x$ is clear so we continue by applying the General Power Rule to the last term:

$$f'(x)=2x \cdot (3x+5)^5+(x^2-1) \cdot 5 \cdot (3x+5)^4 \cdot (3x+5)'$$
$$=2x \cdot (3x+5)^5+(x^2-1) \cdot 5 \cdot (3x+5)^4 \cdot 3$$
$$=2x(3x+5)^5+15(x^2-1)(3x+5)^4.$$

Finally, simplify the answer by factoring:

$$f'(x)=(3x+5)^4[2x(3x+5)+15(x^2-1)]=(3x+5)^4(21x^2+10x-15).$$

#

Your Practice 4.14 Find y' if $y=(2x-1)^3(x^2+2)^2$.

Example 4.15 Differentiate $y(t)=\left(\dfrac{t-2}{2t+1}\right)^9$.

Solution First apply the General Power Rule to get

$$y'(t)=9\left(\frac{t-2}{2t+1}\right)^8 \cdot \frac{d}{dt}\left(\frac{t-2}{2t+1}\right).$$

Now use the Quotient Rule to find that

$$\frac{d}{dt}\left(\frac{t-2}{2t+1}\right)=\frac{1 \cdot (2t+1)-(t-2) \cdot 2}{(2t+1)^2}=\frac{5}{(2t+1)^2}$$

and substitute the result into the equation for $y'(t)$:

$$y'(t)=9\left(\frac{t-2}{2t+1}\right)^8 \cdot \frac{5}{(2t+1)^2}=\frac{45(t-2)^8}{(2t+1)^{10}}. \qquad \#$$

Your Practice 4.15　Find y' if $y=\dfrac{(2x+1)^3}{3x}$.

We summarize the differentiation formulas we have learned so far as follows:

Differentiation Formulas

$$\frac{d}{dx}c=0; \qquad \frac{d}{dx}x^n=nx^{n-1}; \qquad \frac{d}{dx}[g(x)]^n=n[g(x)]^{n-1}g'(x);$$

$$[cf(x)]'=cf'; \qquad [f(x)\pm g(x)]'=f(x)'\pm g'(x); \qquad (uv)'=u'v+uv';$$

$$\left(\frac{u}{v}\right)'=\frac{u'v-uv'}{v^2}; \qquad \{f[g(x)]\}'=f'[g(x)]g'(x).$$

Exercise 4.2

　1.　Given $f(x)=x^2+1$, $g(x)=2x-1$, find the functions $f\circ g$, $g\circ f$, $f\circ f$, and $g\circ g$.

　2.　Given $f(x)=x-3$, $g(x)=x^2+4x+5$, find the functions $f\circ g$, $g\circ f$, $f\circ f$, and $g\circ g$.

　3.　Express the function in the form $f\circ g$.

(1) $F(x)=(x^3-5)^6$;

(2) $F(x)=\dfrac{\sqrt{x}}{1+\sqrt{x}}$;

(3) $F(x)=\sqrt{\dfrac{x}{1+x}}$;

(4) $F(x)=e^{2\sqrt{x}-1}$.

4.　Find $f'(x)$.

(1) $f(x)=(3x^2+2)^4$;

(2) $f(x)=(x^3+5x+2)^7$;

(3) $f(x)=\dfrac{1}{(x^2+x+2)^3}$;

(4) $f(x)=\sqrt{3-x}$;

(5) $f(x)=\dfrac{x^3}{(2-3x)^5}$;

(6) $f(x)=\dfrac{4}{(x^2+7)^3}$;

(7) $f(x)=\sqrt{(2x-3)^3(x+1)^5}$;

(8) $f(x)=\sqrt{\dfrac{2x+5}{x^2+3}}$;

(9)　Suppose that $f'(x)=e^x+x$, find $\dfrac{d}{dx}f(x^3)$ at $x=1$.

5.　Suppose that $f'(x)=e^x+x$, find:

(1) $\dfrac{d}{dx}f(x^3)$ at $x=1$;

(2) $\dfrac{d}{dx}f(\sqrt{x})$ at $x=4$;

(3) $\dfrac{d}{dx}f\left(\dfrac{1}{\sqrt{x}}\right)$ at $x=1$;

(4) $\dfrac{d}{dx}f\left(\dfrac{x-1}{x^2+1}\right)$ at $x=0$.

6.　Suppose $L(x)$ is a function with the property that $L'(x)=\dfrac{1}{x}$. Use the Chain Rule to find the derivatives of the following functions and simplify your answers.

(1) $f(x)=L(x^3+2)$;

(2) $f(x)=L\left(\dfrac{1}{x}\right)$;

(3) $f(x)=L\left(\dfrac{3}{4\sqrt{x}}\right)$;

(4) $f(x)=L\left(\dfrac{x^4+1}{x^2+3}\right)$.

7.　Assume that $f(x)$ and $g(x)$ are

differentiable, find:

(1) $\dfrac{d}{dx}\sqrt{f(x)+g(x)}$;

(2) $\dfrac{d}{dx}\left[\dfrac{f(x)}{g(x)}+1\right]^3$;

(3) $\dfrac{d}{dx}f\left[\dfrac{1}{g(x)}\right]$;

(4) $\dfrac{d}{dx}\dfrac{[f(x)]^2}{g(3x)+3x}$.

8. Let $f(x)=(4x-3)^{1/2}$. Find $f'(x)$ and the equation of the line tangent to the graph of f at $x=3$. Find the value(s) of x where the tangent line is horizontal.

9. Find the equation of the line tangent to the graph of f at $x=2$ for $f(x)=x^2\sqrt{2x+12}$.

10. Find the value(s) of x where the tangent line is horizontal for $f(x)=\dfrac{x^3}{(3x-2)^2}$.

11. Find the value(s) of x where the tangent line is horizontal for $f(x)=\dfrac{x-1}{(x-3)^3}$.

12. The number y of bacteria in a certain colony after x days is given approxi-mately by

$$y=(3\times10^6)\dfrac{1}{\sqrt[3]{(x^2-1)^2}}.$$

Find $y'(x)$.

13. An environmental study of a certain suburban community states that the average daily level of carbon monoxide in the air will be $c(p)=\sqrt{0.5p^2+17}$ parts per million when the population is p thousand. It is estimated that t years from now, the population of the community will be $p(t)=3.1+0.1t^2$ thousand. At what rate will the carbon monoxide level be changing with respect to time 3 years from now?

14. It has been determined that the flow of blood from an artery into a small capillary is given by the formula

$$F=kD^2\sqrt{A-C}\ (\text{cm}^3/\text{second})$$

where D is the diameter of the capillary, A is the pressure in the artery, C is the pressure in the capillary, and k is a positive constant.

(1) By how much is the flow of blood F changing with respect to pressure C in the capillary if A and D are kept constant? Does the flow increase or decrease with increasing C?

(2) What is the percentage rate of change of flow F with respect to A if C and D are kept constant?

4.3 Logarithmic Function

4.3.1 Inverse Function

Before we introduce logarithmic functions, we need to know the concept of inverse functions. As shown in Figure 4.5, the function f maps a to 2, the inverse function, denoted by f^{-1} (read as "f inverse"), takes 2 and maps it back into a.

Not every function has an inverse; because an inverse function is a function itself, we require that every value y in the range of f be mapped into exactly one value of x. In other words, we need that whenever $x_1\neq x_2$, then $f(x_1)\neq f(x_2)$, or, equivalently, that $f(x_1)=f(x_2)$ implies $x_1=x_2$.

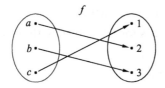 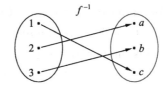

Figure 4.5

Consider $y=x^3$ and $y=x^2$, for $x \in \mathbf{R}$. The function $y=x^3$ has an inverse function, because $x_1^3 \neq x_2^3$ whenever $x_1 \neq x_2$, whereas $y=x^2$ does not have an inverse function, because $x_1 \neq x_2$ does not suggest $x_1^2 \neq x_2^2$. For example, both 2 and -2 are mapped into 4, and we find that $f(2)=f(-2)$ but $2 \neq -2$. In other words, there are two different values of x that produce the same value of y.

More generally, a function f have an inverse on its domain D if $x_1 \neq x_2$ implies $f(x_1) \neq f(x_2)$ (or, equivalently, $f(x_1)=f(x_2)$ implies $x_1=x_2$). Functions that have this property are called ***one-to-one***. A function is a one-to-one function if and only if each second element corresponds to one and only one first element. (Each x and y value is used only once)

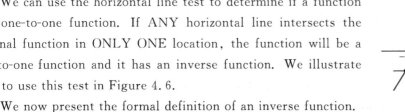

We can use the horizontal line test to determine if a function is a one-to-one function. If ANY horizontal line intersects the original function in ONLY ONE location, the function will be a one-to-one function and it has an inverse function. We illustrate how to use this test in Figure 4.6.

We now present the formal definition of an inverse function.

Figure 4.6

Definition 4.2

Let $f: D \rightarrow S$ be one-to-one function with domain D and range S. Then the inverse function f^{-1} has domain S and range D and is defined by

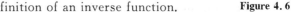

$$f^{-1}(y)=x \text{ if and only if } y=f(x)$$

for all y in S.

Note that the "-1" is ***not*** an exponent despite the fact that it sure does look like one! When dealing with inverse functions we should remember that

$$f^{-1}(x) \neq \frac{1}{f(x)}.$$

The inverse function is uniquely determined by f. To find the inverse function there are four steps:

(1) First, replace $f(x)$ with y. This is done to make the rest of the process easier.

(2) Solve the equation for x.

(3) Interchange x and y. This is done because we usually write functions as functions of x.

(4) Replace y with $f^{-1}(x)$.

Example 4.16 Find the inverse of $f(x)=x^2+3$, $x\geqslant0$.

Solution Note that $f(x)$ is one-to-one. To show it, start with $f(x_1)=f(x_2)$ and demonstrate that this implies $x_1=x_2$:

$$f(x_1)=f(x_2),$$
$$x_1^2+3=x_2^2+3,$$
$$x_1^2=x_2^2.$$

Note that both x_1 and x_2 are nonnegative, then we get $x_1=x_2$ by taking the square root on both sides. Now we apply the four steps to find $f^{-1}(x)$.

(1) Write $y=x^2+3$.

(2) Solve for x:

$$x^2+3=y,$$
$$x=\sqrt{y-3}.$$

The range of f is $[3,+\infty)$, and which is the possible values for y, so we get

$$x=\sqrt{y-3},\ y\geqslant3.$$

(3) Interchange x and y:

$$y=\sqrt{x-3},\ x\geqslant3.$$

(4) Replace y with $f^{-1}(x)$:

$$f^{-1}(x)=\sqrt{x-3},\ x\geqslant3. \qquad\#$$

There is an interesting relationship between the graph of a function and the graph of its inverse. Basically speaking, the process of finding an inverse is simply the swapping of the x and y coordinates. Note that switching x and y corresponds to reflecting the graph of $y=f(x)$ about the line $y=x$. Figure 4.7 shows the graphs of f and f^{-1}. We can see that the graph of the inverse is a reflection of the actual function about the line $y=x$. This will always be the case with the graphs of a function and its inverse.

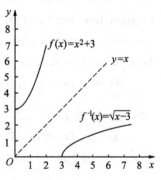

Figure 4.7

Your Practice 4.16 Find the inverse function of $f(x)=x^3+1$, $x\geqslant0$.

4.3.2 Differentiability of Inverses

We obtain some geometric observation about the graphs of $f(x)$ and $f^{-1}(x)$: in one coordinate system, they are reflection about the line $y=x$. An interesting thing to notice is that the slopes of the graphs of f and f^{-1} are multiplicative inverses of each other. For instance, if $f(x)=2x+1$, then f has an inverse function given by $f^{-1}(x)=(x-1)/2$. The slope of the graph of f is 2 and the slope of the graph of f^{-1} is 1/2. When you reflect across $y=x$, you take the reciprocal of the slope. This is a general feature of inverse functions (Figure 4.8). This

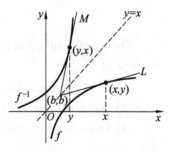

Figure 4.8

geometric observation is of great help in explaining the general differential formula of the inverse function.

The point (y, x) is on the graph of f^{-1}, which means that $f^{-1}(y)=x$. Assuming that f^{-1} is differentiable at y, we denote the tangent line to the graph f^{-1} at (y, x) by M. The slope of M is equal to the value of the derivative of f^{-1} at y:

$$\text{slope of } M=(f^{-1})'(y).$$

We denote the tangent line to f at (x, y) by L. The slope of L will be given by the value of the derivative of f at x:

$$\text{slope of } L=f'(x).$$

Since the graph of f^{-1} is obtained from the graph of f by reflection across $y=x$, the same is true for the tangent lines. M is obtained from L by reflection across the line $y=x$. This implies that the slopes of L and M are reciprocals,

$$(f^{-1})'(y)=\text{slope of } M=\frac{1}{\text{slope of } L}=\frac{1}{f'(x)}.$$

Here is the actual result.

Theorem 4.2 (Derivative of the Inverse Function)

Suppose that f is invertible. If f is differentiable at x and $f'(x)$ is not equal to zero, then the inverse function f^{-1} is differentiable at $y=f(x)$ and the following differentiation formula

$$(f^{-1})'(y)=\frac{1}{f'(x)} \tag{4.10}$$

holds.

Proof By definition, for each y in the domain of f^{-1}, there is one and only one x in the domain of f such that $y=f(x)$. Then

$$f^{-1}[f(x)]=x.$$

Differentiate with respect to x on both sides

$$\frac{\mathrm{d}}{\mathrm{d}x}f^{-1}[f(x)]=\frac{\mathrm{d}}{\mathrm{d}x}x.$$

Apply the Chain Rule to the left side

$$(f^{-1})'[f(x)]f'(x)=1.$$

If $f'(x)\neq0$, then

$$(f^{-1})'[f(x)]=\frac{1}{f'(x)},$$

$$(f^{-1})'(y)=\frac{1}{f'(x)}. \qquad\qquad \#$$

Example 4.17 Given $f(x)=x^3-2x$, find $(f^{-1})'(4)$.

Solution Note that f is one-to-one and

$$(f^{-1})'(y)=\frac{1}{f'(x)}, \quad f(x)=y.$$

To compute $(f^{-1})'(y)$ at $y=4$, we find a number x such that $f(x)=4$:

$$f(x)=4 \Rightarrow x^3-2x=4 \Rightarrow x=2.$$

Since $f'(2)=3\times 2^2-2=10$, then

$$(f^{-1})'(4)=\frac{1}{f'(2)}=\frac{1}{10}.$$

Note that to calculate $(f^{-1})'(4)$ we only need the value of x such that $f(x)=4$, not the inverse function f^{-1}.   #

Your Practice 4.17   If $f(x)=x^3+x$, find $(f^{-1})'(10)$.

Example 4.18   Use the derivative of the inverse function to find the derivative of $f(x)=\dfrac{x-2}{x}$.

Solution   The inverse of $f(x)=\dfrac{x-2}{x}$ is $f^{-1}(y)=\dfrac{2}{1-y}$.

We will use Equation (4.10) and begin by finding $(f^{-1})'(y)$. Thus,

$$(f^{-1})'(y)=\frac{2}{(1-y)^2}$$

and

$$f'(x)=\frac{1}{(f^{-1})'(y)}=\frac{(1-y)^2}{2}=\frac{\left(1-\dfrac{x-2}{x}\right)^2}{2}=\frac{2}{x^2}.$$

We can verify that this is the correct derivative by applying the Quotient Rule to $g(x)$ to obtain

$$f'(x)=\frac{2}{x^2}.$$ #

Your Practice 4.18   Use the derivative of the inverse function to find the derivative of $f(x)=\dfrac{1}{x+2}$.

4.3.3 Logarithmic Functions

Although we have built exponential models and used them to make predictions, how to solve exponential equations has not yet been discussed. The reason is simple: none of the algebraic tools mentioned so far are sufficient to solve exponential equations.

Consider the equation $2^x=6$. We know that $2^2=4$ and $2^3=8$, so it is clear that x must be some value between 2 and 3 since $f(x)=2^x$ is increasing. We could use graph to better estimate the solution. From the graph in Figure 4.9, we could better estimate the solution to be around 2.7. This result is still fairly unsatisfactory, and since the exponential function is one-to-one, it would be great to have an inverse function. None of the functions we have already discussed would serve as an inverse function and so we must introduce a new function, named logarithm (log) as the inverse of an exponential function. Since exponential functions have

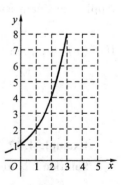

Figure 4.9

different bases, we will define corresponding logarithms of different bases as well.

Definition 4.3

The logarithm to base b function, written as $\log_b x$, is the inverse of the exponential function to the same base b^x.

Since log is a function, it is most correctly written as $\log_b x$, using parentheses to denote function evaluation, just as we would do with $f(x)$. However, when the input is a single variable or number, it is common to drop the parentheses and write the expression as $\log_b x$.

The domain of $f(x) = b^x$ is the set of all real numbers, and its range is the set of all positive numbers. Since the range of f is the domain of its inverse, we find that the domain of $f^{-1}(x) = \log_b x$ is the set of positive numbers. It is important to remember that the logarithm is only defined for positive numbers, that is, $y = \log_b x$ is only defined for $x > 0$.

Since the logarithm and exponential are inverses, we can now summarize the relationship between them:

Properties of Logs (Inverse Properties)
$$b^{\log_b x} = x \ for \ x > 0,$$
$$\log_b b^x = x \ for \ x \in \mathbf{R}.$$

By utilizing the Exponential Rule and the Inverse Property, we can prove the following properties of the logarithm:

$$\log_b(st) = \log_b s + \log_b t, \qquad (product \ Property)$$
$$\log_b\left(\frac{s}{t}\right) = \log_b s - \log_b t, \qquad (quotient \ Property)$$
$$\log_b s^r = r\log_b s. \qquad (exponent \ Property)$$

The Exponent Property allows us to find a method for changing the base of a logarithmic expression:

$$\log_b A = \frac{\log_c A}{\log_c b}.$$

Also recall from the definition of an inverse function that if $f(x) = y$, then $f^{-1}(y) = x$. Applying this to the exponential and logarithmic functions, we have that logarithm is equivalent to an exponential: The statement $b^x = y$ is equivalent to the statement $\log_b y = x$.

Alternatively, we could show this by starting with the exponential function $y = b^x$, then taking the log base b of both sides, giving $\log_b y = \log_b b^x$. Using the Inverse Property of logs we see that $\log_b y = x$.

4.3.3.1   Natural logarithms

The natural log is the logarithm with base e, and is typically written as $\ln x$. Thus, ln

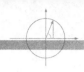

x is the inverse of the exponential function with the natural base e. The graphs of $y=e^x$ and $y=\ln x$ are shown in Figure 4.10. We see that both e^x and $\ln x$ are increasing functions. However, whereas e^x climbs very quickly for large values of x, $\ln x$ increases very slowly for large values of x. Note that each can be obtained as the reflection of the other about the line $y=x$.

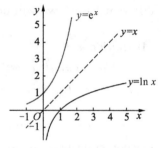

Figure 4.10

4.3.3.2 Common logarithms

The logarithm to base 10 is typically written as $\lg x$ and is called the Common Logarithms.

Example 4.19 Simplify the following expression.

(1) $\log_2(x^2-9)$;

(2) $\log_3 9^x$;

(3) $\ln e^{3x^2+1}$.

Solution

(1) We write x^2-9 as a product then simplify the expression:
$$\log_2(x^2-9)=\log_2(x+3)(x-3)=\log_2(x+3)+\log_2(x-3).$$

(2) Simplifying yields
$$\log_3 9^x=x\log_3 9=x\log_3 3^2=x\cdot 2=2x.$$

The fact that $\log_3 3^2=2$ can be explained in two ways: we can write $9=3^2$ and say that $\log_3 9$ undoes raising 3 to the second power, or we say that $\log_3 9$ denotes the exponent to which we must raise 3 in order to get 9.

(3) We use the fact that $\ln x$ and e^x are inverse functions, and find that
$$\ln e^{3x^2+1}=3x^2+1.$$

Any exponential function with base b can be written as an exponential function with base e. Likewise, any logarithmic function to base b can be written in terms of the natural logarithm. The following two identities illustrate this:

$$b^x=e^{x\ln b},$$
$$\log_b x=\frac{\ln x}{\ln b}.$$

The first identity follows from the fact that **exp** and **ln** are inverse functions, which implies that $b^x=\exp(\ln b^x)$, and the fact that $\ln b^x=x\ln b$. To understand the second identity, note that

$$y=\log_b x \text{ is equivalent to } b^y=x.$$

Taking logarithms to base e on both sides of $b^y=x$, we obtain

$$\ln b^y=\ln x$$

or
$$y\ln b=\ln x,$$

hence,

$$y = \frac{\ln x}{\ln b}.$$

Example 4.20　Write the following expressions in terms of base e.

(1) $3x$;

(2) $4x^3 + 2$;

(3) $\log_5 x$;

(4) $\log_2(4x - 3)$.

Solution

(1) $3^x = \exp(\ln 3^x) = \exp(x\ln 3) = e^{x\ln 3}$;

(2) $4^{x^3+2} = \exp(\ln 4^{x^3+2}) = \exp[(x^3+2)\ln 4] = e^{(x^3+2)\ln 4}$;

(3) $\lg(5x) = \dfrac{\ln 5x}{\ln 10}$;

(4) $\log_2(4x-3) = \dfrac{\ln(4x-3)}{\ln 2}$.　　　　　　　　#

We can use the definition of a logarithm to solve logarithmic equations.

Example 4.21　Using algebra to solve a logarithmic equation $2\ln x + 7 = 11$.

Solution　Subtract 7:

$$2\ln x = 4.$$

Divide by 2:

$$\ln x = 2.$$

Rewrite in exponential form:

$$x = e^2.$$　　　　　　　　#

Example 4.22　Use the one-to-one properties of logarithms to solve the logarithmic equation $\ln(3x-2) - \ln 2 = \ln(x+4)$.

Solution　Apply the Quotient Rule of logarithms,

$$\ln\left(\frac{3x-2}{2}\right) = \ln(x+4).$$

Apply the one-to-one property of a logarithm,

$$\frac{3x-2}{2} = x + 4.$$

Multiply both sides of the equation by 2

$$3x - 2 = 2x + 8.$$

Subtract $2x$ and add 2

$$x = 10.$$　　　　　　　　#

Example 4.23　Radioactive iodine is used by doctors as a tracer in diagnosing certain thyroid gland disorders. This type of iodine decays in such a way that the mass remaining after t days is given by the function

$$m(t) = 6e^{-0.087t}$$

where $m(t)$ is measured in grams.

(1) Find the mass at time $t = 0$.

(2) How much of the mass remains after 20 days?

(3) How many days will it take for iodine to be half of its original mass?

Solution

(1) The mass at time $t=0$ is
$$m(0)=6 \cdot e^0=6 \text{ (grams)}.$$

(2) After 20 days, the mass is
$$m(20)=6 \cdot e^{-0.087 \times 20} \approx 1.053 \text{ (grams)}.$$

(3) Suppose that t days later the mass will be half of its original mass, that is $m(t)=\dfrac{m(0)}{2}=\dfrac{6}{2}=3$. Then
$$3=6e^{-0.087t}.$$

Divide by 6:
$$0.5=e^{-0.087t}$$

Take ln on both sides:
$$\ln 0.5=-0.087t.$$

Use a calculator to find $t \approx 7.967$ (days).

Exercise 4.3

1. Which of the following function is one-to-one?

(1) $f(x)=x^2$;

(2) $f(x)=x^2$, $x \geqslant 0$;

(3) $f(x)=\dfrac{1}{x^3}$;

(4) $f(x)=\dfrac{1}{x^2}$;

(5) $f(x)=x^2-x$;

(6) $f(x)=e^{x+1}$.

2. Show that $f(x)=x^3+1$ is one-to-one, and find its inverse together with its domain. Then graph $f(x)$ and $f^{-1}(x)$ in one coordinate system, together with the line $y=x$, and convince yourself that the graph of $f^{-1}(x)$ can be obtained by reflecting the graph of $f(x)$ about the line $y=x$.

3. Show that $f(x)=x^2-1$, $x \geqslant 0$ is one-to-one, and find its inverse together with its domain. Then graph $f(x)$ and $f^{-1}(x)$ in one coordinate system, together with the line $y=x$, and convince yourself that the graph of $f^{-1}(x)$ can be obtained by reflecting the graph of $f(x)$ about the line $y=x$.

4. Find the inverse of the function $f(x)=\dfrac{x+1}{x}$ (given that x is not equal to 0).

5. Find the inverse of the function $f(x)=(3x-5)^3$.

6. Use the derivative of the inverse function to find the derivative of $f(x)=\sqrt[3]{x}$.

7. Use the derivative of the inverse function to find the derivative of $f(x)=\sqrt[5]{x}$.

8. Write the following expressions in terms of base e.

(1) $2x^2+1$;

(2) 5^{3x};

(3) $\log(x+1)$;

(4) $\log_2(3x^2-4)$.

9. Simplify the following expressions.

(1) $\ln x^2+\ln x^3$;

(2) $e^{2\ln x}$;

(3) $\ln(x^2-4)-\ln(x+2)$;

(4) $\ln e^{x^2+1}$.

10. The graphs of the functions e^x, e^{-x}, $\ln x$ are displayed in Figure 4. 11. Match each equation with the corresponding graph.

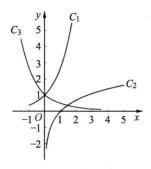

Figure 4. 11

11. Solve equation $e^{2x}=4.304$ (to four decimal places). If you have no calculators, use explicit expression.

12. Solve equation $e^x=0.3059$ to four decimal places.

13. Find the domain and range of the function defined by $y=1+\ln(x+1)$.

14. Show that if $0<b<1$, the function $y=b^x$ can be written in the form $y=e^{-kx}$, where k is a positive constant. Write k in terms of b.

15. Because of the extraordinary range of sensitivity of the human ear (a range of over 1000 million million to 1), it is helpful to use a logarithmic scale, rather than an absolute scale, to measure sound intensity over this range. The unit of measure is called the decibel, after the inventor of the telephone, Alexander Graham Bell. Denote the number of decibel by N and the power of the sound in question by I (in watts per square centimeter), and the power sound just below the threshold of hearing by I_0 (approximately 10^{-16} watt per square centimeter). Then

$$I=I_0 10^{N/10}.$$

Show that this formula can be written in the form

$$N=10\lg\frac{I}{I_0}.$$

16. The relationship between the number of decibel N and the power of sound I can be given as

$$N=10\lg\frac{I}{I_0}.$$

where $I_0 = 10^{-16}$ watt per square centimeter (W/cm^2). Find the decibel of the following sounds:

(1) Whisper: 10^{-13} W/cm^2;

(2) Normal conversation: 3.16×10^{-10} W/cm^2;

(3) Heavy traffic: 10^{-8} W/cm^2;

(4) Jet plane with afterburner: 10^{-1} W/cm^2.

17. How many years will it take an investment of 35000 Yuan to grow to 50000 Yuan if it is invested at 4.75% compounded continuously (to two decimal places)? If you have no calculators, use explicit expression.

4.4 Derivative of e^x and $\ln x$

4.4.1 Derivative of the Natural Exponential Functions

In this section we discuss derivative formula for e^x. Out of all the possible selections for bases of the exponential functions b^x, the simplest derivative formulas appear when the base is selected as e.

In the process of finding the derivative of e^x, we will apply the fact that

$$\lim_{h \to 0} \frac{e^h - 1}{h} = 1. \qquad \text{(Definition 2.13)} \qquad (4.11)$$

Using the definition of the derivative

$$f'(x) = \lim_{h \to 0} \frac{f(x+h) - f(x)}{h},$$

we now apply the three-step process to the natural exponential function $f(x) = e^x$.

Step 1　Calculate the difference:

$$
\begin{aligned}
f(x+h) - f(x) &= e^{x+h} - e^x && \text{(substituting } e^{x+h} \text{ for } f(x+h) \text{ and } e^x \text{ for } f(x)) \\
&= e^x e^h - e^x && \text{(use } e^{a+b} = e^a e^b) \\
&= e^x(e^h - 1). && \text{(factoring)}
\end{aligned}
$$

Step 2　Simplify the quotient:

$$\frac{f(x+h) - f(x)}{h} = e^x \left(\frac{e^h - 1}{h} \right).$$

Step 3　Find the limit:

$$
\begin{aligned}
f'(x) = (e^x)' &= \lim_{h \to 0} \frac{f(x+h) - f(x)}{h} && \text{(definition of the derivative)} \\
&= \lim_{h \to 0} e^x \left(\frac{e^h - 1}{h} \right) \\
&= e^x \lim_{h \to 0} \frac{e^h - 1}{h} && \text{(limit property, note } e^x \text{ is a constant with respect to } h) \\
&= e^x \cdot 1 && \text{(use the limit (4.11))} \\
&= e^x.
\end{aligned}
$$

Thus,

$$\frac{\mathrm{d}}{\mathrm{d}x} e^x = e^x.$$

We have shown that if $f(x) = e^x$, then $f'(x) = e^x$.

> **The Derivative of e^x**
>
> *The derivative of the natural exponential function is itself.*
>
> $$(e^x)' = e^x \ or \ \frac{\mathrm{d}}{\mathrm{d}x} e^x = e^x.$$

The derivative of the natural exponential function indicates that on the graph of $y = e^x$, the slope of the tangent at x (the derivative) is equal to the height of the curve (the function value) at that point. Figure 4.12 shows the fact. That is, at the point $(0, 1)$, the slope is $m=1$; at the point $(1, e)$, the slope is $m=e$; at the point (x, e^x), the slope is $m=e^x$. This correlation between the function and its derivative holds true only for the natural exponential function.

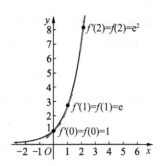

Example 4.24   Find $f'(x)$ for:

(1) $f(x)=(x^3+2)e^x$;   (2) $f(x)=\dfrac{e^x}{x^2}$.

Figure 4.12

Solution

(1) $f'(x)=(x^3+2)'e^x+(x^3+2)(e^x)'$ (Product Rule)

$\qquad =3x^2e^x+(x^3+2)e^x$

$\qquad =e^x(x^3+3x^2+2)$;

(2) $f'(x)=\dfrac{(e^x)'x^2-e^x(x^2)'}{(x^2)^2}$ (Quotient Rule)

$\qquad =\dfrac{e^xx^2-e^x\cdot 2x}{x^4}=\dfrac{e^x(x-2)}{x^3}.$ (canceling x) ♯

Your Practice 4.19   Find $f'(x)$ for:

(1) $f(x)=3x^2+2e^x$;   (2) $f(x)=e^xx^2$.

Example 4.25   Find an equation of the tangent line to the curve $y=\dfrac{e^x}{1+x^2}$ at the point $\left(1, \dfrac{e}{2}\right)$.

Solution   According to the Quotient Rule, we have

$$\frac{d}{dx}f(x)=\frac{\dfrac{d}{dx}e^x\cdot(1+x^2)-e^x\cdot\dfrac{d}{dx}(1+x^2)}{(1+x^2)^2}$$

$$=\frac{e^x\cdot(1+x^2)-e^x\cdot 2x}{(1+x^2)^2}$$

$$=\frac{e^x(1-x)^2}{(1+x^2)^2}.$$

So the slope of the tangent line at $\left(1, \dfrac{e}{2}\right)$ is

$$\frac{d}{dx}f(x)\bigg|_{x=1}=0.$$

This means that the tangent line at $\left(1, \dfrac{e}{2}\right)$ is horizontal (Figure 4.13) and its equation is $y=\dfrac{e}{2}$. We can see that the function is increasing and crosses its tangent line at $\left(1, \dfrac{e}{2}\right)$. ♯

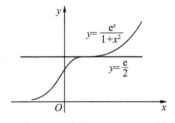

Figure 4.13

Your Practice 4.20   At what point on the curve $y=e^x$ the tangent line is parallel to the line $y=2x$?

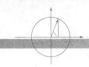

Example 4.26 Find the derivative of $f(x) = e^{-x^3/3}$.

Solution Use the Chain Rule, we obtain

$$f'(x) = e^{-x^3/3} \cdot (-x^3/3)' = e^{-x^3/3} \cdot \left(-\frac{3x^2}{3}\right) = -x^2 e^{-x^3/3}.$$ #

4.4.2 Derivative of Exponential Functions

We will find the derivative of any exponential functions $f(x) = b^x$, $x \in \mathbf{R}$ where b is a positive constant other than 1. Using the identity

$$b^x = e^{\ln b^x}$$

and the fact that $\ln b^x = x \ln b$, we can obtain the derivative of b^x with the help of the Chain Rule, namely,

$$\frac{\mathrm{d}}{\mathrm{d}x} b^x = \frac{\mathrm{d}}{\mathrm{d}x} e^{\ln b^x} = \frac{\mathrm{d}}{\mathrm{d}x} e^{x \ln b}$$
$$= e^{x \ln b} (x \ln b)' = (\ln b) b^x.$$

That is, we find

$$\frac{\mathrm{d}}{\mathrm{d}x} b^x = (\ln b) b^x. \tag{4.12}$$

Example 4.27 Find the derivative of $f(x) = 4^{\sqrt{x}}$.

Solution We use Equation (4.12) and the Chain Rule to get

$$\frac{\mathrm{d}}{\mathrm{d}x} 4^{\sqrt{x}} = (\ln 4) 4^{\sqrt{x}} \cdot \frac{\mathrm{d}\sqrt{x}}{\mathrm{d}x} = \frac{\ln 4}{2\sqrt{x}} 4^{\sqrt{x}}.$$

Another way is to rewrite the exponential function in terms of e. This is often easier since the differential rule for e^x is particularly simple and we do not need to remember the derivative formula of b^x. That is, we write

$$4^{\sqrt{x}} = e^{\ln 4^{\sqrt{x}}} = e^{\sqrt{x} \ln 4}.$$

Then, using the Chain Rule, we find

$$\frac{\mathrm{d}}{\mathrm{d}x} 4^{\sqrt{x}} = e^{\sqrt{x} \ln 4} \cdot (\sqrt{x} \ln 4)' = e^{\sqrt{x} \ln 4} \cdot \left(\ln 4 \frac{1}{2\sqrt{x}}\right) = \frac{\ln 4}{2\sqrt{x}} 4^{\sqrt{x}}.$$ #

Your Practice 4.21 Find the derivative of $f(x) = 3^{\sqrt{x}}$.

4.4.3 Exponential Growth and Decay

Most natural phenomena grow continuously. For example, bacteria will continue to grow within 24 hours, producing new bacteria which will also grow. The bacteria do not wait until the end of the 24 hours, and then all reproduce immediately.

The exponential e is used when modeling continuous growth that occurs naturally such as populations, bacteria, radioactive decay, etc. If a quantity (let us call it $P(t)$ for now) grows continuously by a fixed percent, the pattern can be depicted by the Exponential Growth model as

$$P(t) = P_0 e^{kt}, \; k > 0$$

where

$P =$ ending value (quantity after growth or decay);

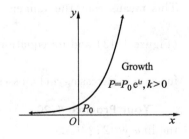

Figure 4.14

P_0 = initial value (quantity before measuring growth or decay);

k = relative growth rate (also called constant of proportionality) ($k>0$, the quantity is increasing (growing); $k<0$, the quantity is decreasing (decaying));

t = time that has passed.

The differential form of the exponential growth is

$$\frac{dP(t)}{dt} = kP(t).$$

This statement can be written as "the rate of growth of quantity at a time is directly proportional to the quantity at that time". In other words, with exponential growth the more you have of something, the faster it grows (which can lead to some ridiculous numbers after some time has elapsed).

Example 4.28　A strain of bacteria growing on your desktop doubles every 5 minutes. Assuming that you start with only one bacterium, how many bacteria will appear at the end of 100 minutes?

Solution　We apply an exponential growth model $P(t) = e^{kt}$ with the initial value to be 1. We find the value of k by

$$2 = e^{5k}.$$

Taking ln on both sides to get ln $2 = 5k$ and $k = \ln(2/5) \approx 0.1386294361$. Now, using this k value and the time of 100 minutes we have

$$P(100) = e^{0.1386294361 \times 100} = 1048576. \qquad \#$$

Exponential decay (Figure 4.15) describes a function of time of a quantity that decreases exponentially. The basic formula that describes exponential decay is

$$P(t) = P_0 e^{-kt}, \quad k>0.$$

As you can see, the exponential decay formula is almost the same as the exponential growth, with the sole exception being that the scale constant is negative.

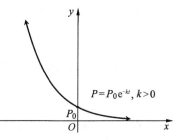

Figure 4.15

Accordingly, the differential form of the exponential decay is

$$\frac{dP(t)}{dt} = -kP(t).$$

Example 4.29　A common example of exponential decay is radioactive decay. Radioactive materials, and some other substances, decompose according to a formula for exponential decay. A radioactive substance is often described in terms of its half-life, which is the time required for half the material to decompose. Radium-226 is a kind of Radioactive material. After 500 years, a sample of radium-226 has decayed to 80.4% of its original mass. Find the half-life of radium-226.

Solution　Let A be the mass of radium present at time t ($t=0$ corresponds to 500 years ago), then $A = A_0 e^{-kt}$.

First we determine k. We are given that when $t = 500$, $A = 0.804A_0$. Substituting these values into the formula for exponential decay, we obtain $0.804A_0 = A_0 e^{-500k}$. Dividing through by A_0 gives us $0.804 = e^{-500k}$. Taking natural logs (i. e. ln) of both sides (common logs could be used as well) to get $\ln 0.804 = \ln e^{-500k}$ and $\ln 0.804 = -500k$. Then

$$k = -(\ln 0.804)/500 \approx 0.000436.$$

Now, we set

$$\frac{A_0}{2} = A_0 e^{-0.000436t}.$$

Dividing through by A_0 again, we get $0.5 = e^{-0.000436t}$. To solve for t, take natural logs: $\ln 0.5 = \ln e^{-0.000436t}$. Then applying the Cancellation Property for logarithms yields $\ln 0.5 = -0.000436t$. So

$$t = (\ln 0.5)/(-0.000436)$$

or $t \approx 1590$. The half-life is approximately 1590 years.   #

4.4.4 Derivative of Logarithmic Functions

We will find the derivative of the logarithmic functions by the Chain Rule. Recall that
$$f(x) = \log_b x \text{ if and only if } b^{f(x)} = x.$$
Differentiate with respect to x on both sides of $b^{f(x)} = x$ then we get
$$(\ln b)b^{f(x)} \cdot f'(x) = 1.$$
Using the fact $b^{f(x)} = x$, $f(x) = \log_b x$ we have
$$(\ln b)x \cdot (\log_b x)' = 1.$$
Solving the equation we get
$$\frac{d}{dx}\log_b x = \frac{1}{(\ln b)x}.$$

If the base is taken as the exponential, that is, $b = e$, then
$$\frac{d}{dx}\ln x = \frac{1}{x}.$$

We summarize this in the following box.

Derivative of Logarithmic Functions
$$\frac{d}{dx}\ln x = \frac{1}{x},$$
$$\frac{d}{dx}\log_b x = \frac{1}{(\ln b)x}.$$

Example 4.30 Differentiate $y = \ln(3x^2 - 5x)$.

Solution We use the Chain Rule with $u = g(x) = 3x^2 - 5x$ and $f(u) = \ln u$:
$$\frac{dy}{dx} = \frac{dy}{du}\frac{du}{dx} = \frac{1}{u}(6x - 5) = \frac{6x - 5}{3x^2 - 5x}.$$ #

The preceding example is of the form $y = \ln g(x)$. We will frequently come across such functions. Use the Chain Rule, we find their derivatives as shown in the following box:

The General Logarithmic Rule

$$\frac{\mathrm{d}}{\mathrm{d}x}\ln\,g(x)=\frac{g'(x)}{g(x)}.$$

Example 4.31　Differentiate $y=3x\ln\,x^2$.

Solution　We first apply the Product Rule

$$y'=\frac{\mathrm{d}}{\mathrm{d}x}(3x)\cdot\ln\,x^2+3x\cdot\left(\frac{\mathrm{d}}{\mathrm{d}x}\ln\,x^2\right).$$

Then we use the general logarithmic rule:

$$y'=3\ln\,x^2+3x\cdot\frac{(x^2)'}{x^2}=3\ln\,x^2+3x\cdot\frac{2x}{x^2}=3\ln\,x^2+6.$$

Your Practice 4.22　Differentiate $y=\ln(8x^3-3x+1)$.

Logarithmic differentiation

Logarithmic differentiation is powerful in finding the derivatives of functions of the form $y=[u(x)]^{v(x)}$. The basic idea is simply to take logarithms on both sides and then differentiate. In 1695, Leibniz introduced this method, following a suggestion from Johann Bernoulli. Bernoulli generalized this method and published his results two years later.

Example 4.32　Find $\dfrac{\mathrm{d}y}{\mathrm{d}x}$ when $y=(x^2+1)^{x^2}$.

Solution　We take logarithms on both sides of the equation $y=(x^2+1)^{x^2}$,

$$\ln\,y=\ln(x^2+1)^{x^2}.$$

Applying properties of the logarithm, we can simplify the right-hand side as $\ln\,(x^2+1)^{x^2}=x^2\ln(x^2+1)$. We can now differentiate both sides with respect to x:

$$\frac{\mathrm{d}}{\mathrm{d}x}\ln\,y=\frac{\mathrm{d}}{\mathrm{d}x}[x^2\ln(x^2+1)],$$

$$\frac{1}{y}\frac{\mathrm{d}y}{\mathrm{d}x}=2x\cdot\ln(x^2+1)+x^2\cdot\frac{2x}{x^2+1},$$

$$\frac{\mathrm{d}y}{\mathrm{d}x}=y\left[2x\ln(x^2+1)+\frac{2x^3}{x^2+1}\right],$$

$$\frac{\mathrm{d}y}{\mathrm{d}x}=(x^2+1)^{x^2}\left[2x\ln(x^2+1)+\frac{2x^3}{x^2+1}\right].$$

We can also differentiate this function without using logarithmic differentiation. Write the function as

$$y=(x^2+1)^{x^2}=\exp[\ln(x^2+1)^{x^2}]=\exp[x^2\ln(x^2+1)].$$

Here $\exp[x]$ is an alternative notation for e^x. Now we apply the Chain Rule:

$$\frac{\mathrm{d}y}{\mathrm{d}x}=\exp[x^2\ln(x^2+1)]\frac{\mathrm{d}}{\mathrm{d}x}[x^2\ln(x^2+1)]$$

$$=\exp[x^2\ln(x^2+1)]\left[2x\,\ln(x^2+1)+x^2\,\frac{2x}{x^2+1}\right]$$

$$=(x^2+1)^{x^2}\left[2x\,\ln(x^2+1)+\frac{2x^3}{x^2+1}\right]. \qquad\#$$

Either approach will give us the correct answer.

Your Practice 4.23 Find the derivative of $y = x^x$.

Example 4.33 Find the derivative of

$$y = \frac{e^x x^{3/2} \sqrt{1+x}}{(x^2-3)^3 (3x+2)^4}.$$

Solution It would be rather difficult to apply the Quotient Rule. Taking logarithms on both sides, however, we see that the expression simplifies. It is very important that we simplify the expression by applying the properties of the logarithm before differentiating.

$$\ln y = \ln \frac{e^x x^{3/2} \sqrt{1+x}}{(x^2-3)^3 (3x+2)^4}$$

$$= \ln e^x + \ln x^{3/2} + \ln \sqrt{1+x} - \ln(x^2-3)^3 - \ln(3x+2)^4$$

$$= x + \frac{3}{2}\ln x + \frac{1}{2}\ln(1+x) - 3\ln(x^2-3) - 4\ln(3x+2).$$

This no longer look so scary, and we can differentiate both sides:

$$\frac{d}{dx}\ln y = \frac{d}{dx}\left[x + \frac{3}{2}\ln x + \frac{1}{2}\ln(1+x) - 3\ln(x^2-3) - 4\ln(3x+2) \right],$$

$$\frac{1}{y}\frac{dy}{dx} = 1 + \frac{3}{2}\frac{1}{x} + \frac{1}{2}\frac{1}{1+x} - 3\frac{2x}{x^2-3} - 4\frac{3}{3x+2}.$$

Finally, solving for dy/dx yields

$$\frac{dy}{dx} = \left[1 + \frac{3}{2x} + \frac{1}{2(1+x)} - \frac{6x}{x^2-3} - \frac{12}{3x+2} \right] \frac{e^x x^{3/2} \sqrt{1+x}}{(x^2-3)^3 (3x+2)^4}. \qquad \#$$

We can also use logarithmic differentiation to prove the General Power Rule:

Power Rule

Let $f(x) = x^r$ where r is any real number, then

$$\frac{d}{dx}x^r = rx^{r-1}.$$

Proof We set $y = x^r$ and use logarithmic differentiation to get

$$\frac{d}{dx}\ln y = \frac{d}{dx}(\ln x^r),$$

$$\frac{1}{y}\frac{dy}{dx} = \frac{d}{dx}(r \ln x),$$

$$\frac{1}{y}\frac{dy}{dx} = r\frac{1}{x}.$$

Solving for dy/dx yields

$$\frac{dy}{dx} = r\frac{1}{x}y = r\frac{1}{x}x^r = rx^{r-1}. \qquad \#$$

Exercise 4.4

1. Find $f'(x)$ and simplify.

(1) $f(x)=3e^x-4x^e$;

(2) $f(x)=-5e^x+6x^e$;

(3) $f(x)=(x^3-2x+5)e^x$;

(4) $f(x)=(2x^5+x^3+6)e^x$;

(5) $f(x)=\dfrac{x^2-1}{e^x}$;

(6) $f(x)=\dfrac{x+2020}{e^x}$;

(7) $f(x)=\dfrac{1-xe^x}{x+e^x}$;

(8) $f(x)=\dfrac{e^x+3}{x^2+7}$.

2. Find the equation of the line tangent to the graph of $y=f(x)$ at the indicated values of x.

(1) $f(x)=3-e^x$, $x=1$;

(2) $f(x)=\dfrac{e^x}{x}$, $x=1$;

(3) $f(x)=e^x g(x)$ where $g(0)=2$ and $g'(0)=-3$, $x=0$.

3. A student draws the tangent line to the graph of $f(x)=e^x$ at $x=4$ as shown in Figure 4.16. Is he correct? Explain.

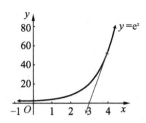

Figure 4.16

4. A student draws the tangent line to the graph of $f(x)=e^x$ at $x=3$ as shown in Figure 4.17. Is she correct? Explain.

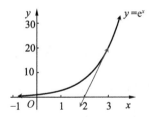

Figure 4.17

5. If $f(x)=e^x-x$ then $f'(x)=e^x-1$. Indicate which curve corresponding to them in Figure 4.18. Find the interval where

(1) f is increasing;

(2) $f'(x)>0$;

(3) f is decreasing;

(4) $f'(x)<0$.

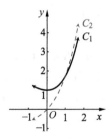

Figure 4.18

6. Find $f'(x)$ and simplify.

(1) $f(x)=(3x^2+5)^4$;

(2) $f(x)=(2x^4+5x-3)^3$;

(3) $f(x)=e^{4x}$;

(4) $f(x)=e^{3x^2+5x+4}$;

(5) $f(x)=\ln(x+2e^x-3x^2)$;

(6) $f(x)=3\ln(x^2-1)$;

(7) $f(x)=(1-\ln x)^3$;

(8) $f(x)=\ln(3+x^2)^3$;

(9) $f(x)=\sqrt{\ln x}$;

(10) $f(x)=[\ln(1+x^2)]^3$.

7. Let $f(x)=(4x-3)^{1/2}$. Find $f'(x)$ and the equation of the line tangent to the

graph of f at $x=3$. Find the value(s) of x where the tangent line is horizontal.

8. Find the indicated derivative and simplify.

(1) $\dfrac{d}{dt}2(t^2+3t)^{-3}$;

(2) $\dfrac{dg}{dw}$ if $g(w)=\sqrt{3w-7}$;

(3) $h'(x)$ if $h(x)=\dfrac{e^{2x}}{x^2+9}$;

(4) $F'(x)$ if $F(x)=(e^{x^2+1})^3$.

9. A yeast culture at room temperature (68 °F) is placed in a refrigerator set at a constant temperature of 38 °F. After t hours, the temperature T of the culture is given approximately by

$$T=30e^{-0.58t}+38, \quad t\geqslant 0.$$

What are the rate of change of temperature of the culture at the end of 1 hour and at the end of 4 hours?

10. A student claims that the line tangent to the graph of $g(x)=\ln x$ at $x=3$ passes through the origin. Is he correct? Will the line tangent at $x=4$ pass through the origin? Explain.

11. An experiment was set up to find a relationship between weight and systolic blood pressure in children. Using hospital records for 5000 children, the experimenters found that the systolic blood pressure was given approximately by

$$P(x)=17.5(1+\ln x), \quad 10\leqslant x\leqslant 100,$$

where $P(x)$ is measured in millimeters of mercury and x is measured in pounds. What are the rate of change of blood pressure with respect to weight at the 40-pound weight level and at the 90-pound weight level?

12. A research group using hospital records developed the following approximate mathematical model relating systolic blood pressure and age:

$$P(x)=40+25\ln(x+1), \quad 0\leqslant x\leqslant 65$$

where $P(x)$ is pressure, measured in millimeters of mercury and x is age in years. What are the rate of change of pressure at the end of 10 years, at the end of 30 years and at the end of 60 years?

13. A single cholera bacterium divides every 0.5 hour to produce two complete cholera bacteria. If we start with a colony of 5000 bacteria, after t hours there will be

$$A(t)=5000 \cdot 2^{2t}$$

bacteria. Find $A'(t)$, $A'(1)$, and $A'(5)$, and interpret the results.

14. A single cholera bacterium divides every 0.25 hour to produce two complete cholera bacteria. If we start with a colony of 1000 bacteria, after t hours there will be

$$A(t)=5000 \cdot 2^{2t}$$

bacteria. Find $A'(t)$, $A'(1)$, and $A'(5)$, and interpret the results.

15. Let $f(x)=\ln x$.

(1) Use the definition of the derivative to show that

$$f'(1)=\lim_{h\to 0}\frac{\ln(1+h)}{h};$$

(2) Show that

$$\ln\left[\lim_{h\to 0}(1+h)^{1/h}\right]=1.$$

16. Use logarithmic differentiation to find the derivative.

(1) $f(x)=x^x$;

(2) $f(x)=(\ln x)^x$;

(3) $f(x)=x^{\ln x}$;

(4) $f(x)=x^{1/x}$;

(5) $f(x)=x^{x^x}$;

(6) $f(x)=(x^x)^x$.

17. Differentiate
$$y=\frac{e^{3x}(4x-3)^2}{\sqrt{(x^2+1)(x^4+9)}}.$$

18. Differentiate
$$y=\frac{e^{-2x}x^2}{(x^2+1)^{2x}}.$$

4.5　Implicit Differentiation

So far, we have worked with functions given by equations of the form $y=f(x)$, where the dependent variable y on the left is given clearly by the expression on the right involving the independent variable x. A function in this form is said to be in explicit form. It is also possible to define y implicitly as a function of x, as in the following equation

$$(x^2+y^2-1)^3=x^2y^3.$$

Here, y is given as a function of x, that is, y is the dependant variable. The equation cannot be solved explicitly for y in terms of x or can be done so only with great effort. If our interest is to find the derivative $\dfrac{dy}{dx}$, we can apply a very useful technique called *implicit differentiation*, which consists of differentiating both sides of the defining equation with respect to x and then solving algebraically for $\dfrac{dy}{dx}$.

Example 4.34　Suppose $y=f(x)$ is a differentiable function of x that satisfies the equation $x^2+y^2=4$. Find the derivative $\dfrac{dy}{dx}$. What is the slope at the point $(1,\sqrt{3})$?

Solution　We are going to differentiate both sides of the given equation term by term with respect to x. We need to remember that y is actually a function of x.

$$\frac{d}{dx}(x^2+y^2)=\frac{d}{dx}4.$$

Apply the Sum Rule:

$$\frac{d}{dx}x^2+\frac{d}{dx}y^2=\frac{d}{dx}4.$$

Starting with the left-hand side and using the Power Rule, we find $\dfrac{d}{dx}x^2=2x$. To differentiate y^2 with respect to x, we must apply the Chain Rule. We find $\dfrac{d}{dx}y^2=2y\dfrac{dy}{dx}$ and $\dfrac{d}{dx}4=0$. Therefore we have

$$2x+2y\frac{dy}{dx}=0.$$

Solve for $\dfrac{dy}{dx}$:

$$\frac{dy}{dx}=\frac{-2x}{2y}=-\frac{x}{y}.$$

The slope at the point $(1,\sqrt{3})$ is $m=-\dfrac{1}{\sqrt{3}}=-\dfrac{\sqrt{3}}{3}$. Figure 4.19 shows the result.　#

We can solve y from the equation in the previous example rather than differentiate y directly. We find

$$y = \begin{cases} \sqrt{4-x^2}, & \text{for } y \geq 0, \\ -\sqrt{4-x^2}, & \text{for } y < 0. \end{cases}$$

Then

$$\frac{dy}{dx} = \begin{cases} -\dfrac{2x}{2\sqrt{4-x^2}} = -\dfrac{x}{y}, & \text{for } y > 0, \\ \dfrac{2x}{2\sqrt{4-x^2}}, & \text{for } y < 0. \end{cases}$$

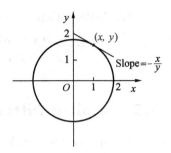

Figure 4. 19

This example shows the advantage of using implicit differentiation. Even though we were able to solve for y and thus y becomes an explicit function, implicit differentiation was actually quicker.   #

Example 4.35   Given $x^3 + y^3 = 9xy$, find $\dfrac{dy}{dx}$ and the slope of the tangent line at $(4, 2)$.

Solution   We differentiate both sides with respect to x:

$$\frac{d}{dx}(x^3 + y^3) = \frac{d}{dx}(9xy).$$

Applying the Sum Rule we see

$$\frac{d}{dx}x^3 + \frac{d}{dx}y^3 = \frac{d}{dx}(9xy).$$

The first term is $\dfrac{d}{dx}x^3 = 3x^2$. Apply the Chain Rule to the second term:

$$\frac{d}{dx}y^3 = 3y^2\frac{dy}{dx}.$$

To the right-hand side term, we use the Product Rule:

$$\frac{d}{dx}(9xy) = 9\frac{d}{dx}(xy) = 9\left(y + x\frac{dy}{dx}\right).$$

Putting the pieces together we are left with the equation

$$3x^2 + 3y^2\frac{dy}{dx} = 9y + 9x\frac{dy}{dx}.$$

We solve for $\dfrac{dy}{dx}$:

$$3y^2\frac{dy}{dx} - 9x\frac{dy}{dx} = 9y - 3x^2,$$

$$(3y^2 - 9x)\frac{dy}{dx} = 9y - 3x^2,$$

$$\frac{dy}{dx} = \frac{9y - 3x^2}{3y^2 - 9x} = \frac{3y - x^2}{y^2 - 3x}.$$

For the second part of the problem, we simply plug $x = 4$ and $y = 2$ into the equation above, hence the slope of the tangent line at $(4, 2)$ is $5/4$. Figure 4. 20 shows the curve and the tangent line.   #

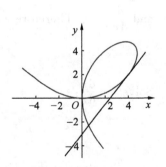

Figure 4. 20

Your Practice 4.24   Given $e^y + xy - e = 0$, find $\left.\dfrac{dy}{dx}\right|_{x=0}$.

Exercise 4.5

1. Use implicit differentiation to find $\dfrac{dy}{dx}$ and evaluate $\dfrac{dy}{dx}$ at the indicated point.

   (1) $y^2 = 1 + x^2$, $(0, 1)$;

   (2) $y^2 + 2y + 3x = 0$, $(0, -2)$;

   (3) $\ln y = 2y^2 - x$, $(2, 1)$;

   (4) $xe^y - y = x^2 - 2$, $(2, 0)$.

2. A hyperbola passing through $(8,6)$ consists of all points whose distance from the origin is a constant more than its distance from the point $(5, 2)$. Find the slope of the tangent line to the hyperbola at $(8,6)$.

3. In biophysics, the equation $(L+m)(V+n) = k$ is called the fundamental equation of muscle contraction, where m, n, and k are constants and V is the velocity of the shortening of muscle fibers for a muscle subjected to a load L. Find dL/dV by implicit differentiation.

4. The graph of the equation $x^2 - xy + y^2 = 9$ is an ellipse. Find the lines tangent to this curve at the two points where it intersects the x-axis. Show that these lines are parallel.

5. The graph of the equation $x^2 - xy + y^2 = 9$ is an ellipse. Find the lines tangent to this curve at the two points where it intersects the y-axis. Show that these lines are parallel.

6. Find an equation for the tangent line to $x^4 = y^2 + x^2$ at $(2, \sqrt{12})$. (This curve is the **Kampyle of Eudoxus**)

7. Find an equation for the tangent line to $x^{2/3} + y^{2/3} = 4$ at the point $(-1, 3\sqrt{3})$. (This curve is an **astroid**)

8. Find an equation for the tangent line to $y^2 = x^2 - x^4$ at $(1/2, \sqrt{3}/4)$. (This curve is a **lemniscate**)

4.6   Related Rates

Related rates is an important application of implicit differentiation. We begin with a motivating example.

Example 4.36   Suppose an object is moving along a path described by $y = x^2$, that is, it is moving on a parabolic path. At a particular time $t = 5$, the x coordinate is 6 and we measure the speed at which the x coordinate of the object is changing and find that $dx/dt = 3$. At the same time, how fast is the y coordinate changing?

Solution   We have two variables x and y which are both changing with time. We know one of the rates of change at a given instant dx/dt, and we want to find the other rate dy/dt at that instant. Since $y = x^2$, using the Chain Rule we have

$$\frac{dy}{dt} = 2x \frac{dx}{dt}.$$

At $t=5$ we know that $x=6$ and $dx/dt=3$, so $dy/dt=2\times6\times3=36$. #

In a typical related problems, there are at least two changing quantities. You are asked to figure out the rate at which one is changing given sufficient information on all of the others. We can apply the following key steps to set up and solve related rates problems:

> 1. *Draw a picture or otherwise make a mathematical model of the situation.*
> 2. *Label all quantities which can change as variables.*
> 3. *Identify the underlying independent variable in the problem. This is usually time but it need not be.*
> 4. *Identify in terms of the variables and their derivatives what is being asked and what is given.*
> 5. *Use the mathematical model to write down a relation among the variables.*
> 6. *Differentiate this relation with respect to the underlying independent variable, usually making heavy use of the Chain Rule.*
> 7. *Solve for the quantity wanted.*
> 8. *Go back over your work and write up a presentable solution.*

In short, related rates problems combine word problems together with implicit differentiation.

Example 4.37 A plane is flying directly away from you at 500 kilometers per hour at an altitude of 3 kilometers. How fast is the plane's distance from you increasing at the moment when the plane is flying over a point on the ground 4 kilometers from you?

Solution We first draw a schematic representation of the situation, as in Figure 4.21. Because the plane is in level flight directly away from you, the rate at which x changes is the speed of the plane, $\dfrac{dx}{dt}=500$. The distance between you and the plane is y; it is $\dfrac{dy}{dt}$ that we wish to know. By the Pythagorean

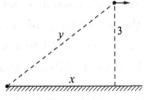

Figure 4. 21

Theorem we know that

$$x^2+9=y^2.$$

Taking the derivative:

$$2x\frac{dx}{dt}+0=2y\frac{dy}{dt}.$$

We are interested in the time at which $x=4$; at this time we know that $4^2+9=y^2$, so $y=5$. Putting together all the information we get

$$2\times4\times500=2\times5\frac{dy}{dt}.$$

Thus, $\dfrac{dy}{dt}=400$ km/h. #

Example 4. 38 A light is on the top of a 12 feet tall pole and a 5 feet 6 inch tall person is walking away from the pole at a rate of 2 feet per second.

(1) At what rate is the tip of the shadow moving away from the pole when the person is 25 feet from the pole?

(2) At what rate is the tip of the shadow moving away from the person when the person is 25 feet from the pole?

Solution　We start off with putting all the relevant quantities into the sketch (Figure 4.22).

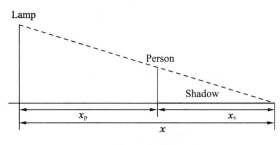

Figure 4.22

Here x is the distance of the tip of the shadow from the pole, x_p is the distance of the person from the pole and x_s is the length of the shadow. Also note that we converted the person's height over to 5.5 feet since all the other measurements are in feet.

The tip of the shadow is defined by the rays of light just getting past the person and so we can see they form a set of similar triangles. This will be useful down the road.

(1) In this case we want to determine $\dfrac{dx}{dt}$ when $x_p = 25$ given that $\dfrac{dx_p}{dt} = 2$. We have $x = x_p + x_s$ but we will need to eliminate x_s from the equation in order to get an answer. To do this we can again make use of the fact that the two triangles are similar to get, $\dfrac{5.5}{12} = \dfrac{x_s}{x}$. From this we can see that, $x_s = \dfrac{11}{24}x$. We can then plug this into the equation above and solve for x:

$$x = x_p + x_s = x_p + \frac{11}{24}x,$$

$$x = \frac{24}{13}x_p.$$

Differentiate:

$$\frac{dx}{dt} = \frac{24}{13}\frac{dx_p}{dt}.$$

When $\dfrac{dx_p}{dt} = 2$, $\dfrac{dx}{dt} = \dfrac{24}{13} \times 2 \approx 3.6923$ feet per second.

The tip of the shadow is then moving away from the pole at a rate of 3.6923 feet per second.

(2) In this case we want to determine $\dfrac{dx_s}{dt}$ when $x_p = 25$.

Again, we can use $x = x_p + x_s$, however unlike the first part we now know that $\dfrac{dx_p}{dt} = 2$ and $\dfrac{dx}{dt} = 3.6923$ feet per second, so in this case all we need to do is to differentiate the equation and plug in for all the known quantities.

$$\frac{dx}{dt} = \frac{dx_p}{dt} + \frac{dx_s}{dt},$$

$$3.6923 = 2 + \frac{dx_s}{dt},$$

$$\frac{dx_s}{dt} = 1.6923 \text{ feet per second.}$$

The tip of the shadow is then moving away from the person at a rate of 1.6923 feet per second.　　　　　　#

Exercise 4.6

1. Assume that $x = x(t)$ and $y = y(t)$. Find dx/dt if $x^2 - 2xy - y^2 = 7$; $dy/dt = -1$ when $x = 2$ and $y = -1$.

2. Assume that $x = x(t)$ and $y = y(t)$ are differentiable. Find dy/dt when $x^2 + y^2 = 1$; $dx/dt = 2$ for $x = 1/2$ and $y > 0$.

3. Assume that $x = x(t)$ and $y = y(t)$ are differentiable. Find dy/dt when $y^2 = x^2 - x^4$; $dx/dt = 1$ for $x = 1/2$ and $y > 0$.

4. Assume that $x = x(t)$ and $y = y(t)$ are differentiable. Find dy/dt when $x^2 y = 1$; $dx/dt = 3$ for $x = 2$.

5. A spherical balloon is being inflated at a constant rate of 20 cubic inches per second. How fast is the radius of the balloon changing at the instant the balloon's diameter d is 12 inches? Is the radius changing more rapidly when $d = 12$ or when $d = 16$?

6. A police helicopter is flying at 150 kilometers per hour at a constant altitude of 0.5 kilometers above a straight road. The pilot uses radar to determine that an oncoming car is at a distance of exactly 1 kilometer from the helicopter, and that this distance is decreasing at 190 kilometers per hour. Find the speed of the car.

7. A police helicopter is flying at 200 kilometers per hour at a constant altitude of 1 kilometres above a straight road. The pilot uses radar to determine that an oncoming car is at a distance of exactly 2 kilometers from the helicopter, and that this distance is decreasing at 250 kilometers per hour. Find the speed of the car.

8. Water is poured into a conical container at the rate of 10 cm^3/s. The cone points directly down, it has a height of 30 cm and a base radius of 10 cm (Figure 4.23). How fast is the water level rising when the water is 4 cm deep (at its deepest point)?

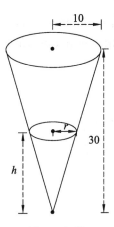

Figure 4.23

9. Nutria (Myocastor coypus), or river rats, are a large, herbivorous, semiaquatic rodent. The average daily metabolic rate for infant nutria can be expressed as a function of weight by $m/86=w^{0.5}$ where w is the weight of the nutria (in kg) and m is the metabolic rate (in kcal/day). Suppose that the weight of the nutria is changing with respect to time at the rate $\mathrm{d}w/\mathrm{d}t$. Find $\mathrm{d}m/\mathrm{d}t$ then determine $\mathrm{d}m/\mathrm{d}t$ for a 0.5 kg infant nutria gaining weight at a rate of 0.1 kg/day.

Summary and Review

Important Terms, Symbols, and Concepts

- Given two functions, the composite function $f\circ g$ (also called the composition of f and g) is defined by
$$(f\circ g)(x)=f[g(x)]$$
for each x in the domain of g for which $g(x)$ is in the domain of f.

- A function is called one-to-one if $x_1\neq x_2$ implies $f(x_1)\neq f(x_2)$ (or, equivalently, $f(x_1)=f(x_2)$ implies $x_1=x_2$).

- Let $f: D\to S$ be one-to-one function with domain D and range S. Then the inverse function f^{-1} has domain S and range D and is defined by
$$f^{-1}(y)=x \text{ if and only if } y=f(x)$$
for all y in S.

- Suppose that f is invertible. If f is differentiable at x and $f'(x)$ is not equal to zero, then the inverse function f^{-1} is differentiable at $y=f(x)$ and the following differentiation formula holds
$$(f^{-1})'(y)=\frac{1}{f'(x)}.$$

- The logarithm to base b function, written as $\log_b x$, is the inverse of the exponential function to the same base b.

- The exponential growth is modelled by $P(t)=P_0 e^{kt}$, $k>0$ or $\dfrac{\mathrm{d}P(t)}{\mathrm{d}t}=kP(t)$.

- The exponential decay is modelled by $P(t)=P_0 e^{-kt}$, $k>0$ or $\dfrac{\mathrm{d}P(t)}{\mathrm{d}t}=-kP(t)$.

- Implicit differentiation: finding the derivative of a dependent variable in an implicit function by differentiating each term separately, and expressing the derivative of the dependent variable as a symbol, and solving the resulting expression for the symbol.

- When two or more related quantities are changing as implicit functions of time, their rates of change can be related by implicitly differentiating the equation that relates the quantities themselves.

Summary of Rule of Differentiation

$$[u(x)v(x)]' = u'(x)v(x) + u(x)v'(x),$$

$$\left(\frac{u}{v}\right)' = \frac{u'v - uv'}{v^2}, \quad \frac{\mathrm{d}}{\mathrm{d}x}\left(\frac{u}{v}\right) = \frac{\dfrac{\mathrm{d}u}{\mathrm{d}x}v - u\dfrac{\mathrm{d}v}{\mathrm{d}x}}{v^2}.$$

$$\frac{\mathrm{d}y}{\mathrm{d}x} = \frac{\mathrm{d}y}{\mathrm{d}u}\frac{\mathrm{d}u}{\mathrm{d}x},$$

$$\frac{\mathrm{d}x^n}{\mathrm{d}x} = nx^{n-1}, \quad \frac{\mathrm{d}[g(x)]^n}{\mathrm{d}x} = ng(x)^{n-1}g'(x).$$

$$\frac{\mathrm{d}e^x}{\mathrm{d}x} = e^x, \quad \frac{\mathrm{d}e^{g(x)}}{\mathrm{d}x} = e^{g(x)}g'(x),$$

$$\frac{\mathrm{d}\ln x}{\mathrm{d}x} = \frac{1}{x}, \quad \frac{\mathrm{d}\ln g(x)}{\mathrm{d}x} = \frac{g'(x)}{g(x)}.$$

Guideline for Implicit Differentiation

Given an implicitly defined relation $f(x, y) = C$ for some constant C, we apply the following steps to implicitly find $\dfrac{\mathrm{d}y}{\mathrm{d}x}$:

(1) Apply the differentiation operator $\dfrac{\mathrm{d}}{\mathrm{d}x}$ to both sides of the equation $f(x, y) = C$;

(2) Follow through with the differentiation by keeping in mind that y is a function of x, and so the Chain Rule applies;

(3) Solve $\dfrac{\mathrm{d}y}{\mathrm{d}x}$.

Steps for Solving Related Rates Problems

(1) Sketch and label a diagram of the problem if applicable.

(2) Identify the independent variable (often, but not always, time).

(3) Unless already introduced, use a let statement to introduce dependent variables.

(4) State the known and unknown rate(s) and value(s) using your variable name(s).

(5) Find an equation relating the known and unknown variables.

(6) Differentiate the equation implicitly w. r. t the independent variable.

(7) Use substitution of known values to solve the new equation.

Chapter 5　Graphing and Optimization

Introduction

- Local Extrema and the Mean Value Theorem
- the First Derivatives and Graphs
- the Second Derivatives and Graphs
- Optimization
- L'Hôspital's Rule
- Periodicity and Trigonometric Functions
- Graphing of Functions

This chapter showes how derivatives affect the graph shape of a function and, in particular, how they help us locate maximum and minimum values of functions.

5.1　Local Extrema and the Mean Value Theorem

5.1.1　Local Extrema

Many of our applications in this chapter will revolve around minimum and maximum values of a function. Let us first explain exactly what we mean by maximum and minimum values.

Figure 5.1 shows the graph of a function with absolute minimum at a and absolute maximum at d. Note that $(a, f(a))$ is the lowest point on the graph and $(c, f(c))$ is the highest point. If we consider only values of x near b (for example, if we restrict our attention to the interval (a, c)), then $f(b)$ is the largest of those values of $f(x)$ and is called a **local maximum value** of f. Likewise, $f(c)$ is called a **local minimum value** of f because $f(c) \leqslant f(x)$ for x near c (for instance, in the interval (b, d)). The function f also has a local minimum at e. In general, we have the following definition.

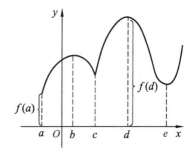

Figure 5.1

Definition 5.1 (Local Extrema)

A function f has a local maximum (or relative maximum) at c if $f(x) \leqslant f(c)$ for all x near c. f has a local minimum at c if $f(x) \geqslant f(c)$ for all x near c.

Example 5.1   The function $f(x)=x^2$ has an absolute (and local) minimum value $f(0)=0$ because $f(x)\geqslant f(0)=0$ for all x. This corresponds to the fact that the origin is the lowest point on the parabola (Figure 5.2). However, there is no highest point on the parabola and so this function has no maximum value.　　　　　　　　　　　　　　#

Example 5.2   For the function $f(x)=x^3$ shown in Figure 5.3. We see that this function has neither an absolute maximum value nor an absolute minimum value. In fact, it has no local extreme values either.　　　　　　　　　　　　　　　　　　#

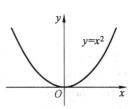

Figure 5.2

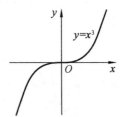

Figure 5.3

5.1.2　Critical Numbers

When looking at Local Maxima and Minima, and Absolute Maxima and Minima, we assumed that if the point $(c, f(c))$ is an extreme (that is, the point is either a local maximum or local minimum), then $f'(c)=0$. This theorem is commonly known as one of Fermat's theorems.

Theorem 5.1 (Fermat's Theorem)

　　If f has a local maximum or minimum at c, and $f'(c)$ exists, then $f'(c)=0$.

Proof   Suppose that f has a local maximum at $(c,$ $f(c))$. By the definition of a local maximum, we know that $f(c)\geqslant f(x)$ when x is close to c, that is $f(c)\geqslant f(c+h)$ as $h\to 0$ and thus $f(c+h)-f(c)\leqslant 0$. Dividing both sides by $h>0$ and taking the right-hand limit of both sides we obtain that:

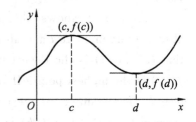

Figure 5.4

$$\lim_{h\to 0^+}\frac{f(c+h)-f(c)}{h}\leqslant \lim_{h\to 0^+}0,$$

$$\lim_{h\to 0^+}\frac{f(c+h)-f(c)}{h}\leqslant 0.$$

Since $f'(c)$ exists, we know that $f'(c)\leqslant 0$.

Now suppose that $h<0$, we therefore get that $\dfrac{f(c+h)-f(c)}{h}\geqslant 0$, and taking the left-hand limit of both sides we get that:

$$\lim_{h\to 0^-}\frac{f(c+h)-f(c)}{h}\geqslant \lim_{h\to 0^-}0,$$

$$\lim_{h\to 0^-}\frac{f(c+h)-f(c)}{h}\geqslant 0.$$

Once again, since $f'(c)$ exists, we know that $f'(c) \geqslant 0$. Since $f'(c) \geqslant 0$ and $f'(c) \leqslant 0$, then $f'(c) = 0$.   #

It is important to note that the converse of this theorem is not necessarily true, that is, $f(c) = 0$ does not imply that $(c, f(c))$ is an extrema. For example, consider the function $f(x) = x^3$ whose derivative is $f'(x) = 3x^2$. Clearly, $f'(x) = 0$ at $x = 0$, however, as we have shown in Example 5.2, the point $(0, 0)$ is neither local maxima or local minima. It is also important that there may be an extreme value even when $f'(c)$ does not exist. For example, if $f(x) = |x|$, then $f(0) = 0$ is a minimum value, but $f'(0)$ does not exist.

Fermat's Theorem does suggest that we should at least start looking for extreme values of f at the numbers where $f'(c) = 0$ or where $f'(c)$ does not exist. Such numbers are given a special name, **Critical Number**.

Definition 5.2 (Critical Number)

   The function $f(x)$ has a critical number at $x = c$ if $f(c)$ is defined and either $f'(c) = 0$ (Type 1) or $f'(c)$ does not exist (Type 2).

Type 1 critical numbers correspond to horizontal tangent lines in the graph of the function. Type 2 critical numbers typically correspond to corner points or vertical tangent lines (Figure 5.5).

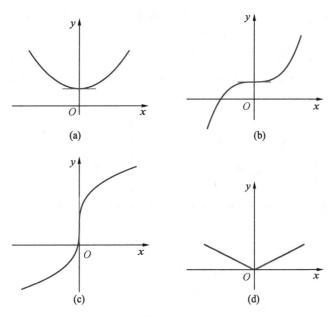

(a)   (b)

(c)   (d)

Figure 5.5

Example 5.3   Find the critical numbers of the function $f(x) = 2x^3 - 3x^2 - 72x + 15$.

Solution   We need to compute $f'(x)$. We have $f'(x) = 6x^2 - 6x - 72$.

Noting that $f'(x)$ exists for every x, there are no Type 2 critical numbers. To find

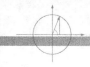

the Type 1 critical numbers, we solve the equation $f'(x)=0$ and have

$$6(x+3)(x-4)=0,$$

$$x=-3 \text{ or } x=4.$$

Therefore, $x=-3$ and $x=4$ are the critical numbers of f; these are the only places where local extrema could possibly occur. #

Example 5.4 Find the critical numbers of the function $f(x)=3x^{4/3}-12x^{1/3}$.

Solution Note that f is defined for all real number x. We then compute $f'(x)$. We have

$$f'(x)=3 \cdot \frac{4}{3}x^{1/3}-12 \cdot \frac{1}{3}x^{-2/3}=4x^{1/3}-\frac{4}{x^{2/3}}$$

$$=\frac{4x^{1/3} x^{2/3}}{x^{2/3}}-\frac{4}{x^{2/3}}=\frac{4x-4}{x^{2/3}}.$$

The derivative fails to exist when $x=0$. Since the original function f is defined when $x=0$, 0 is a Type 2 critical number of f.

If $x\neq0$, then $f'(x)=0$ only when the numerator $4x-4=0$; that is, $f'(x)=0$ when $x=1$. Therefore, $x=1$ is a Type 1 critical number. So the critical numbers of f are 0 and 1. These numbers are the possible locations for local extrema. #

Your Practice 5.1 Find the critical numbers for the function $f(x)=2x^3-3x^2-36x+7$.

Your Practice 5.2 Find the critical numbers for the function $g(x)=x^2 e^{3x}$.

5.1.3 The Mean Value Theorem

The Mean Value Theorem is one of the most important theorems in calculus. First, let us start with a special case of the Mean Value Theorem, called Rolle's theorem.

Informally, Rolle's theorem states that if a differentiable function f takes on the same values at the two end points of an interval, then there must be an interior point c where $f'(c)=0$. Figure 5.6 illustrates this theorem.

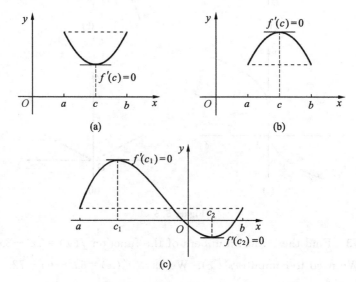

Figure 5.6

Theorem 5. 2 (Rolle's Theorem)

Suppose $f(x)$ is continuous over the closed interval $[a, b]$ and differentiable in the open interval (a, b). If $f(a)=f(b)$, then there exists at least one $c\in(a, b)$ such that $f'(c)=0$.

Proof   Let $k=f(a)=f(b)$. If f is a constant function, then $f'(x)=0$ for all $x\in(a, b)$ and the result is trivially true. We assume in the following that f is not constant.

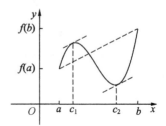

Figure 5. 7

Since f is a continuous function over the closed interval $[a, b]$, it follows from the Extreme Value Theorem that f has an absolute maximum and an absolute minimum. If f is not a constant function, then there exists $x_0\in(a, b)$ so that either $f(x_0)>f(a)$ or $f(x_0)<f(a)$. The absolute maximum is greater than k and the absolute minimum is less than k. Since $f(a)=f(b)=k$, f attains a global extremum at an interior point c. This global extremum is also a local extremum. Since f is differentiable at c, by Fermat's Theorem, $f'(c)=0$.   #

An important point about Rolle's Theorem is that the differentiability of the function f is critical. If f is not differentiable, even at a single point, the result may not hold. For example, the function $f(x)=|x|$ is continuous over $[-1, 1]$ and $f(-1)=f(1)=1$, but $f'(c)\neq0$ for any $c\in(-1, 1)$.

The Mean Value Theorem states that if f is continuous over the closed interval $[a, b]$ and differentiable over the open interval (a, b), then there exists a point $c\in(a, b)$ such that the tangent line to the graph of f at c is parallel to the secant line connecting $(a, f(a))$ and $(b, f(b))$.

Rolle's Theorem is a special case of the Mean Value Theorem. In Rolle's Theorem, we consider differentiable functions f that are equal at the end points. The Mean Value Theorem generalizes Rolle's Theorem by considering functions that are not necessarily equal at the end points. Consequently, we can view the Mean Value Theorem as a slanted version of Rolle's Theorem (Figure 5. 7): the secant and tangent lines are no longer necessarily horizontal but "tilled" and still parallel.

Theorem 5. 3 (the Mean Value Theorem)

If $f(x)$ is continuous over the closed interval $[a, b]$ and differentiable on the open interval (a, b), then there exists at least one $c\in(a, b)$ such that

$$f'(c)=\frac{f(b)-f(a)}{b-a}.$$

Proof   The proof follows from Rolle's Theorem by introducing an appropriate function that satisfies the criteria of Rolle's Theorem. Consider the line connecting $(a,$

$f(a))$ and $(b, f(b))$. Since the slope of that line is

$$\frac{f(b)-f(a)}{b-a}$$

and the line passes through the point $(a, f(a))$, the equation of that line can be written as

$$y=\frac{f(b)-f(a)}{b-a}(x-a)+f(a).$$

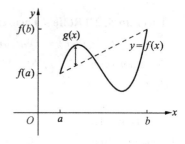

Figure 5. 8

Let $g(x)$ denote the vertical difference between the point $(x, f(x))$ and the point (x, y) on that line. Therefore,

$$g(x)=f(x)-\frac{f(b)-f(a)}{b-a}(x-a)-f(a).$$

We see that $g(a)=g(b)=0$. Since f is a differentiable function over (a, b), g is also a differentiable function over (a, b). Furthermore, since f is continuous over $[a, b]$, g is also continuous over $[a, b]$. Therefore, g satisfies the criteria of Rolle's Theorem. Consequently, there exists a point $c \in (a, b)$ such that $g'(c)=0$. Since

$$g'(x)=f'(x)-\frac{f(b)-f(a)}{b-a},$$

we see that

$$g'(c)=f'(c)-\frac{f(b)-f(a)}{b-a}.$$

Since $g'(c)=0$, we conclude that

$$f'(c)=\frac{f(b)-f(a)}{b-a}. \qquad \#$$

One application that helps us illustrate the Mean Value Theorem involves velocity. If the average speed of a car between two locations was v km/h, then there was at least one instant when the speed indicator displayed v km/h. For example, suppose we drive a car for 1 h down a straight road with an average velocity of 50 m/h. Let $s(t)$ and $v(t)$ denote the position and velocity of the car, respectively, for $0 \leqslant t \leqslant 1$. Assuming that the position function $s(t)$ is differentiable, we can apply the Mean Value Theorem to conclude that, at some time $c \in (0, 1)$, the speed of the car was exactly

$$v(c)=s'(c)=\frac{s(1)-s(0)}{1-0}=50 \text{ m/h}.$$

We now get an important corollary of the Mean Value Theorem. At this point, we know the derivative of any constant function is zero. The Mean Value Theorem allows us to conclude that the converse is also true. In particular, if $f'(x)=0$ for all x in some interval I, then $f(x)$ is constant over that interval.

Corollary 5. 1 (Functions with a Derivative of Zero)

If f is differentiable over the interval I and $f'(x)=0$ for every $x \in I$, then $f(x)$ is constant on I.

Proof　Since f is differentiable over I, f must be continuous over I. Suppose $f(x)$ is not constant for every x in I. Then there exist a, $b \in I$, where $a \neq b$ and $f(a) \neq f(b)$. Choose the notation so that $a < b$. Therefore,

$$\frac{f(b)-f(a)}{b-a} \neq 0.$$

Since f is a differentiable function, by the Mean Value Theorem, there exists $c \in (a, b)$ such that

$$f'(c) = \frac{f(b)-f(a)}{b-a}.$$

Therefore, there exists $c \in (a, b)$ such that $f'(c) \neq 0$, which contradicts the assumption that $f'(x) = 0$ for every $x \in I$.　　　　　　　#

Example 5.5　Assume that f is continuous over $[-1, 1]$ and differentiable on $(-1, 1)$, with $f(0) = 3$ and $f'(x) = 0$ for every $x \in (-1, 1)$. Find $f(x)$.

Solution　Corollary 5.1 tells us that f is a constant. Since we know that $f(0) = 3$, this implies that $f(x) = 3$ for every $x \in (-1, 1)$.　　　　　　　#

Exercise 5.1

1. Find all critical points for

(1) $f(x) = x^3 - 12x + 8$;

(2) $f(x) = x^3 - 12x^2 - 2x + 1$;

(3) $f(x) = \dfrac{5}{x-4}$;

(4) $f(x) = \dfrac{1}{3}x^3 - \dfrac{5}{2}x^2 + 4x$;

(5) $f(x) = (x^2 - 1)^3$;

(6) $f(x) = \dfrac{4x}{1+x^2}$.

2. Verify that the function $f(x) = x^2 + 2x$ over $[-2, 0]$ satisfies the criteria stated in Rolle's Theorem and find all values c in the given interval where $f'(c) = 0$.

3. Verify that the function $f(x) = x^3 - 4x$ over $[-2, 2]$ satisfies the criteria stated in Rolle's Theorem and find all values c in the given interval where $f'(c) = 0$.

4. For $f(x) = \sqrt{x}$ over the interval $[0, 9]$, show that f satisfies the hypothesis of the Mean Value Theorem, and therefore there exists at least one value $c \in (0, 9)$ such that $f'(c)$ is equal to the slope of the line connecting $(0, f(0))$ and $(9, f(9))$. Find these values c guaranteed by the Mean Value Theorem.

5. Suppose that we know that $f(x)$ is continuous and differentiable on $[6, 15]$. We also know that $f(6) = 2$ and $f'(x) \leqslant 5$. What is the largest possible value for $f(15)$?

6. Suppose that we know that $f(x)$ is continuous and differentiable everywhere. Let us also suppose that $f(x)$ has two roots. Show that $f'(x)$ must have at least one root.

5.2 The First Derivatives and Graphs

In this section, we use the derivative to determine intervals on which a given function is increasing or decreasing. We will also determine the local extremes of the function.

5.2.1 The First Derivatives and Monotonicity

When the function f is differentiable, then the derivative is used to determine the intervals where a function is either increasing or decreasing.

To see how the derivative can tell us where a function is increasing or decreasing, look at Figure 5.9. Between A and B and between C and D, the tangent lines have positive slope and so $f'(x) > 0$. Between B and C, the tangent lines have negative slope and so $f'(x) < 0$. Thus it appears that f increases when $f'(x)$ is positive and decreases when $f'(x)$ is negative. We summarize these important results in the box.

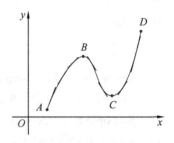

Figure 5.9

> **Theorem 5.4 (Increasing/Decreasing Test)**
>
> *Suppose $f(x)$ is a differentiable function on an open interval I.*
> *(1) If $f'(x) > 0$ on an interval, then f is increasing on that interval.*
> *(2) If $f'(x) < 0$ on an interval, then f is decreasing on that interval.*

Proof We will prove (1); the proof of (2) is similar. Suppose f is not an increasing function on I. Then there exist a and b in I such that $a < b$, but $f(a) \geq f(b)$. Since f is a differentiable function over I, by the Mean Value Theorem there exists $c \in (a, b)$ such that

$$f'(c) = \frac{f(b) - f(a)}{b - a}.$$

Since $f(a) \geq f(b)$, we know that $f(b) - f(a) \leq 0$. Also, $a < b$ tells us that $b - a > 0$. We conclude that

$$f'(c) = \frac{f(b) - f(a)}{b - a} \leq 0.$$

However, $f'(x) > 0$ for every $x \in I$. This is a contradiction, and therefore f must be an increasing function over I. #

Example 5.6 Determine whether the function $f(x) = 4x + x^3$ is increasing or decreasing on $(-\infty, +\infty)$.

Solution The function is increasing on $(-\infty, +\infty)$ because $f'(x) = 4 + 3x^2 > 0$ for any x. #

Example 5.7 Determine whether the function $f(x) = e^{-2x}$ is increasing or decreasing on $(-\infty, +\infty)$.

Solution The function is decreasing on $(-\infty, +\infty)$ because $f'(x) = -2e^{-2x} < 0$ for any x. #

Example 5.8　Find where the function $f(x) = x^3 + 3x^2 - 9x - 8$ is increasing and where it is decreasing.

Solution　We have $f'(x) = 3x^2 + 6x - 9 = 3(x^2 + 2x - 3) = 3(x+3)(x-1)$. To use the Increasing/Decreasing Test we have to know where $f'(x) > 0$ and where $f'(x) < 0$.

Solving the equation $f'(x) = 0$, which is equivalent to $(x+3)(x-1) = 0$, we get $x = -3$ or $x = 1$.

These solutions divide the x-axis into three intervals: $(-\infty, -3), (-3, 1)$, and $(1, +\infty)$. Determine the sign of $f'(x)$ on each interval by testing a number in that interval.

Let -4 be the test number in $(-\infty, -3)$. Then $f'(-4) = 3(-4)^2 + 6(-4) - 9 = 15 > 0$, so $f'(x) > 0$ when x is in $(-\infty, -3)$ and, hence, f is increasing in $(-\infty, -3)$. choosing $x = 0$ in $(-3, 1)$, we have $f'(0) = -9$, so that $f'(x) < 0$ and f is decreasing in $(-3, 1)$. Choosing $x = 2$ in $(1, +\infty)$, we have $f'(2) = 15$, which means that $f'(x) > 0$ and f is increasing in $(1, +\infty)$.

We arrange our work in a chart (Table 5.1). A plus sign indicates that the given expression is positive, and a minus sign indicates that it is negative. The last row of the chart gives the conclusion based on the Increasing/Decreasing Test. For instance, $f'(x) < 0$ for $(-3, 1)$, so $f(x)$ is decreasing on $(-3, 1)$. (It would also be true to say that f is decreasing on the closed interval $[-3, 1]$)

The graph of f shown in Figure 5.10 confirms the information in the chart.　#

Table 5.1

x	$(-\infty, -3)$	-3	$(-3, 1)$	1	$(1, +\infty)$
test number	-4		0		2
$f'(x)$	$+$	0	$-$	0	$+$
$f(x)$	↗		↘		↗

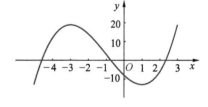

Figure 5.10

We summarize the procedure to find increasing/decreasing intervals as the following.

1. *Compute the derivative f'.*
2. *Find the critical numbers of f.*
3. *Solve the inequalities $f'(x) > 0$ and $f'(x) < 0$ by testing a number in each of the intervals determined by the critical numbers.*
   The solutions of $f'(x) > 0$ are intervals on which f is increasing and the solutions of $f'(x) < 0$ are intervals on which f is decreasing.

Your Practice 5.3　Find where the function $f(x) = x^3 + \dfrac{7}{2}x^2 - 10x - 4$ is increasing and where it is decreasing.

5.2.2　The First Derivative Test

Recall that if f has a local maximum or minimum at $x = c$, then $x = c$ must be a critical number of f, but not every critical number gives rise to a maximum or a minimum. We therefore need a test that will tell us whether or not f has a local maximum or minimum at a critical number.

We can see from Figure 5.10 that at $x = -3$ there exist a local maximum value of f because f increases on $(-\infty, -3)$ and decreases on $(-3, 1)$. Or, in terms of derivatives, $f'(x) > 0$ for $x < -3$ and $f'(x) < 0$ for $-3 < x < 1$. In other words, the sign of $f'(x)$ changes from positive to negative at $x = -3$. This observation is the basis of the following test.

Theorem 5.5 (the First Derivative Test)

Suppose that c is a critical number of a continuous function f.

(1) If f' changes from positive to negative at c, then f has a local maximum at c.

(2) If f' changes from negative to positive at c, then f has a local minimum at c.

(3) If f' does not change sign at c, then f has no local maximum or minimum at c.

The First Derivative Test is a consequence of the Increasing/Decreasing Test. In part (1), for instance, since the sign of $f'(x)$ changes from positive to negative at c, f is increasing to the left of c and decreasing to the right of c. It follows that f has a local maximum at c.

It is easy to remember the First Derivative Test by visualizing diagrams such as those in Figure 5.11.

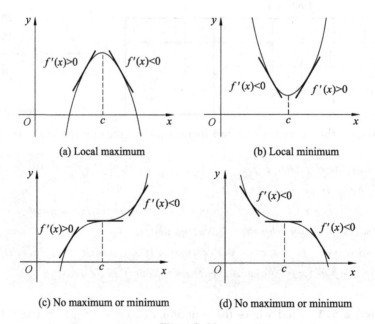

Figure 5.11

Example 5.9   Find all local maxima or local minima for $f(x) = x^3 + 3x^2 - 9x - 8$.

Solution   We have found the increasing and decreasing intervals in Example 5.8, and have $f'(x) = 3x^2 + 6x - 9$. Solving the equation $f'(x) = 0$ yields $x = -3$ or $x = 1$. These numbers divide the x-axis into three intervals: $(-\infty,-3)$, $(-3,1)$, and $(1,+\infty)$. Using $x=-4,0,2$ as the test number in each interval, we make Table 5.2:

Table 5.2

x	$(-\infty,-3)$	-3	$(-3,1)$	1	$(1,+\infty)$
test number	-4		0		2
$f'(x)$	$+$	0	$-$	0	$+$
$f(x)$	↗	LMA	↘	LMI	↗

We get that $f(-3)=19$ is a local maximum value and $f(-1)=-13$ is a local minimum value.　　#

Example 5.10　Find all local maxima or local minima for $f(x)=3x^{4/3}-12x^{1/3}$.

Solution　In Example 5.4, we have found that $f'(x)=\dfrac{4x-4}{\sqrt[3]{x^2}}$ and the critical numbers of f are 0 and 1.

Use $-1,-1/2$ and 2 to apply the first derivative test and form Table 5.3:

Table 5.3

x	$(-\infty,0)$	0	$(0,1)$	1	$(1,+\infty)$
test number	-1		$1/2$		2
$f'(x)$	$-$	not exist	$-$	0	$+$
$f(x)$	↘	0	↘	LMI	↗

Therefore, $f(1)=-9$ is the local minimum value.　　#

Exercise 5.2

1. The graph of the derivative of a function is given in Figure 1.24. Determine the intervals on which the function increases and decreases.

2. This problem is about some function. All we know about the function is that it exists everywhere and we also know the information given below about the derivative of the function.

$f'(-5)=0$, $f'(-1)=0$, $f'(4)=0$, $f'(9)=0$, $f'(x)<0$ on $(-5,-1)\cup(-1,4)\cup(9,+\infty)$, $f'(x)>0$ on $(-\infty,-5)\cup$

$(4,9)$.

Answer each of the following questions about this function.

(1) Identify the critical points of the function;

(2) Determine the intervals on which the function increases and decreases;

(3) Classify the critical points as local maximums, local minimums or neither.

3. Find the intervals on which $f(x)$ is increasing (decreasing) and the local extrema (if any).

(1) $f(x)=x^3+4x-5$;

(2) $f(x)=x^4-2x^2+3$;

(3) $f(x)=\dfrac{x^2}{x-2}$;

(4) $f(x)=x^2+\dfrac{1}{x^2}$;

(5) $f(x)=xe^{2-x^2/2}$;

(6) $f(x)=x-2\ln(1+x^2)$.

4. Let $r>0$. Find the local maxima and minima of the function $f(x)=\sqrt{r^2-x^2}$ on its domain $[-r, r]$.

5. Let $f(x)=ax^2+bx+c$ with $a\neq0$. Show that f has exactly one critical point. Give conditions on a and b which guarantee that the critical point will be a maximum. It is possible to see this without using calculus at all, explain.

6. Answer each of the following questions.

(1) What is the minimum degree of a polynomial that has exactly one local extrema?

(2) What is the minimum degree of a polynomial that has exactly two local extrema?

(3) What is the minimum degree of a polynomial that has exactly three local extrema?

(4) What is the minimum degree of a polynomial that has exactly n local extrema?

7. For some function $f(x)$, it is known that there is a local minimum at $x=-4$. Answer each of the following questions about this function.

(1) What is the simplest form for the derivative of this function?

Note: There are really many possible forms of the derivative, so to make the rest of this problem as simple as possible you want, use the simplest form of the derivative.

(2) Using your answer from (1) to determine the most general form that the function itself can take.

(3) Given that $f(-4)=6$, find a function that will have a local minimum at $x=-4$.

Note: There are many possible answers here so just give one of them.

8. For some function $f(x)$, it is known that there is a critical point at $x=4$ that is neither a local minimum or a local maximum. Answer each of the following questions about this function.

(1) What is the simplest form for the derivative of this function?

Note: There are really many possible forms of the derivative, so to make the rest of this problem as simple as possible you can, use the simplest form of the derivative.

(2) Using your answer from (1) to determine the most general form that the function itself can take.

(3) Given that $f(4)=3$, find a function that will have a critical point at $x=4$ that is neither a local minimum nor a local maximum.

Note: There are many possible answers here, so just give one of them.

9. For some function $f(x)$, it is known that there is a local maximum at $x=2$ and a local minimum at $x=5$. Answer each of the following questions about this function.

(1) What is the simplest form for the derivative of this function?

Note: There are really many possible forms of the derivative, so to make the rest of this problem as simple as possible you can, use the simplest form of the derivative.

(2) Using your answer from (1) to determine the most general form that the function itself can take.

(3) Given that $f(2)=4$ and $f(5)=-6$, find a function that will have a local maximum at $x=2$ and a local minimum at $x=5$.

Note: There are many possible answers here, so just give one of them.

10. Given that $f(x)$ and $g(x)$ are increasing functions. Show that $f(x)+g(x)$ is an increasing function.

11. Given that $f(x)$ and $g(x)$ are increasing functions. Show that $h(x)=f[(g(x)]$ will also be an increasing function.

12. Given that $f(x)$ is an increasing function. Will $h(x)=[f(x)]^2$ be an increasing function? If yes, prove it. If no, can you determine any other conditions needed on the function $f(x)$ that will guarantee that $h(x)$ will also increase?

13. A drug is injected into the bloodstream of a patient through the right arm. The drug concentration in the bloodstream of the left arm t hours after the injection is approximated by

$$C(t)=\frac{0.28t}{t^2+4}, \ 0<t<24.$$

Find the critical numbers of $C(t)$, the intervals on which the drug concentration is increasing, the intervals on which the concentration of the drug is decreasing, and the local extrema.

14. The concentration $C(t)$, in milligrams per cubic centimeter, of a particular drug in a patient's bloodstream is given by

$$C(t)=\frac{0.16t}{t^2+6t+6}, \ 0<t<12$$

where t is the number of hours after the drug is taken orally. Find the critical values of $C(t)$, the intervals where the drug concentration increases, the intervals where the concentration decreases, and the local extrema.

5.3　The Second Derivatives and Graphs

5.3.1　Higher Derivatives

Let the function $f(x)$ be differentiable in a certain interval, then its derivative $f'(x)$ is also a function in this interval. If this function may have a derivative of its own, denoted by $(f')'=f''$. This new function is called the **second derivative** of f because it is the derivative of the derivative of f. The second derivative is denoted by various notations as

$$f''=(f')'=\frac{d}{dx}\left(\frac{dy}{dx}\right)=\frac{d^2y}{dx^2}.$$

Example 5.11　If $f(x)=x^3-x$, find $f'(x)$ and $f''(x)$.

Solution　Apply the Sum Rule:

$$f'(x)=3x^2-1.$$

So the second derivative is

$$f''(x)=[f'(x)]'=(3x^2-1)'=6x. \qquad \text{\#}$$

We can interpret $f''(x)$ as the slope of the curve $y=f'(x)$ at the point $(x, f'(x))$. In other words, it is the rate of change of the slope of the original curve $y=f(x)$.

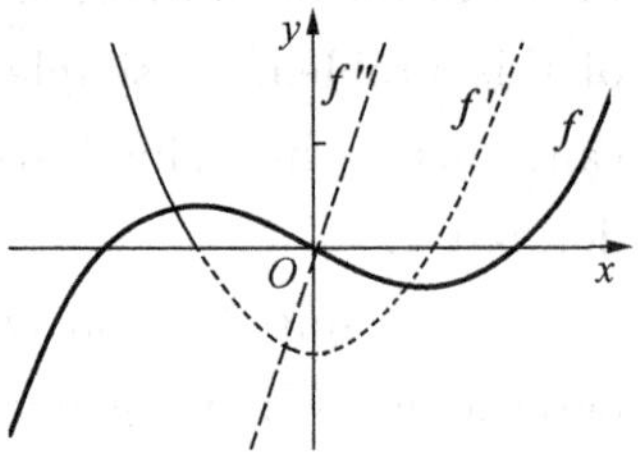

Notice from Figure 5.12 that $f''(x)$ is negative when $y=f'(x)$ has negative slope and positive when $y=f'(x)$ has positive slope. So the graphs serve as a check on our calculations.

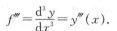

Figure 5.12

Similarly, if f'' exists and is differentiable, we can calculate the third derivative of the function $f(x)$:

$$f'''=\frac{\mathrm{d}^3 y}{\mathrm{d}x^3}=y'''(x).$$

The result of taking the derivative n times is called the nth derivative of $f(x)$ with respect to x and is denoted as

$$\frac{\mathrm{d}^n f}{\mathrm{d}x^n}=\frac{\mathrm{d}^n y}{\mathrm{d}x^n}$$

or
$$f^{(n)}(x)=y^{(n)}(x).$$

Thus, the notion of the nth order derivative is introduced inductively by sequential calculation of n derivatives starting from the first order derivative. Transition to the next higher-order derivative is performed using the recurrence formula

$$y^{(n)}(x)=[y^{(n-1)}(x)]'.$$

Example 5.12 Given the function $f(x)=(2x-1)^3(x+1)$. Find all derivatives of the nth order from $n=1$ to $n=5$.

Solution First we convert the given function into a polynomial: $f(x)=(2x-1)^3(x+1)=8x^4-4x^3-6x^2+5x-1$. Now we successively calculate the derivatives from 1st to 5th order:

$$y'=(8x^4-4x^3-6x^2+5x-1)'=32x^3-12x^2-12x+5,$$
$$y''=(y')'=(32x^3-12x^2-12x+5)'=96x^2-24x-12,$$
$$y'''=(y'')'=(96x^2-24x-12)'=192x-24,$$
$$y^{(4)}=(y''')'=(192x-24)'=192,$$
$$y^{(5)}=(y^{(4)})'=(192)'=0. \qquad \text{\#}$$

If $f(x)$ represents the position of a particle at time x, then $f'(x)$ will represent the velocity (rate of change of the position) of the particle and $f''(x)$ will represent the acceleration (the rate of change of the velocity) of the particle.

You are probably familiar with acceleration from driving or riding in a car. The speedometer tells you your velocity (speed). When you leave from a stop and press down on the accelerator, you are accelerating your speed.

Example 5.13 Find the nth order derivative of the natural logarithm function $y=\ln x$.

Solution We compute several successive derivatives of the given function:

$$y' = (\ln x)' = \frac{1}{x},$$

$$y'' = (y')' = \left(\frac{1}{x}\right)' = (x^{-1})' = -x^{-2} = -\frac{1}{x^2},$$

$$y''' = (y'')' = \left(-\frac{1}{x^2}\right)' = 2x^{-3} = \frac{2}{x^3},$$

$$y^{(4)} = (y''')' = \left(\frac{2}{x^3}\right)' = -6x^{-4} = -\frac{6}{x^4},$$

$$y^{(5)} = (y^{(4)})' = \left(-\frac{6}{x^4}\right)' = 24x^{-5} = \frac{24}{x^5}.$$

We get the derivative of an arbitrary nth order

$$y^{(n)} = \frac{(-1)^{n-1}(n-1)!}{x^n}. \qquad\qquad \#$$

This formula can be rigorously demonstrated using the method of mathematical induction.

5.3.2　Concavity

The sign of the first derivative of a function gives us information about its monotonicity. The sign of the second derivative gives us information about its concavity.

In general, the graph of a function is curved with different bending directions. Figure 5.13 shows the graphs of two increasing functions in (a, b). Both graphs start from point A and end at point B but they look different because they bend in different directions. In Figure 5.13 (a), the curve opens up while the curve opens down. Thus they can be distinguished by their concavity. We say a function is concave up if its graph is curved with the opening upward. Similarly, a function is concave down if its graph opens downward. Notice that a function can be concave up regardless of whether it is increasing or decreasing. A function can be concave up and either increasing or decreasing. Similarly, a function can be concave down and either increasing or decreasing.

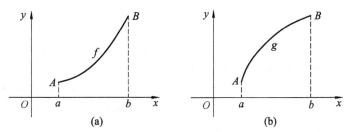

Figure 5.13

Let us see how the second derivative helps determine the intervals of concavity. Take an epidemic as an example. Suppose an epidemic has started, and you, as a member of congress, must decide whether the current methods are effectively fighting the spread of the disease or whether more drastic measures and more money are needed. In Figure 5.14, $f(x)$ is the number of people who are infected at time x, and two different situations are shown. In both Figure 5.14 (a) and (b), the number of people with the disease, $f(\text{now})$, and the rate at which new people are getting sick, $f'(\text{now})$, are the same. The difference in the two situations is the concavity of f, and that difference in concavity might have a big effect on your decision.

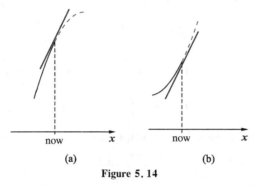

Figure 5.14

In Figure 5.14(a), f is concave down at "now", the slopes are decreasing, and it looks as if it is tailing off. We can say "f is increasing at a decreasing rate". It appears that the current methods are starting to bring the epidemic under control. In Figure 5.14(b), f is concave up, the slopes are increasing, and it looks as if it will keep increasing faster and faster. It appears that the epidemic is still out of control.

The differences between the graphs come from whether the derivative is increasing or decreasing. As the derivative tells us if the original function is increasing or decreasing, the second derivative gives us a mathematical way to tell how the graph of a function is curved. Thus the second derivative tells us if the original function is concave up or down.

Definition 5.3

We say that a function f is concave up on an open interval I if it is differentiable there and the derivative f' is increasing on the interval. We say that a function f is concave down on an interval I if f' exists and decreasing on the interval.

In general, without having the graph of a function f, how can we determine its concavity? By definition, a function f is concave up if f is increasing. From the increasing/decreasing test theorem, we know that if f is a differentiable function, then f is increasing if its derivative $f''(x) > 0$. Therefore, a function f that is twice differentiable is concave up when $f''(x) > 0$. Similarly, a function f is concave down if f is decreasing. We know that a differentiable function f is decreasing if its derivative $f''(x) < 0$. Therefore, a twice-differentiable function f is concave down when $f''(x) < 0$.

Applying this logic is known as the concavity test.

Theorem 5.6 (Test for Concavity)

Suppose that f is twice differentiable over an interval I.
(1) If $f''(x) > 0$ for every $x \in I$, then f is concave up over I.
(2) If $f''(x) < 0$ for every $x \in I$, then f is concave down over I.

We conclude that we can determine the concavity of a function f by looking at the second derivative of f. In addition, we observe that a function f can switch concavity (Figure 5.14). However, a continuous function can switch concavity only at a point x if $f''(x)=0$ or $f''(x)$ is undefined. Consequently, to determine the intervals where a function f is concave up and concave down, we look for those values of x where $f''(x)=0$ or $f''(x)$ is undefined. When we have determined these points, we divide the domain of f into smaller intervals and determine the sign of f'' over each of these smaller intervals. If f'' changes sign as we pass through a point x, then f changes concavity. It is important to remember that a function f may not change concavity at a point x even if $f''(x)=0$ or $f''(x)$ is undefined. If, however, f does change concavity at a point a and f is continuous at a, we say the point $(a, f(a))$ is an inflection point of f.

Figure 5.15 shows the concavity of a function at several points. The graph is concave upward (abbreviated $\cup$) on the intervals (b, c), (d, e), and (e, p) and concave downward (abbreviated $\cap$) on the intervals (a, b), (c, d), and (p, q). B, C, D and P are points of inflection. If a curve has a tangent at a point of inflection, then the curve crosses its tangent there.

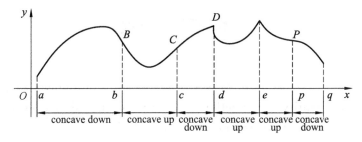

Figure 5.15

From the definition we know that if f'' is positive on an interval, the graph of $y=f(x)$ is concave up on that interval. We can say that f is increasing (or decreasing) at an increasing rate. If f'' is negative on an interval, the graph of $y=f(x)$ is concave up on that interval. We can say that f is increasing (or decreasing) at a decreasing rate.

Inflection points happen when the concavity changes. Because we know the connection between the concavity of a function and the sign of its second derivative, we can use this to find inflection points.

Example 5.14   Find all intervals where $f(x) = x^4 - 4x^3$ is concave upward or downward and find any points of inflection.

Solution   The concept is very similar to that of finding intervals of increase and decrease. We still set a derivative equal to 0, and we still plug in values of testing numbers to check the signs of the derivatives in those intervals. The main difference is that instead of working with the first derivative to find intervals of increase and decrease, we work with the second derivative to find intervals of concavity.

We have

$$f'(x)=4x^3-12x^2=4x^2(x-3),$$
$$f''(x)=12x^2-24x=12x(x-2).$$

To find the inflection points we set $f''(x)=0$ and obtain $x=0$ or $x=2$. We divide the domain of f into three intervals $(-\infty, 0)$, $(0, 2)$ and $(2, +\infty)$. Using test numbers -1, 1, 3 in those intervals to determine the sign of $f''(x)$ and make Table 5.4:

Table 5.4

x	$(-\infty, 0)$	0	$(0, 2)$	2	$(2, +\infty)$
test number	-1		1		3
$f''(x)$	$+$	0	$-$	0	$+$
$f(x)$	U	0	∩	-16	U

Therefore, f is concave upward on $(-\infty, 0)$ and $(2, +\infty)$, concave downward on $(0, 2)$. The points $(0, 0)$ and $(2, -16)$ are inflection points.   #

Your Practice 5.4 Find all intervals where $f(x)=x^3-5x^2+3x-6$ is concave upward or downward and find any points of inflection.   #

Exercise 5.3

1. Each quotation in this problem is a statement about a quantity of something changing over time. Let $f(t)$ represent the quantity at time t. For each quotation, tell what f represents and whether the first and the second derivatives of f are positive or negative.

(1) "Unemployment rose again, but the rate of increase is smaller than last month."

(2) "Our profits declined again, but at a slower rate than last month."

(3) "The population is still rising at a faster rate than last year."

(4) "The child's temperature is still rising, but slower than it was a few hours ago."

(5) "The number of whales is decreasing, but at a slower rate than last year."

(6) "The number of people with the flu is rising and at a faster rate than last month."

2. On which intervals is the function in Figure 5.16

(1) concave up?

(2) concave down?

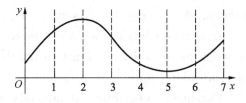

Figure 5.16

3. On which intervals is the function in Figure 5.17

(1) concave up?

(2) concave down?

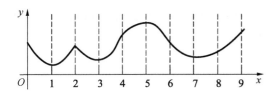

Figure 5.17

4. Which of the labeled points in Figure 5.18 are inflection points?

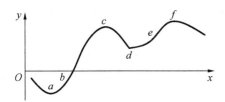

Figure 5.18

5. Which of the labeled points in Figure 5.19 are inflection points?

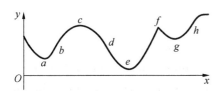

Figure 5.19

6. How many inflection points can a

(1) quadratic polynomial have?

(2) cubic polynomial have?

(3) polynomial of degree n have?

7. Fill in Table 5.5 with "$+$", "$-$", or "0" for the function shown in Figure 5.20.

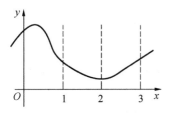

Figure 5.20

Table 5.5

x	0	1	2	3
f				
$f'(x)$				
$f''(x)$				

8. Fill in Table 5.6 with "$+$", "$-$", or "0" for the function shown in Figure 5.21.

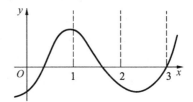

Figure 5.21

Table 5.6

x	0	1	2	3
f				
$f'(x)$				
$f''(x)$				

9. Let $f(x) = x^3 + 30x^2$. Find the x and y coordinates of all inflection points.

10. Find the intervals on which the graph of $f(x) = \ln(x^2 - 2x + 10)$ is concave upward (concave downward), and the x coordinates of the inflection points.

11. One hour after x milligrams of a particular drug are given to a person, the change in body temperature $T(x)$, in degrees Fahrenheit, is given by

$$T(x) = x^2 \left(1 - \frac{x}{9}\right), \quad 0 \leqslant x \leqslant 6.$$

The rate $T'(x)$ at which $T(x)$ changes with respect to the size of the dosage x is called the sensitivity of the body to the dosage.

(1) When is $T'(x)$ increasing/decreasing?

(2) Where does the graph of T have inflection points?

(3) Sketch the graphs of T and T' on the same coordinate system.

(4) What is the maximum value of $T'(x)$?

5.4 Optimization

5.4.1 Locating Absolute Extrema

The Extreme Value Theorem states that a continuous function over a closed, bounded interval has an absolute maximum and an absolute minimum. These absolute extrema could occur at an endpoint or at an interior point. If an absolute extremum does not occur at an endpoint, however, it must occur at an interior point, in which case the absolute extremum is a local extremum. Therefore, by Fermat's Theorem, the point c at which the local extremum occurs must be a critical point. We summarize this result in the following theorem.

> **Theorem 5.7 (Location of Absolute Extrema)**
>
> *Suppose that f is a continuous function over a closed, bounded interval I. The absolute maximum of f over I and the absolute minimum of f over I must occur at endpoints of I or at critical points of f in I.*

To find the absolute maximum and minimum of a continuous function on a closed interval, we simply identify the endpoints and critical numbers in the interval, evaluate the function at each of them, and choose the largest and smallest values. With this idea in mind, let us examine a procedure for locating absolute extrema.

> **Locating Absolute Extrema Over a Closed Interval**
>
> *Step 1   Check to make certain that f is continuous over $[a, b]$.*
>
> *Step 2   Find the critical numbers in the interval (a, b).*
>
> *Step 3   Evaluate f at the endpoints a and b and at the critical numbers found in step 2.*
>
> *Step 4   The absolute maximum of f on $[a, b]$ is the largest value found in step 3*
>
> *Step 5   The absolute minimum of f on $[a, b]$ is the smallest value found in step 3.*

Now let us discuss how to use this strategy to find the absolute maximum and absolute minimum values of a continuous function.

Example 5.15　Find the absolute maximum and absolute minimum of $f(x) = x^3 + 3x^2 - 9x - 7$ on the interval $[-6, 4]$.

Solution　Step 1　Since $f(x)$ is a polynomial, it is continuous over $[-6, 4]$.

Step 2　Find the critical numbers in the interval $(-6, 4)$. Since $f'(x) = 3x^2 + 6x - 9$, f' is defined for all real numbers x. There are no critical points where the derivative is undefined. It remains to check where $f'(x) = 0$. Since $f'(x) = 3x^2 + 6x - 9 = 3(x^2 + 2x - 3) =$

$3(x+3)(x-1)=0$ at $x=-3$ and $x=1$, and the two points is in the interval $[-6, 4]$, $f(-3)$ and $f(1)$ are candidates for an absolute extremum of f over $[-6, 4]$.

Step 3   We evaluate function values and find

$$f(-6)=-61, \ f(-3)=20 \text{ and } f(1)=-12, \ f(4)=69. \tag{5.1}$$

Step 4   We find that the absolute maximum of f over the interval $[-6, 4]$ is 69, and it occurs at $x=4$.

Step 5   The absolute minimum of f over the interval $[-6, 4]$ is -61, and it occurs at $x=-6$.

Note that in this example the absolute maximum and the absolute minimum occur at the endpoint. The graph of $f(x)$ is sketched in Figure 5.22.   #

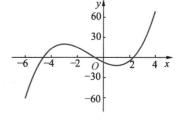

Figure 5.22

Your Practice 5.5   Find the absolute maximum and absolute minimum of $f(x)=x^3-12x$ on the interval $[-5, 5]$.

5.4.2   The Second Derivative and Extrema

The second derivative provides sometimes a simpler way than using the first derivative to locate extreme values.

We know that if a continuous function has a local extremum, it must occur at a critical point. However, a function need not have a local extremum at a critical point. Here we examine how the second derivative test can be used to determine whether a function has a local extremum at a critical point. Let f be a twice-differentiable function such that $f(a)=0$

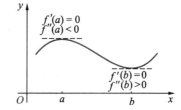

Figure 5.23   The second derivative test

and f'' is continuous over an open interval I containing a. Suppose $f''(a)<0$. Since f'' is continuous over I, $f''(a)<0$ for every $x \in I$ (Figure 5.23). Then, f' is a decreasing function over I. Since $f'(a)=0$, we conclude that for every $x \in I$, $f'(x)>0$ if $x<a$ and $f'(x)<0$ if $x>a$. Therefore, by the first derivative test, f has a local maximum at $x=a$.

Theorem 5.8 (the Second Derivative Test for Local Extrema)

Let c be a critical number of $f(x)$ such that $f'(c)=0$.

(1) If the second derivative $f''(c)>0$, then $f(c)$ is a local minimum.

(2) If $f''(c)<0$, then $f(c)$ is a local maximum.

(3) If $f''(c)=0$, then the test is inconclusive.

Note that for case (3) when $f''(c)=0$, then f may have a local maximum, local minimum, or neither at c. For example, the functions $f(x)=x^3$, $f(x)=x^4$, and $f(x)=-x^4$ all have critical points at $x=0$. In each case, the second derivative is zero at $x=0$. However, the function $f(x)=x^4$ has a local minimum at $x=0$ whereas the function $f(x)=-x^4$ has a local maximum at $x=0$, and the function $f(x)=x^3$ does not have a local extremum at $x=0$.

Let us discuss how to use the second derivative test to determine whether f has a local maximum or local minimum at a critical point c where $f'(c)=0$.

Example 5.16　Find the local maxima and minima for the function $f(x)=x^3-6x^2+9x+1$. Use the Second Derivative Test for Local Extrema when it applies.

Solution　If $f(x)=x^3-6x^2+9x+1$, then

$$f'(x)=3x^2-12x+9=3(x-3)(x-1),$$
$$f''(x)=6x-12=6(x-2).$$

To find the critical numbers, we set $f'(x)=0$ and obtain $x=1$ and $x=3$. To use the Second-Derivative Test, we evaluate f'' at these critical numbers:

$$f''(1)=-6,\ f''(3)=6.$$

Since $f'(1)=0$ and $f''(1)<0$, $f(1)=5$ is a local maximum. Since $f'(3)=0$ and $f''(1)>0$, $f(3)=1$ is a local minimum.　　　　　#

Your Practice 5.6　Find the local maxima and minima for the function $f(x)=x^3-9x^2+24x-10$. Use the Second Derivative Test for Local Extrema when it applies.

5.4.3　The Second Derivative Test for Absolute Extrema

Now, suppose that a function is continuous on an interval that is not closed and we want to find its absolute maximum or minimum value. Since the Extreme Value Theorem no longer applies, we cannot be certain that the absolute maximum or minimum value exists.

In general, the best procedure to take when the interval is not closed is to sketch the graph of the function. However, one special case that occurs frequently in applications can be analyzed without drawing a graph. It often happens that f is continuous on an interval I and has only one critical value c in the interval I (here, I can be any type of interval—open, closed, or half-closed). If this is the case and if f'' exists, we have the Second Derivative Test for Absolute Extrema.

> **the Second-Derivative Test for Absolute Extrema on an Open Interval**
>
> *Suppose f'' is continuous near c. Let c be the only one critical number in an open interval I.*
>
> *(1) If $f'(c)=0$ and $f''(c)>0$, then $f(c)$ is the absolute minimum of f on I.*
>
> *(2) If $f'(c)=0$ and $f''(c)<0$, then $f(c)$ is the absolute maximum of f on I.*

Example 5.17　Find the absolute extrema of $f(x)=x+\dfrac{4}{x}$ in $(0,+\infty)$.

Solution　If $f(x)=x+\dfrac{4}{x}$, then

$$f'(x)=1-\frac{4}{x^2}=\frac{(x-2)(x+2)}{x^2},\ f''(x)=\frac{8}{x^3}.$$

The only critical value in the interval $(0,+\infty)$ is $x=2$. Since $f''(2)=1>0$, $f(2)=4$ is the absolute minimum value of f on $(0,+\infty)$.　　　　　#

Your Practice 5.7　Find the absolute extrema of $f(x)=12-x-\dfrac{5}{x}$ on $(0,+\infty)$.

5.4.4　Optimization Problems

The methods we have learned for finding extreme values have practical applications in many areas of life. For instance, a business person wants to minimize costs and maximize profits; a traveler wants to minimize transportation time; Fermat's Principle in optics states that light follows the path that takes the least time.

In solving such practical problems the greatest challenge is often to convert the word problem into a mathematical optimization problem by setting up the function that is to be maximized or minimized. We point out that in a real application optimal problem, the critical point is the optimal point if there is only one critical point.

We outline the steps to follow in solving this type of problems.

Steps in Solving Optimization Problems

　　Step 1　*Understand the Problem. The first step is to read the problem carefully until it is clearly understood. Ask yourself: What is the unknown? What are the given quantities? What are the given conditions?*

　　Step 2　*Draw a Diagram. In most problems it is useful to draw a diagram and identify the given and required quantities on the diagram.*

　　Step 3　*Introduce Notation. Assign a symbol to the quantity that is to be maximized or minimized (let's call it Q for now). Also select symbols (a, b, c,···; x, y, z, ···) for other unknown quantities and label the diagram with these symbols.*

　　Step 4　*Express Q in terms of some of the other symbols from Step 3.*

　　Step 5　*If Q has been expressed as a function of more than one variable in Step 4, use the given information to find relationships (in the form of equations) among these variables. Then use these equations to eliminate all but one of the variables in the expression for Q. Thus Q will be expressed as a function of one variable, say, x. Write the domain of this function.*

　　Step 6　*Use the first derivative test or the second derivative test to find the maximum or minimum value of Q.*

Example 5.18　A rectangle garden is to be constructed against the side of a garage. The gardener has 100 feet of fencing, and will construct a three-sided fence; the side of the garage will form the fourth side. What dimensions will give the garden of greatest area?

Solution　Let x be the side of the garden that is perpendicular to the side of the garage. Then the garden has width x and length $100-2x$ feet. The area is

$$A(x)=x\cdot(100-2x)=100x-2x^2,\ 0<x<50.$$

Then $A'(x)=100-4x$. The only critical point is $x=25$. So $x=25$ must also be the global maximum for the real life problem.

The optimal dimensions for the garden are

$$width=25 \text{ feet}, \quad length=50 \text{ feet}. \qquad \#$$

Example 5. 19 A box is to be made from a sheet of cardboard that measures 12×12. The construction will be achieved by cutting a square from each corner of the sheet and then folding up the sides. What is the box of greatest volume that can be constructed in this fashion?

Solution Let x be the side length of the square that are to be cut. Then the side length of the resulting box will be $12-2x$. The height of the box will be x.

The volume of the box will be

$$V=x \cdot (12-2x) \cdot (12-2x)=144x-48x^2+4x^3, \ 0<x<6.$$

Now $V'(x)=144-96x+12x^2=12(x-2)(x-6)$.

Let $V'(x)=0$ then we have $x=2$ or $x=6$. But $x=6$ is not in the domain. So $x=2$ is the only critical point.

We conclude that $x=2$ is the optimal number for the problem. If squares of side 2 are cut from the sheet of cardboard then a box of maximum volume will result. $\qquad \#$

Your Practice 5.8 The sum of two positive numbers is 60. How can we choose them so as to maximum their product?

Exercise 5.4

1. Find the absolute maximum and absolute minimum of $f(x)=x^2-4x+3$ over the interval $[1, 4]$.

2. Find the absolute maximum and minimum, if either exists, for $f(x)=\dfrac{2x}{x^2+1}$ on the indicated intervals.

   (1) $[-1, 5]$;

   (2) $[-1, 3]$;

   (3) $[2, 5]$.

3. Use the second derivative to find the location of all local extrema for $f(x)=x^5-5x^3$.

4. Consider the function $f(x)=x^3-\dfrac{3}{2}x^2-18x$. The points $c=3, -2$ satisfy $f'(c)=0$. Use the second derivative test to determine whether f has a local maximum or local minimum at those points.

5. A walnut grower estimates from records that if 20 trees are planted per acre, each tree will yield average 60 pounds of nuts per year. If for each additional tree planted per acre (up to 15) the average yield per tree drops 2 pounds, how many trees should be planted to maximize the yield per acre? What is the maximum yield?

6. Find the absolute maximum value on $(0, +\infty)$ for

   (1) $f(x)=12-x-\dfrac{5}{x}$;

   (2) $f(x)=5\ln x-x$.

7. A company manufactures and sells x digital cameras per week. The weekly price demand and cost equations are, respectively,

$$P(x)=400-0.4x$$

and

$$C(x) = 2000 + 160x.$$

(1) What price should the company charge for the cameras, and how many cameras should be produced to maximize the weekly revenue? What is the maximum revenue?

(2) What is the maximum weekly profit? How much should the company charge for the cameras, and how many cameras should be produced to realize the maximum weekly profit?

5.5   L'Hôspital's Rule

In this section, we examine a powerful tool for evaluating limits. This tool, known as L'Hôspital's Rule, can help us calculate a limit that may otherwise be hard or impossible. Instead of relying on numerical evidence to conjecture that a limit exists, we will be able to show definitively that a limit exists and to determine its exact value.

5.5.1   Indeterminate Forms

Let's compute the following limit

$$\lim_{x \to 1} \frac{e^x - e}{x - 1}.$$

If we use the Quotient Rule (the limit of a quotient is the quotient of the limits), we get $\frac{0}{0}$ which is not defined. The limits does exit but its value is not obvious because both numerator and denominator approach 0.

In general, if we have a limit of the form

$$\lim_{x \to c} \frac{f(x)}{g(x)}$$

where both $f(x) \to 0$ and $g(x) \to 0$ as $x \to c$, then this limit may or may not exist and is called an indeterminate form of type $\frac{0}{0}$. Note that the notation $\frac{0}{0}$ does not mean we are actually dividing zero by zero. Rather, we use the notation $\frac{0}{0}$ to represent a quotient of limits, each of which is zero. An indeterminate form is defined as a limit that does not provide enough information to determine the original limit. L'Hôspital's Rule allows us to simplify the evaluation of limits that involve indeterminate forms.

Theorem 5.9 (L'Hôspital's Rule)

For a real number, if $\lim_{x \to c} f(x) = 0$ *and* $\lim_{x \to c} g(x) = 0$, *then*

$$\lim_{x \to c} \frac{f(x)}{g(x)} = \lim_{x \to c} \frac{f'(x)}{g'(x)}$$

provided that the second limit exists or is ∞.

The idea behind L'Hôspital's Rule can be explained using local linear approximations (Figure 5.24) The image above shows two differentiable functions f and g, each of which approaches 0 as $x \to c$. If we zoom in toward the point $(c, 0)$, the graphs would start to look almost linear. But if the functions actually were linear, as in the second graph, then their ratio would be

$$\frac{m_1(x-c)}{m_2(x-c)} = \frac{m_1}{m_2},$$

which is the ratio of their derivatives. This suggests that

$$\lim_{x \to c} \frac{f(x)}{g(x)} = \lim_{x \to c} \frac{f'(x)}{g'(x)}.$$

We now give an explanation for the case in which f' and g' are continuous. Using the alternative form of the definition of a derivative, we have

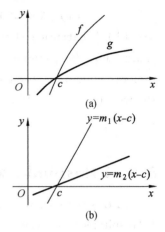

Figure 5.24

$$\lim_{x \to c} \frac{f'(x)}{g'(x)} = \frac{f'(c)}{g'(c)} = \frac{\lim\limits_{x \to c} \dfrac{f(x)-f(c)}{x-c}}{\lim\limits_{x \to c} \dfrac{g(x)-g(c)}{x-c}} = \lim_{x \to c} \frac{\dfrac{f(x)-f(c)}{x-c}}{\dfrac{g(x)-g(c)}{x-c}}$$

$$= \lim_{x \to c} \frac{f(x)-f(c)}{g(x)-g(c)} = \lim_{x \to c} \frac{f(x)}{g(x)}.$$

Example 5.20 Evaluate

$$\lim_{x \to 1} \frac{e^x - e}{x-1}.$$

Solution Since

$$\lim_{x \to 1}(e^x - e) = e^1 - e = 0, \quad \lim_{x \to 1}(x-1) = 0,$$

we can apply L'Hôspital's Rule:

$$\lim_{x \to 1} \frac{e^x - e}{x-1} \overset{\frac{0}{0}}{=\!=\!=} \lim_{x \to 1} \frac{(e^x - e)'}{(x-1)'} = \lim_{x \to 1} \frac{e^x}{1} = e. \qquad \#$$

Example 5.21 Evaluate

$$\lim_{x \to 0} \frac{\ln(1+x^2)}{x^4}.$$

Solution We have $\lim\limits_{x \to 0} \ln(1+x^2) = \ln 1 = 0$, $\lim\limits_{x \to 0} x^4 = 0$, so L'Hôspital's Rule gives

$$\lim_{x \to 0} \frac{\ln(1+x^2)}{x^4} \overset{\frac{0}{0}}{=\!=\!=} \lim_{x \to 0} \frac{[\ln(1+x^2)]'}{(x^4)'} = \lim_{x \to 0} \frac{\dfrac{2x}{1+x^2}}{4x^3}$$

$$= \lim_{x \to 0} \frac{1}{2x^2(1+x^2)} = +\infty. \qquad \#$$

L'Hôspital's Rule can be applied several times provided that all the conditions are satisfied, for instance,

$$\lim_{x \to 0} \frac{x^2}{e^x - 1 - x} \overset{\frac{0}{0}}{=\!=\!=} \lim_{x \to 0} \frac{(x^2)'}{(e^x - 1 - x)'} = \lim_{x \to 0} \frac{2x}{e^x - 1}$$

$$\overset{\frac{0}{0}}{=\!=\!=} \lim_{x \to 0} \frac{2}{e^x} = 2.$$

Your Practice 5.9　Evaluate $\lim\limits_{x\to0}\dfrac{e^{2x}-1-2x}{x^2}$.

L'Hôspital's Rule says that the limit of a quotient of functions is equal to the limit of the quotient of their derivatives, provided that the given conditions are satisfied. It is especially important to verify the conditions regarding the limits of both the numerator and denominator before using L'Hôspital's Rule. For example, the following is not correct:

$$\lim_{x\to1}\frac{\ln x}{x}=\lim_{x\to1}\frac{(\ln x)'}{x'}=\lim_{x\to1}\frac{1/x}{1}=1.$$

This is because $\lim\limits_{x\to1}\ln x=0$ but the denominator $\lim\limits_{x\to1}x=1$, so it is not a $\dfrac{0}{0}$ type and the L'Hôspital's Rule cannot be applied.

Your Practice 5.10　Show that the limit $\lim\limits_{x\to1}\dfrac{3x^2+5}{x^2+1}$ cannot be evaluated by applying L'Hôspital's rule.

L'Hôspital's Rule remains valid for one-sided limits and for limits at infinity or negative infinity; that is, "$x\to c$" can be replaced by any of the symbols: $x\to c^+$, $x\to c^-$, $x\to+\infty$, or $x\to-\infty$.

Example 5.22　Find $\lim\limits_{x\to1^+}\dfrac{\ln x}{(x-1)^2}$.

Solution　We have $\lim\limits_{x\to1^+}\ln x=0$ and $\lim\limits_{x\to1^+}(x-1)^2=0$. Apply the L'Hôspital's Rule:

$$\lim_{x\to1^+}\frac{\ln x}{(x-1)^2}\overset{\tfrac{0}{0}}{=\!=\!=}\lim_{x\to1^+}\frac{(\ln x)'}{[(x-1)^2]'}=\lim_{x\to1^+}\frac{1/x}{2(x-1)}=\frac{1}{2x(x-1)}=+\infty.\qquad\#$$

Example 5.23　Find $\lim\limits_{x\to+\infty}\dfrac{\ln(1+e^{-x})}{e^{-x}}$.

Solution　Since $\lim\limits_{x\to+\infty}\ln(1+e^{-x})=0$ and $\lim\limits_{x\to+\infty}e^{-x}=0$, L'Hôspital's Rule applies:

$$\lim_{x\to+\infty}\frac{\ln(1+e^{-x})}{e^{-x}}\overset{\tfrac{0}{0}}{=\!=\!=}\lim_{x\to+\infty}\frac{[\ln(1+e^{-x})]'}{(e^{-x})'}$$

$$=\lim_{x\to+\infty}\frac{\dfrac{-e^{-x}}{1+e^{-x}}}{-e^{-x}}$$

$$=\lim_{x\to+\infty}\frac{1}{1+e^{-x}}=1.\qquad\#$$

5.5.2　L'Hôspital's Rule in Other Cases

We can also use L'Hôspital's Rule to evaluate limits of quotients $\dfrac{f(x)}{g(x)}$ in which $f(x)\to\pm\infty$ and $g(x)\to\pm\infty$. Limits of this form are classified as indeterminate forms of type $\dfrac{\infty}{\infty}$. Again, note that we are not actually dividing ∞ by ∞. Since ∞ is not a real number, that is impossible; rather, $\dfrac{\infty}{\infty}$ is used to represent a quotient of limits, each of which is $+\infty$ or $-\infty$.

> **Theorem 5. 10 (L'Hôspital's Rule of $\frac{\infty}{\infty}$ case)**
>
> *Suppose f and g are differentiable functions over an open interval containing c, except possibly at c. Suppose $\lim\limits_{x\to c} f(x) = +\infty\ (or\ -\infty)$ and $\lim\limits_{x\to c} g(x) = +\infty\ (or\ -\infty)$. Then*
>
> $$\lim_{x\to c}\frac{f(x)}{g(x)} = \lim_{x\to c}\frac{f'(x)}{g'(x)}.$$
>
> *Provided that the limit on the right exists or is $+\infty$ or $-\infty$. This result also holds if $c = +\infty$ or $c = -\infty$, or the limit is one-sided.*

Example 5. 24 Evaluate $\lim\limits_{x\to +\infty}\dfrac{\ln x}{x^2}$.

Solution Here $\lim\limits_{x\to +\infty}\ln x = +\infty$ and $\lim\limits_{x\to +\infty} x^2 = +\infty$. Therefore, we can apply L'Hôspital's Rule and obtain

$$\lim_{x\to +\infty}\frac{\ln x}{x^2}\overset{\frac{\infty}{\infty}}{=\!=\!=}\lim_{x\to +\infty}\frac{(\ln x)'}{(x^2)'} = \lim_{x\to +\infty}\frac{1/x}{2x} = \lim_{x\to +\infty}\frac{1}{2x^2} = 0. \qquad \#$$

Your Practice 5.11 Evaluate $\lim\limits_{x\to +\infty}\dfrac{e^{3x}}{x^3}$.

5.5.3 Other Indeterminate Forms

The expressions $0\cdot\infty$, $\infty - \infty$, 1^∞, ∞^0, and 0^∞ are all considered indeterminate forms. These expressions are not real numbers. Rather, they represent forms that arise when trying to evaluate certain limits. Next we realize why these are indeterminate forms and then understand how to use L'Hôspital's Rule in these cases. The key idea is that we must rewrite the indeterminate forms in such a way that we arrive at the indeterminate form $\dfrac{0}{0}$ or $\dfrac{\infty}{\infty}$.

Example 5. 25 Evaluate $\lim\limits_{x\to 0^+} x\ln x$.

Solution First, we rewrite the function $x\ln x$ as a quotient to apply L'Hôspital's Rule. If we write $x\ln x = \dfrac{\ln x}{1/x}$, we see that $\ln x \to -\infty$ and $\dfrac{1}{x}\to +\infty$ as $x\to 0^+$. Therefore, we can apply L'Hôspital's Rule and obtain

$$\lim_{x\to 0^+}\frac{\ln x}{1/x} = \lim_{x\to 0^+}\frac{(\ln x)'}{(1/x)'} = \lim_{x\to 0^+}\frac{1/x}{-1/x^2} = \lim_{x\to 0^+}(-x) = 0.$$

We conclude that

$$\lim_{x\to 0^+} x\ln x = 0. \qquad \#$$

Example 5. 26 Evaluate $\lim\limits_{x\to 0}(1+x)^{\frac{1}{x}}$.

Solution We use the natural logarithm function and its properties to reduce the problem to a related problem involving a limit of a quotient.

Let $y = (1+x)^{\frac{1}{x}}$, then

$$\ln y = \ln (1+x)^{\frac{1}{x}} = \frac{1}{x}\ln (1+x) = \frac{\ln (1+x)}{x}.$$

We need to evaluate $\lim\limits_{x \to 0} \dfrac{\ln (1+x)}{x}$. Applying L'Hôspital's Rule, we obtain

$$\lim_{x \to 0} \frac{\ln (1+x)}{x} = \lim_{x \to 0} \frac{[\ln(1+x)]'}{x'} = \lim_{x \to 0} \frac{1}{1+x} = 1.$$

Therefore, $\lim\limits_{x \to 0} \ln y = 1$. Since the natural logarithm function is continuous, we conclude that

$$\ln(\lim_{x \to 0} y) = 1,$$

which leads to

$$\lim_{x \to 0} y = e^1 = e.$$

Hence,

$$\lim_{x \to 0} (1+x)^{\frac{1}{x}} = e.$$

This procedure can be applied when evaluating limits involves exponents.   #

Your Practice 5.12   Evaluate $\lim\limits_{x \to 0} x^x$.

We have shown that

$$e = \lim_{x \to 0} (1+x)^{1/x}.$$

Make a table of values for small values of x, we get the value of e correct to seven decimal places,

$$e \approx 2.7182818.$$

Exercise 5.5

Find the limit.

1. $\lim\limits_{x \to 3} \dfrac{x^2 - 9}{x - 3}.$

2. $\lim\limits_{x \to 0^+} \dfrac{\sqrt{x+1} - 1}{x^3}.$

3. $\lim\limits_{x \to +\infty} \dfrac{e^x - 1}{x^3}.$

4. $\lim\limits_{x \to 0} \dfrac{e^{4x} - 1 - 4x}{x^2}.$

5. $\lim\limits_{x \to +\infty} \dfrac{\ln x}{x}.$

6. $\lim\limits_{x \to 0^+} \dfrac{x\ln x}{x^2 - 1}.$

7. $\lim\limits_{x \to 2} \dfrac{\ln (x-1)}{x-1}.$

8. $\lim\limits_{x \to 0} \dfrac{\ln (1+x^2)}{x^3}.$

9. $\lim\limits_{x \to -1} \dfrac{x^3 + x^2 - x - 1}{x^3 + 4x^2 + 5x + 2}.$

10. $\lim\limits_{x \to +\infty} \dfrac{3x^2 + x^2 - x - 1}{x^3 + 5x + 2}.$

11. $\lim\limits_{x \to +\infty} \dfrac{1 - x^2}{5x}.$

12. $\lim\limits_{x \to +\infty} \dfrac{1 - x^2}{5x^2}.$

13. $\lim\limits_{x \to +\infty} \dfrac{1 + x^2}{1 + e^x}.$

14. $\lim\limits_{x \to +\infty} \dfrac{e^{-x}}{\ln (1+4e^{-x})}.$

15. $\lim\limits_{x \to +\infty} x^2 \ln x.$

5.6 Periodicity and Trigonometric Functions

We encounter many periodic phenomena in our physical world. The London Eye (Figure 5.25) completes one rotation every 30 miniutes. When we look at the behavior of this Ferris wheel it is clear that it completes 1 cycle, or 1 revolution, and then repeats this revolution over and over again. This is an example of a periodic function, because the Ferris wheel repeats its revolution or one cycle every 30 miniutes, and so we say it has a period of 30 miniutes. In mathematics, a function is periodic if

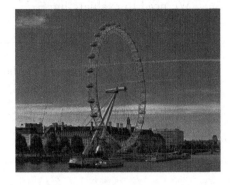

Figure 5.25

its function values repeats with respect to the independent variable. The periodicity of a function is no longer limited to time.

5.6.1 Definition of Periodic Function

> **Definition 5.4**
>
> A function is said to be periodic if there exists a positive real number T such that
> $$f(x+T)=f(x) \text{ for every } x \in D$$
> where D is the domain of the function $f(x)$.

The least positive real number T ($T>0$) is known as the **fundamental period** or simply the period of the function. The T is not a unique positive number. All integral multiple of T within the domain of the function is also the period of the function. Hence,
$$f(x+nT)=f(x); \; n \text{ is an integer, for every } x \in D.$$
Thus, the graph of periodic functions can be made by repeating a specific smallest part of the graph. In the context of periodic function, an "aperiodic" function is one, which is not periodic.

In order to determine periodicity and period of a function, we can follow the algorithm as:

(i) Put $f(x+T)=f(x)$.

(ii) If there exists a positive number T satisfying equation in (i) and it is independent of x, then $f(x)$ is periodic. Otherwise, function $f(x)$ is aperiodic. The least value of T is the period of the periodic function.

Example 5.27 Let $f(x)$ be a function and k be a positive real number such that
$$f(x+k)+f(x)=0 \text{ for every } x \in \mathbf{R}.$$
Prove that $f(x)$ is periodic and determine its period.

Proof The given equation can be rewritten as
$$f(x+k)=-f(x) \text{ for every } x \in \mathbf{R}.$$
Here, our objective is to convert its right-hand side as $f(x)$. For this, replacing "x" by

"$x+k$", we have

$$f(x+2k)=-f(x+k) \text{ for every } x \in \mathbf{R}.$$

Combining two equations, we get

$$f(x+2k)=-f(x+k)=-[-f(x)]=f(x) \text{ for every } x \in \mathbf{R}.$$

It means that $f(x)$ is a periodic function and its period is $2k$.   #

Example 5.28   The function f has a period of 3. Figure 5.26 represents part of its graph. What would the graph look like for the interval $[-8,8]$?

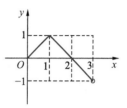

Solution   This graph covers an interval of 3 units. Because the period is given as 3, this graph represents one complete cycle of the function. Therefore, simply replicate the graph segment to the left and to the right (Figure 5.27).   #

Figure 5.26

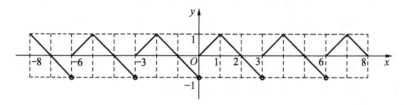

Figure 5.27

5.6.2　Trigonometric Functions

5.6.2.1　Angle

An angle is a measure of rotation. Angles can be measured in one of two units: degrees or radians. The relationship between these two measures may be expressed as follows: One complete rotation is measured as $360°$ in degrees or 2π in radians. Angle measure can be positive or negative, depending on the direction of rotation. Angle measure is the amount of rotation between the two rays forming the angle. Rotation is measured from the initial side to the terminal side of the angle. Positive angles (Figures 5.28(a) and (c)) result from counterclockwise rotation, and negative angles (Figures 5.28(b) and (d)) result from clockwise rotation. An angle with its initial side on the x-axis is said to be in standard position.

Angles that are in standard position are said to be quadrantal if their terminal side coincides with a coordinate axis. Angles in standard position that are not quadrantal fall in one of the four quadrants, as shown in Figure 5.28.

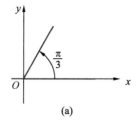

(a)

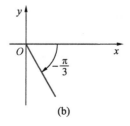

(b)

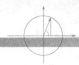

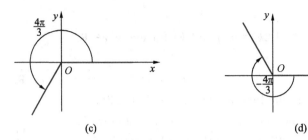

Figure 5. 28

5.6.2.2   Functions of acute angles

The characteristics of similar triangles, originally formulated by Euclid, are the building blocks of trigonometry. Euclid's theorems state if two angles of one triangle have the same measure as two angles of another triangle, then the two triangles are similar. Also, in similar triangles, angle measure and ratios of corresponding sides are preserved. Because all right triangles contain a 90° angle, all right triangles that contain another angle of equal measure must be similar. Therefore, the ratio of the corresponding sides of these triangles must be equal in value. These relationships lead to the trigonometric ratios.

The following ratios are defined using a circle $x^2 + y^2 = r^2$ and refer to Figure 5. 29:

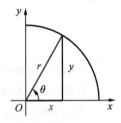

$$\text{sine of } \theta = \sin \theta = \frac{y}{r} = \frac{\text{length of side opposite } \theta}{\text{length of hypotenuse}}$$

$$\text{cosine of } \theta = \cos \theta = \frac{x}{r} = \frac{\text{length of side adjacent to } \theta}{\text{length of hypotenuse}}$$

$$\text{tangent of } \theta = \tan \theta = \frac{y}{x} = \frac{\text{length of side opposite } \theta}{\text{length of side adjacent to } \theta}.$$

Figure 5. 29

The cosecant, secant, and cotangent are trigonometric functions that are the reciprocals of the sine, cosine, and tangent, respectively:

$$\text{cosecant of } \theta = \csc \theta = \frac{r}{y} = \frac{\text{length of hypotenuse}}{\text{length of side opposite } \theta}$$

$$\text{secant of } \theta = \sec \theta = \frac{r}{x} = \frac{\text{length of hypotenuse}}{\text{length of side adjacent to } \theta}$$

$$\text{cotangent of } \theta = \cot \theta = \frac{x}{y} = \frac{\text{length of side adjacent to } \theta}{\text{length of side opposite } \theta}.$$

If trigonometric ratios of angle θ are combined in an equation and the equation is valid for all values of θ, then the equation is known as a trigonometric identity. Using the trigonometric ratios shown in the preceding equation, the following trigonometric identities can be constructed:

$$\frac{\sin \theta}{\cos \theta} = \tan \theta,$$

$$\frac{\cos \theta}{\sin \theta} = \cot \theta,$$

$$\sin^2 \theta + \cos^2 \theta = 1.$$

Example 5.29   Find $\sin \theta$ and $\tan \theta$ if θ is an acute angle ($0 \leqslant \theta \leqslant \pi$) and $\cos \theta = \dfrac{\sqrt{3}}{2}$.

Solution   Using $\sin^2 \theta + \cos^2 \theta = 1$ we get

$$\sin^2 \theta + \left(\frac{\sqrt{3}}{2} \right)^2 = 1.$$

Thus

$$\sin^2 \theta = 1 - \left(\frac{\sqrt{3}}{2} \right)^2 = 1 - \frac{3}{4} = \frac{1}{4}.$$

Because θ is an acute angle,

$$\sin \theta = \sqrt{\frac{1}{4}} = \frac{1}{2}.$$

Then

$$\tan \theta = \frac{\sin \theta}{\cos \theta} = \frac{\dfrac{1}{2}}{\dfrac{\sqrt{3}}{2}} = \frac{1}{\sqrt{3}} = \frac{\sqrt{3}}{3}. \qquad \#$$

Your Practice 5.13   Find $\sin \theta$ and $\tan \theta$ if θ is an acute angle ($0 \leqslant \theta \leqslant \pi$) and $\cos \theta = \dfrac{1}{4}$.

5.6.2.3   Trigonometric functions

Remember, if the angles of a triangle remain the same, but the sides increase or decrease in length proportionally, these ratios remain the same. Therefore, trigonometric ratios in right triangles are dependent only on the size of the angles, not on the lengths of the sides. Now we use the unite circle and let the angle be x, then the length of hypotenuse (Figure 5.30(a)) is the sine function $y = \sin x$. For each angle, we use the y-value of the point on the circle to determine the output value of the sine function (Figure 5.30(b)).

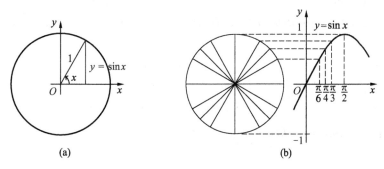

(a)   (b)

Figure 5.30

Since the point on the circle repeat itself every full rotation, the sine function has period 2π. Plotting more points gives the full shape of the sine functions as shown in Figure 5.31.

Like the sine function we can track the value of the cosine function through the 4 quadrants of the unit circle as we place it on a graph (Figure 5.31).

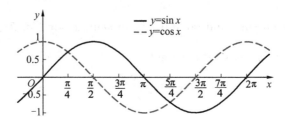

Figure 5. 31

Both of these functions are defined on a domain of all real numbers, since we can evaluate the sine and cosine of any angle. By thinking of sine and cosine as points on a unit circle, it becomes clear that the range of both functions must be the interval $[-1, 1]$.

Both graphs are considered sinusoidal graphs. Sinusoidal functions are a specific type of periodic function.

In both graphs, the shape of the graph begins repeating after 2π. In other words, if you were to shift either graph horizontally by 2π, the resulting shape would be identical to the original function.

The sine function is continuous everywhere, as we see in the graph above, therefore, $\lim\limits_{x\to c} \sin x = \sin c$.

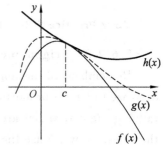

5.6.2.4   The Squeeze Theorem

The Squeeze Theorem proved very useful for establishing basic trigonometric limits. This theorem allows us to calculate limits by "squeezing" a function, with a limit at point c that is unknown, between two functions having a common known limit at c. Figure 5. 32 illustrates this idea.

Figure 5. 32

the Squeeze Theorem

Let $f(x)$, $g(x)$, and $h(x)$ be defined for every $x \neq c$ over an open interval containing c. If

$$f(x) \leqslant g(x) \leqslant h(x)$$

for every $x \neq c$ in an open interval containing c and

$$\lim_{x\to c} f(x) = L = \lim_{x\to c} h(x)$$

where L is a real number, then $\lim\limits_{x\to c} g(x) = L$.

Example 5.30   Apply the Squeeze Theorem to evaluate $\lim\limits_{x\to 0} x\cos x$.

Solution   Because $-1 \leqslant \cos x \leqslant 1$ for every x, we have $-x \leqslant x \cdot \cos x \leqslant x$ for $x \geqslant 0$ and $x \leqslant x \cdot \cos x \leqslant -x$ for $x \leqslant 0$ (if x is negative the direction of the inequalities changes when we multiply). Since

$$\lim_{x\to 0} (-x) = 0 = \lim_{x\to 0} x,$$

from the Squeeze Theorem, we obtain

$$\lim_{x \to 0} x \cos x = 0.$$

The graphs of $f(x) = -x$, $g(x) = x \cos x$, and $h(x) = x$ are shown in Figure 5.33.   #

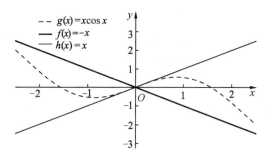

Figure 5.33

Your Practice 5.14   Use the Squeeze Theorem to evaluate $\lim\limits_{x \to 0} x^2 \cos \dfrac{1}{x}$.

5.6.2.5 Limits of two trigonometric functions

We now use the Squeeze Theorem to tackle several very important limits. Although this discussion is somewhat lengthy, these limits prove invaluable for the development of the derivative of the trigonometric functions.

Theorem 5.11

$$\lim_{x \to 0} \frac{\sin x}{x} = 1.$$

Proof   We begin by considering the unit circle (Figure 5.34). Each point B on the unit circle has coordinates $(\cos x, \sin x)$ for some angle x. Using similar triangles, we can extend the line from the origin through the point to point $C(1, \tan x)$. (Here we are assuming that $0 \leqslant x \leqslant \dfrac{\pi}{2}$. Later we will show that we can also consider negative x) The figure shows three regions have been constructed in the first quadrant, two triangles and a sector of a circle. We can find:

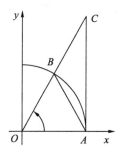

Figure 5.34

area of triangle $AOB <$ area of sector $AOB <$ area of triangle AOC.

The area of the triangle OAC is $\dfrac{1}{2} \tan x$; the area of the sector is $\dfrac{1}{2} x$; the area of the triangle OAB is $\dfrac{1}{2} \sin x$. It is then clear that

$$\frac{1}{2} \sin x < \frac{1}{2} x < \frac{1}{2} \tan x.$$

Divide all terms by $\dfrac{1}{2} \sin x$ giving

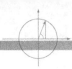

$$1 < \frac{x}{\sin x} < \frac{1}{\cos x}.$$

Taking reciprocals reverses the inequalities, giving

$$\cos x < \frac{\sin x}{x} < 1.$$

(These inequalities hold for all values of x near 0, even negative values, since $\cos(-x) = \cos x$ and $\sin(-x) = -\sin x$)

Now as $x \to 0$ then $\cos x \to 1$.

So $\frac{\sin x}{x}$ lies between 1 and something that is tending towards 1. So as $x \to 0$ then $\frac{\sin x}{x} \to 1$, and

$$\lim_{x \to 0} \frac{\sin x}{x} = 1. \qquad\qquad \#$$

Theorem 5.12

$$\lim_{x \to 0} \frac{1 - \cos x}{x} = 0.$$

Proof When we multiply top and bottom by $1 + \cos x$ we get:

$$\frac{1 - \cos x}{x} \frac{1 + \cos x}{1 + \cos x} = \frac{1 - \cos^2 x}{x(1 + \cos x)}.$$

Using the trigonometric identity $\cos^2 x + \sin^2 x = 1$, we can rewrite this as

$$\frac{\sin^2 x}{x(1 + \cos x)}.$$

And the limit we started with become

$$\lim_{x \to 0} \frac{\sin^2 x}{x(1 + \cos x)}.$$

Rearranged to this form:

$$\lim_{x \to 0} \frac{\sin x}{x} \cdot \frac{\sin x}{1 + \cos x}.$$

We know the first limit $\lim_{x \to 0} \frac{\sin x}{x} = 1$, and the second limit does not need much work because at $x = 0$ we know directly that $\frac{\sin 0}{1 + \cos 0} = 0$, so

$$\lim_{x \to 0} \frac{\sin x}{x} \cdot \frac{\sin x}{1 + \cos x} = \lim_{x \to 0} \frac{\sin x}{x} \cdot \lim_{x \to 0} \frac{\sin x}{1 + \cos x} = 1 \times 0 = 0. \qquad \#$$

Example 5.31 Find

$$\lim_{x \to 0} \sin \frac{\pi}{x}.$$

Solution The graph of $y = \sin \frac{\pi}{x}$ is shown in Figure 5.35. The values of $f(x)$ oscillate often between -1 and 1 as $x \to 0$. We can see why as follows: As $x \to 0^+$, the argument in the sine function goes to positive infinity; likewise, as $x \to 0^-$, the argument in the function goes to negative infinity.

$$\lim_{x \to 0^+} \frac{\pi}{x} = +\infty \text{ and } \lim_{x \to 0^-} \frac{\pi}{x} = -\infty.$$

Since the sine function oscillates between -1 and

1, we see that $\sin \dfrac{\pi}{x}$ oscillates between -1 and 1 as $x \to$

0. This function is called an oscillation function. We

conclude that $\lim\limits_{x \to 0} \sin \dfrac{\pi}{x}$ does not exist.　　　　#

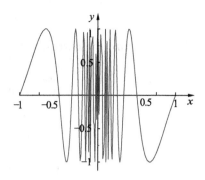

5.6.2.6   Derivative of sin x and cos x

Figure 5.35

Theorem 5.13

The function sin x *and* cos x *are differentiable for every* x, *and*

$$\frac{d}{dx} \sin x = \cos x \text{ and } \frac{d}{dx} \cos x = -\sin x.$$

Proof   We prove the first formula; the second one can be proved in a similar way. We need the trigonometric identity

$$\sin(A+B) = \sin A \cos B + \cos A \sin B.$$

Using the formal definition of derivatives, we find

$$\frac{d}{dx} \sin x = \lim_{h \to 0} \frac{\sin(x+h) - \sin x}{h}$$

$$= \lim_{h \to 0} \frac{\sin x \cos h + \cos x \sin h - \sin x}{h}.$$

Regroup:

$$\lim_{h \to 0} \left(\sin x \frac{\cos h - 1}{h} + \cos x \frac{\sin h}{h} \right).$$

Split it into two limits:

$$\lim_{h \to 0} \left(\sin x \frac{\cos h - 1}{h} \right) + \lim_{h \to 0} \left(\cos x \frac{\sin h}{h} \right).$$

And we can bring sin x and cos x outside the limits because they are functions of x not h,

$$\sin x \lim_{h \to 0} \frac{\cos h - 1}{h} + \cos x \lim_{h \to 0} \frac{\sin h}{h}.$$

We showed in previous subsection that

$$\lim_{h \to 0} \frac{\cos h - 1}{h} = 0 \text{ and } \lim_{h \to 0} \frac{\sin h}{h} = 1.$$

Therefore,

$$\frac{d}{dx} \sin x = \sin x \lim_{h \to 0} \frac{\cos h - 1}{h} + \cos x \lim_{h \to 0} \frac{\sin h}{h} = \sin x \cdot 0 + \cos x \cdot 1 = \cos x. \qquad \#$$

The derivatives of the other trigonometric functions can be found using the following identities:

$$\tan x = \frac{\sin x}{\cos x}, \ \cot x = -\frac{\cos x}{\sin x},$$

$$\sec x = \frac{1}{\cos x}, \quad \csc x = -\frac{1}{\sin x}.$$

We summarize the derivatives of all trigonometric functions in the following box.

$$\frac{\mathrm{d}}{\mathrm{d}x}\sin x = \cos x, \quad \frac{\mathrm{d}}{\mathrm{d}x}\cos x = -\sin x,$$

$$\frac{\mathrm{d}}{\mathrm{d}x}\tan x = \sec^2 x, \quad \frac{\mathrm{d}}{\mathrm{d}x}\cot x = -\csc^2 x,$$

$$\frac{\mathrm{d}}{\mathrm{d}x}\sec x = \sec x \tan x, \quad \frac{\mathrm{d}}{\mathrm{d}x}\csc x = -\csc x \cot x.$$

Exercise 5.6

1. Find all values of θ such that $\sin \theta = 1$; give your answer in radians.

2. Use an angle sum identity to compute $\cos \frac{\pi}{12}$.

3. Verify the identity $\frac{\cos \theta}{1-\sin \theta} = 1 + \sin \theta$.

4. Verify the identity $2\csc 2t = \sec t\csc t$.

5. Verify the identity $\sin 3t\sin t = 2\cos 2t\sin t$.

6. Sketch $y = 2\sin x$.

7. Sketch $y = \sin 2x$.

8. Sketch $y = \sin(-x)$.

9. Find all of the solutions of $2\sin t - 1 - \sin^2 t = 0$ in the interval $[0, 2\pi]$.

10. Differentiate $\sin^2 \sqrt{x}$.

11. Differentiate $\sin x \sqrt{x}$.

12. Differentiate $\frac{1}{\sin x}$.

13. Differentiate $\frac{x^2+x}{\sin x}$.

14. Differentiate $\sqrt{1-\sin^2 x}$.

15. Compute $\lim\limits_{x \to 0} \frac{\sin 3x}{x}$.

16. Compute $\lim\limits_{x \to 0} \frac{\sin 5x}{\sin 3x}$.

17. Compute $\lim\limits_{x \to 0} \frac{\tan x}{x}$.

18. Compute $\lim\limits_{x \to 0} \frac{\csc 3x}{\cot 4x}$.

19. Compute $\lim\limits_{x \to \frac{\pi}{4}} \frac{\sin x - \cos x}{\cos 2x}$.

20. For every $x \geqslant 0$, $4x-5 \leqslant f(x) \leqslant x^2-4x+7$. Find $\lim\limits_{x \to 2} f(x)$.

21. For every x, $2x \leqslant f(x) \leqslant x^2-2x+3$. Find $\lim\limits_{x \to 3} f(x)$.

22. Use the Squeeze Theorem to show that $\lim\limits_{x \to 0} x^4 \cos \frac{2}{x} = 0$.

5.7   Graphing of Functions

It is useful to know what the graph of the function looks like whether we are interested in a function as a purely mathematical object or in connection with some application to the real world. To obtain a good picture of the graph, certain crucial information should be considered: domain, range, symmetry, asymptotes, intervals of increase and decrease, concavity, points of inflection, etc. We can put all of this information together to sketch graphs that reveal the important features of functions.

Guidelines for sketching curves

The following steps are taken in the process of curve sketching. Not every step is relevant to every function. For instance, a given curve might not possess symmetry or have an asymptote.

1. **Domain**   Start by finding the domain D of the function f, and determine the points of discontinuity (if any).

2. **Intercepts**   Determine the x-intercepts and y-intercepts of the function, if possible. To find the x-intercept, we let $y=0$ and solve the equation for x. Similarly, we let $x=0$ to find the y-intercept.

3. **Symmetry**   Determine whether the function is even, odd, or neither, and check the periodicity of the function. If $f(-x)=f(x)$ for every x in the domain, then $f(x)$ is even and symmetric about the y-axis. If $f(-x)=-f(x)$ for every x in the domain, then $f(x)$ is odd and symmetric about the origin.

4. **Asymptotes**   Find the vertical and horizontal asymptotes of the function. Some functions have slant asymptotes.

5. **Intervals of Increase and Decrease**   Calculate the first derivative $f'(x)$ and find the critical points of the function. Determine the intervals where the function is increasing and decreasing using the First Derivative Test.

6. **Local Maximum and Minimum**   Use the First or the Second Derivative Test to classify the critical points as local maximum or local minimum. Calculate the y-values of the local extrema points.

7. **Concavity/Convexity and Points of Inflection**   Using the Second Derivative Test, find the points of inflection. Determine the intervals where the function is convex upward and convex downward.

8. **Graph of the Function**   Sketch a graph of $f(x)$ using all the information obtained above.

Example 5.32   Sketch the graph of $f(x)=\dfrac{x}{x+1}$.

Solution

(1) $f(x)$ is not defined at $x=-1$.

(2) There is a y-intercept $f(0)=0$. Solving the equation $\dfrac{x}{x+1}=0$ we get the x-intercept 0.

(3) No symmetry.

(4) When $x=-1$, the denominator is zero while the numerator is nonzero. We have $\lim\limits_{x\to-1}f(x)=\infty$ so the graph has a vertical asymptote $x=-1$. We also have $\lim\limits_{x\to+\infty}f(x)=1$

so the graph has a horizontal asymptote $y=1$.

(5) $f'(x)=\dfrac{1}{(x+1)^2}$ and $f''(x)=\dfrac{-2}{(x+1)^3}$ are nonzero. There are neither critical points nor inflection points. The domain consists of two regions separated by $x=-1$. We determine the sign of $f'(x)$ and $f''(x)$ by Table 5.7:

Table 5.7

x	$(-\infty,-1)$	$(-1,+\infty)$
$f'(x)$	$+$	$+$
$f''(x)$	$+$	$-$
$f(x)$	⌡	⌐

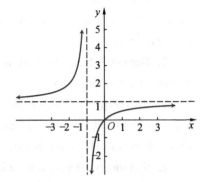

Figure 5.36

(6) We finish the sketch in Figure 5.36.　　#

Your Practice 5.15　Sketch the graph of $f(x)=\dfrac{2x+4}{x-1}$.

Example 5.33　Sketch the graph of $f(x)=e^{-x^2/2}$.

Solution

(1) The domain is **R**.

(2) The y-intercept is $f(0)=1$. There are no x-intercepts.

(3) f is even.

(4) $\lim\limits_{x\to+\infty} f(x)=0$ so the graph has a horizontal asymptote $y=0$.

(5) $f'(x)=-xe^{-x^2/2}$. We have a critical number $x=0$.

(6) $f''(x)=(-1)e^{-x^2/2}+(-x)(-x)e^{-x^2/2}=(x^2-1)e^{-x^2/2}$. Let $f''(x)=0$ we get $x=-1$ and $x=1$.

We determine the sign of $f'(x)$ and $f''(x)$ by Table 5.8:

Table 5.8

x	$(-\infty,-1)$	-1	$(-1,0)$	0	$(0,1)$	1	$(1,+\infty)$
$f'(x)$	$+$		$+$		$-$		$-$
$f''(x)$	$+$		$-$		$-$		$+$
$f(x)$	⌡	inflex	⌐	max	⌐	inflex	⌐

(7) Using this information, we sketch the curve in Figure 5.37.　　#

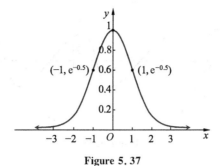

Figure 5.37

Example 5.34　Sketch the graph of $f(x)=\dfrac{\cos x}{2+\sin x}$.

Solution

(1) The domain is **R**.

(2) The y-intercept is $f(0)=\dfrac{1}{2}$. The x-intercepts occur when $\cos x=0$, that is, $x=\dfrac{(2k+1)\pi}{2}$, where k is an integer.

(3) f is neither even nor odd, but $f(x)$ is periodic and has period 2π because $f(x+2\pi)=f(x)$. Thus, in what follows, we need to consider only $0\leqslant x\leqslant 2\pi$ and then extend the curve by translation.

(4) Asymptotes: None.

(5) We get

$$f'(x)=\frac{(2+\sin x)(-\sin x)-\cos x\cos x}{(2+\sin x)^2}=-\frac{2\sin x+1}{(2+\sin x)^2}.$$

Let $f'(x)=0$, we obtain $x=\dfrac{7\pi}{6}$ and $x=\dfrac{11\pi}{6}$.

6. We get

$$f''(x)=-\frac{2\cos x(1-\sin x)}{(2+\sin x)^3}.$$

Let $f''=0$, we obtain $x=\dfrac{\pi}{2}$ and $x=\dfrac{3\pi}{2}$.

(7) Make Table 5.9:

Table 5.9

x	$\left(0,\dfrac{\pi}{2}\right)$	$\dfrac{\pi}{2}$	$\left(\dfrac{\pi}{2},\dfrac{7\pi}{6}\right)$	$\dfrac{7\pi}{6}$	$\left(\dfrac{7\pi}{6},\dfrac{3\pi}{2}\right)$	$\dfrac{3\pi}{2}$	$\left(\dfrac{3\pi}{2},\dfrac{11\pi}{6}\right)$	$\dfrac{11\pi}{6}$	$\left(\dfrac{11\pi}{6},2\pi\right)$
$f'(x)$	$-$		$-$		$+$		$+$		$-$
$f''(x)$	$+$		$-$		$-$		$+$		
$f(x)$	↘	inflex	⌣	min	↗	inflex	⌢	max	↘

(8) The graph of the function restricted to is shown in Figure 5.38(a). Then we extend it, using periodicity, to the complete graph in Figure 5.38(b). #

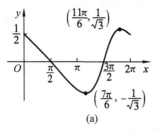

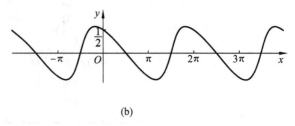

(a) (b)

Figure 5. 38

Exercise 5.7

1. Use the guidelines of this section to sketch the curve.

(1) $f(x)=\dfrac{2x^2+5}{4-x^2}$;

(2) $f(x)=x^3$;

(3) $f(x)=x^2-2x-3$;

(4) $f(x)=x^3+3x^2-9x+6$;

(5) $f(x)=x\sqrt{x+1}$;

(6) $f(x)=x^{2/3}$;

(7) $f(x)=\dfrac{x^3}{3}-4x$;

(8) $f(x)=3\sin x-\sin^3 x$;

(9) $f(x)=\dfrac{\sin x}{1+\cos x}$.

Some curves have asymptotes that are oblique, that is, neither horizontal nor vertical. If

$$\lim_{x\to+\infty}\ [f(x)-(mx+b)]=0,$$

then the line $y=mx+b$ is called a **slant asymptote** because the vertical distance between the curve $y=f(x)$ and the line $y=mx+b$ approaches 0, as in Figure 5. 39. (A similar situation exists if we let $x\to-\infty$)

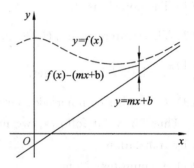

Figure 5. 39

2. Find an equation of the slant asymptote without sketching the curve.

(1) $f(x)=\dfrac{x^3+1}{x^2+2}$;

(2) $f(x)=\dfrac{2x^3+x^2+x+1}{x^2+3x}$.

3. Show that the curve $y=\sqrt{x^2+4x}$ has two slant asymptotes: $y=-x-2$ and $y=x+2$. Use this fact to help sketch the curve.

4. Let $f(x)=\dfrac{x^3+1}{x}$. Show that

$$\lim_{x\to\pm\infty}\ [f(x)-x^2]=0.$$

This shows that the graph of f approaches the graph of $y=x^2$, and we say that the curve is asymptotic to the parabola $y=x^2$. Use this fact to help sketch the graph of f.

Summary and Review

Key Concepts

- A function may have both an absolute maximum and an absolute minimum, or have just one absolute extremum, or have no absolute maximum or absolute minimum.

- If a function has a local extremum, the point at which it occurs must be a critical point. However, a function need not have a local extremum at a critical point.

- If $f'(x) > 0$ over an interval I, then f is increasing over I. If $f'(x) < 0$ over I, then f is decreasing over I. If $f'(x) = 0$ over I, then f is constant over I.

- If c is a critical point of f and $f'(x) > 0$ for $x < c$ and $f'(x) < 0$ for $x > c$, then f has a local maximum at c.

  If c is a critical point of f and $f'(x) < 0$ for $x < c$ and $f'(x) > 0$ for $x > c$, then f has a local minimum at c.

- If $f''(x) > 0$ over an interval I, then f is concave up over I.

  If $f''(x) < 0$ over an interval I, then f is concave down over I.

- If $f'(c) = 0$ and $f''(c) > 0$, then f has a local minimum at c.

  If $f'(c) = 0$ and $f''(c) < 0$, then f has a local maximum at c.

- L'Hôpital's Rule can be used to evaluate the limit of a quotient when the indeterminate form $\dfrac{0}{0}$ or $\dfrac{\infty}{\infty}$ arises.

  L'Hôpital's Rule can also be applied to other indeterminate forms if they can be rewritten in terms of a limit involving a quotient that has the indeterminate form $\dfrac{0}{0}$ or $\dfrac{\infty}{\infty}$.

- To solve an optimization problem, begin by drawing a picture and introducing variables. Find an equation relating the variables. Find a function of one variable to describe the quantity that is to be minimized or maximized. Look for critical points to locate local extrema.

- If $f(x + T) = f(x)$ holds true for every x in the domain of the function $f(x)$, then f is said to be periodic and T is its period.

Key Equations

- $\lim\limits_{x \to 0} \dfrac{\sin x}{x} = 1$.

- $(\sin x)' = \cos x$, $(\cos x)' = -\sin x$.

Important Theorems

- The Squeeze Theorem: If $f(x) \leqslant g(x) \leqslant h(x)$ for all $x \neq c$ and $\lim\limits_{x \to c} f(x) = L = \lim\limits_{x \to c} h(x)$, then $\lim\limits_{x \to c} g(x) = L$, where L is a real number.

- Rolle's Theorem: If f is continuous over $[a, b]$ and differentiable in (a, b) and $f(a) = f(b)$, then there exists a point $c \in (a, b)$ such that $f'(c) = 0$.

- Mean Value Theorem: If f is continuous over $[a, b]$ and differentiable in (a, b), then there exists a point $c \in (a, b)$ such that $f'(c) = \dfrac{f(b) - f(a)}{b - a}$.

- L'Hôspital's Rule: If f and g are differentiable functions over an interval c, except possibly at c, and $\lim\limits_{x \to c} f(x) = \lim\limits_{x \to c} g(x) = 0$ or $\lim\limits_{x \to c} f(x)$ and $\lim\limits_{x \to c} g(x)$ are infinite, then $\lim\limits_{x \to c} \dfrac{f(x)}{g(x)} = \lim\limits_{x \to c} \dfrac{f'(x)}{g'(x)}$, assuming the limit on the right exists or is ∞.

Glossary

- Absolute extremum. If f has an absolute maximum or absolute minimum at c, we say f has an absolute extremum at c.

- Absolute maximum. If $f(c) \geqslant f(x)$ for every x in the domain of f, we say f has an absolute maximum at c.

- Absolute minimum. If $f(c) \leqslant f(x)$ for every x in the domain of f, we say f has an absolute minimum at c.

- Critical point. If $f'(c) = 0$ or $f'(c)$ is undefined, we say that c is a critical point of f.

- Fermat's Theorem. If f has a local extremum at c, then c is a critical point of f.

- Local extremum. If f has a local maximum or local minimum at c, we say f has a local extremum at c.

- Local maximum. If there exists an interval I such that $f(c) \geqslant f(x)$ for every $x \in I$, we say f has a local maximum at c.

- Local minimum. If there exists an interval I such that $f(c) \leqslant f(x)$ for every $x \in I$, we say f has a local minimum at c.

- Concave down. If f is differentiable over an interval I and f' is decreasing over I, then f is concave down over I.

- Concave up. If f is differentiable over an interval I and f' is increasing over I, then f is concave up over I.

- Concavity. The upward or downward curve of the graph of a function.

- Concavity test. Suppose f is twice differentiable over an interval I. If $f'' > 0$ over I, then f is concave up over I; if $f'' < 0$ over I, then f is concave down over I.

- The First Derivative Test. Let f be a continuous function over an interval I containing a critical point c such that f is differentiable over I except possibly at c; if f' changes sign from positive to negative as x increases through c, then f has a local maximum at c; if f' changes sign from negative to positive as x increases through c, then f has a local minimum at c; if f' does not change sign as x increases through c, then f does not have a local extremum at c.

- Inflection point. If f is continuous at c and f changes concavity at c, the point $(c, f(c))$ is an inflection point of f.

- The Second Derivative Test. Suppose $f'(c) = 0$ and f'' is continuous over an interval containing c. If $f'' > 0$, then f has a local minimum at c; if $f'' < 0$, then f

has a local maximum at c. If $f''=0$, then the test is inconclusive.

- Indeterminate forms. When evaluating a limit, the forms $\dfrac{0}{0}$, $\dfrac{\infty}{\infty}$, $0 \cdot \infty$, $\infty - \infty$, 0^∞, ∞^0 and 1^∞ are considered indeterminate because further analysis is required to determine whether the limit exists and, if so, what its value is.

- Optimization problems. Problems that are solved by finding the maximum or minimum of a function.

Chapter 6   Integration

6.1   Antiderivatives and Indefinite Integrals

6.1.1   Antiderivatives

In the past two chapters we have been given a function, $f(x)$, and asked what the derivative of this function was. We have seen how to calculate derivatives of many functions and have been introduced to a variety of their applications. Starting with this section we are going to turn this process around.

We now want to ask what function we differentiated to get the function $f(x)$, and why would we be interested in such a function?

Example 6.1   What function did we differentiate to get the function $f(x) = x^3 - 3x^2 + 5$?

Solution   Let us actually start by getting the derivative of this function to help us see how to approach this problem. The derivative of this function is

$$f(x) = x^3 - 3x^2 + 5.$$

The point of this was to remind us of how differentiation works. When differentiating powers of x, we multiply the term by the original exponent and then drop the exponent by one. Now, let us go back and work the problem. We got x^3 by differentiating a function and since we drop the exponent by one it looks like we must have differentiated x^4. However, if we had differentiated x^4 we would have $4x^3$ and we don't have a 4 in front of the first term, so the 4 needs to cancel out after we've differentiated. Then it looks like we would have to differentiate $\frac{1}{4}x^4$ in order to get x^3. Likewise, for the second term, in order to get $-3x^2$ after differentiating we would have to differentiate $-x^3$. The third term is just a constant and we know that if we differentiate x we get 1. So, it looks like we had to differentiate $5x$ to get the last term.

Putting all of this together gives the following function,

$$F(x) = \frac{1}{4}x^4 - x^3 + 5x.$$

Our answer is easy enough to check. Simply differentiate

$$F'(x) = x^3 - 3x^2 + 5 = f(x).$$

So, it looks like we got the correct function. Or did we? We know that the derivative of a constant is zero and so any of the following will also give $f(x)$ upon differentiating:

$$F(x) = \frac{1}{4}x^4 - x^3 + 5x + 6;$$

$$F(x) = \frac{1}{4}x^4 - x^3 + 5x - \frac{1}{8};$$

$$F(x) = \frac{1}{4}x^4 - x^3 + 5x - \pi;$$

$$\cdots\cdots$$

In fact, any function of the form,

$$F(x) = \frac{1}{4}x^4 - x^3 + 5x + C \ (C \text{ is a constant})$$

will give $f(x)$ upon differentiating.   #

　　There were two points to this example. The first point was to get you thinking about how to solve these problems. First of all, it is important to remember that we are actually only asking what we differentiated to get the given function. Another point is to realize that there are in fact an unlimited number of functions, and each of them will differ by a constant.

　　This example suggests that in order to find the solutions, we reverse the process of differentiation. We begin with a definition.

Definition 6. 1 (Antiderivative)

　　A function F is an antiderivative of the function f if
$$F'(x) = f(x)$$
for all x in the domain of f.

　　If $F(x)$ is an antiderivative of $f(x)$, then any function in the form $F(x) + C$ is also an antiderivative. Are there any others that are not of the form? The answer is "No". From the Mean Value Theorem, we know that if F and G are differentiable functions such that $F'(x) = G'(x)$, then $F(x) - G(x) = C$ for some constant C. This fact leads to the following important theorem.

Theorem 6. 1 (General Form of an Antiderivative)

　　Let F be an antiderivative of f over an interval I. Then,

　　(1) for each constant C, the function $F(x) + C$ is also an antiderivative of f over I;

　　(2) if G is an antiderivative of f over I, there is a constant C for which $G(x) = F(x) + C$ over I.

　　In other words, the most general antiderivative of f over I is $F(x) + C$.

We use Theorem 6.1 and our knowledge of derivatives to find all the antiderivatives for several functions.

Example 6.2 For each of the following functions, find all antiderivatives.

(1) $f(x)=x^2$;

(2) $f(x)=e^x$;

(3) $f(x)=\dfrac{1}{x}$;

(4) $f(x)=\cos x$.

Solution

(1) Because

$$\frac{\mathrm{d}}{\mathrm{d}x}\frac{x^3}{3}=x^2,$$

then $F(x)=\dfrac{x^3}{3}$ is an antiderivative of x^2. Therefore,

every antiderivative of x^2 is of the form $\dfrac{x^3}{3}+C$ for

some constant C, and every function of the form $\dfrac{x^3}{3}+$

C is an antiderivative of x^2. Figure 6.1 shows some of

the antiderivatives.

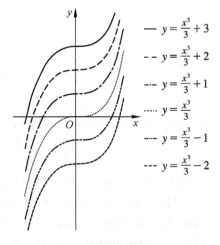

$$— y=\frac{x^3}{3}+3$$
$$-- y=\frac{x^3}{3}+2$$
$$--- y=\frac{x^3}{3}+1$$
$$\cdots y=\frac{x^3}{3}$$
$$--- y=\frac{x^3}{3}-1$$
$$--- y=\frac{x^3}{3}-2$$

Figure 6.1

(2) Since

$$\frac{\mathrm{d}}{\mathrm{d}x}e^x=e^x,$$

then $F(x)=e^x$ is an antiderivative of e^x. Therefore, every antiderivative of e^x is of the form e^x+C for some constant C and every function of the form e^x+C is an antiderivative of e^x.

(3) Let $f(x)=\ln|x|$. For $x>0$, $f(x)=\ln(x)$ and

$$\frac{\mathrm{d}}{\mathrm{d}x}\ln x=\frac{1}{x}.$$

For $x<0$, $f(x)=\ln(-x)$ and

$$\frac{\mathrm{d}}{\mathrm{d}x}\ln(-x)=\frac{-1}{-x}=\frac{1}{x}.$$

Therefore,

$$\frac{\mathrm{d}}{\mathrm{d}x}\ln|x|=\frac{1}{x}.$$

Thus, $F(x)=\ln|x|$ is an antiderivative of $\dfrac{1}{x}$. Therefore, every antiderivative of $\dfrac{1}{x}$ is of

the form $\ln|x|+C$ for some constant C and every function of the form $\ln|x|+C$ is an

antiderivative of $\dfrac{1}{x}$.

(4) We have

$$\frac{\mathrm{d}}{\mathrm{d}x}\sin x=\cos x,$$

so $F(x)=\sin x$ is an antiderivative of $\cos x$. Therefore, every antiderivative of $\cos x$ is of the form $\sin x+C$ for some constant C and every function of the form $\sin x+C$ is an antiderivative of $\cos x$.   #

Your Practice 6.1 Find all antiderivatives of $f(x)=\sqrt{x}$.

6.1.2 Indefinite Integrals

We now discuss the formal notation used to represent antiderivatives and examine some of their properties. These properties allow us to find antiderivatives of more complicated functions.

> **Definition 6.2 (Indefinite Integral)**
>
> *If $F(x)$ is any antiderivative of $f(x)$, then the family of antiderivatives for $f(x)$ is called an indefinite integral and denoted*
>
> $$\int f(x)\mathrm{d}x=F(x)+C,\ C\ is\ any\ constant.$$

In this definition, $\int$ is called the ***integral symbol***, $f(x)$ is called the ***integrand***, x is called the ***integration variable*** and C is called the ***constant of integration***.

For example, since $\dfrac{x^3}{3}$ is an antiderivative of x^2, we write

$$\int x^2\,\mathrm{d}x = \frac{x^3}{3}+C.$$

Figure 6.1 shows the graph of the integral of x^2. Their graphs are vertical translates of one another. (This makes sense because each curve must have the same slope at any given value of x)

Note that often we will just say integrals instead of indefinite integrals (or definite integrals for that matter when we get to those). It will be clear from the context of the problem that we are talking about an indefinite integral (or definite integral).

Given the terminology introduced in this definition, the act of finding the antiderivatives of a function f is usually referred to as integrating f.

Example 6.3 Evaluate

$$\int (x^3-3x^2+5)\mathrm{d}x.$$

Solution Since this is really asking for the most general antiderivative we just need to reuse the final answer from Example 6.1.

The indefinite integral is,

$$\int (x^3-3x^2+5)\mathrm{d}x = \frac{1}{4}x^4-x^3+5x+C.$$

There are a couple of warnings. One of the most common mistakes we make when using integrals (both indefinite and definite) is forgetting $\mathrm{d}x$ at the end of the integral. This is required! Although it is nothing more than a differential, the $\mathrm{d}x$ notation is very important in ending the integral. Without the dx it will not be clear where the integrand ends. Consider the following variations of the above example:

$$\int (x^3 - 3x^2 + 5)dx = \frac{1}{4}x^4 - x^3 + 5x + C,$$

$$\int (x^3 - 3x^2)dx + 5 = \frac{1}{4}x^4 - x^3 + C + 5,$$

$$\int x^3 dx - 3x^2 + 5 = \frac{1}{4}x^4 + C - 3x^2 + 5.$$

We only need to integrate what is between the integral sign and the dx. Each of the above integrals end in a different place and so we get different answers because we integrate a different number of terms each time.

The next point is to note that the integration variable does not really matter. For instance,

$$\int (x^3 - 3x^2 + 5)dx = \frac{1}{4}x^4 - x^3 + 5x + C,$$

$$\int (s^3 - 3s^2 + 5)ds = \frac{1}{4}s^4 - s^3 + 5s + C,$$

$$\int (u^3 - 3u^2 + 5)du = \frac{1}{4}u^4 - u^3 + 5u + C.$$

Changing the integration variable in the integral simply changes the variable in the answer. However, it is important to notice that when we change the integration variable in the integral we also changed the differential (dx, ds, du) to match the new variable. This is more important than we might realize at this point.

Another use of the differential at the end of integral is to tell us what variable we are integrating with respect to. To see why this is important, we take a look at the following two integrals

$$\int 2x dx = x^2 + C,$$

$$\int 2t dx = 2tx + C.$$

The dx tells us that we are integrating x's. That means all other variables in the integrand are considered to be constants. We may get an incorrect answer if we neglect to put in the dx.

6.1.3 Indefinite Integrals List

We can evaluate indefinite integrals of some functions directly from properties of derivatives. For example, for $n \neq -1$,

$$\int x^n dx = \frac{1}{n+1}x^{n+1} + C,$$

which directly comes from

$$\frac{d}{dx}\frac{1}{n+1}x^{n+1} = \frac{1}{n+1}(n+1)x^n = x^n.$$

This fact is known as the Power Rule for integrals.

Power Rule for Integrals

For $n \neq -1$,

$$\int x^n \mathrm{d}x = \frac{1}{n+1} x^{n+1} + C, \ C \text{ is any constant.}$$

Evaluating indefinite integrals for some other functions is also a straightforward calculation. Table 6.1 lists the indefinite integrals for several common functions.

Table 6.1　Integration formulas

Differentiation Formulas	Indefinite Integral
$\dfrac{\mathrm{d}}{\mathrm{d}x} k = 0$	$\displaystyle\int k \mathrm{d}x = \int kx^0 \mathrm{d}x = kx + C$
$\dfrac{\mathrm{d}}{\mathrm{d}x} x^n = nx^{n-1}$	$\displaystyle\int x^n \mathrm{d}x = \frac{1}{n+1} x^{n+1} + C \text{ for } n \neq -1$
$\dfrac{\mathrm{d}}{\mathrm{d}x} \ln|x| = \dfrac{1}{x}$	$\displaystyle\int \frac{1}{x} \mathrm{d}x = \ln|x| + C$
$\dfrac{\mathrm{d}}{\mathrm{d}x} \mathrm{e}^x = \mathrm{e}^x$	$\displaystyle\int \mathrm{e}^x \mathrm{d}x = \mathrm{e}^x + C$
$\dfrac{\mathrm{d}}{\mathrm{d}x} \sin x = \cos x$	$\displaystyle\int \cos x \, \mathrm{d}x = \sin x + C$
$\dfrac{\mathrm{d}}{\mathrm{d}x} \cos x = -\sin x$	$\displaystyle\int \sin x \, \mathrm{d}x = -\cos x + C$

From the definition of indefinite integral of f, we know

$$\int f(x) \mathrm{d}x = F(x) + C$$

if and only if F is an antiderivative of f. Therefore, when claiming that $\int f(x) \mathrm{d}x = F(x) + C$, it is important to check whether this statement is correct by verifying that $F'(x) = f(x)$.

Example 6.4 Verify that

$$\int x \cos x \mathrm{d}x = x \sin x + \cos x + C.$$

Solution Since

$$\frac{\mathrm{d}}{\mathrm{d}x}(x \sin x + \cos x + C) = \sin x + x \cos x - \sin x = x \cos x,$$

the statement

$$\int x \cos x \mathrm{d}x = x \sin x + \cos x + C$$

is correct.　　　　　　　　　　　　　　　　　　　　　　　　　　#

Your Practice 6.2 Verify that

$$\int (x + \mathrm{e}^x) \mathrm{d}x = \frac{1}{2} x^2 + \mathrm{e}^x + C.$$

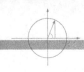

6.1.4 Properties of the Indefinite Integral

Let us now turn our attention to evaluating indefinite integrals for more complicated functions.

If F and G are antiderivatives of any functions f and g respectively, then

$$\frac{\mathrm{d}}{\mathrm{d}x}[F(x)+G(x)]=F'(x)+G'(x)=f(x)+g(x).$$

Therefore, $F(x)+G(x)$ is an antiderivative of $f(x)+g(x)$ and we have

$$\int[f(x)+g(x)]\mathrm{d}x = F(x)+G(x)+C.$$

Similarly,

$$\int[f(x)-g(x)]\mathrm{d}x = F(x)-G(x)+C.$$

Next, we consider the task of finding an antiderivative of $kf(x)$, where k is any real number. Since

$$kf(x)=k\,\frac{\mathrm{d}}{\mathrm{d}x}F(x)=[kF(x)]'$$

for any real number k, we conclude that

$$\int kf(x)\mathrm{d}x = kF(x)+C.$$

These properties are summarized in the following.

Properties of Indefinite Integrals

If functions f and g have antiderivatives, and k is any number, then

(1) $\displaystyle\int kf(x)\mathrm{d}x=k\int f(x)\mathrm{d}x$;

(2) $\displaystyle\int [f(x)\pm g(x)]\mathrm{d}x=\int f(x)\mathrm{d}x\pm\int g(x)\mathrm{d}x.$

In other words, we can factor multiplicative constants out of indefinite integrals; the integral of a sum or difference of functions is the sum or difference of the individual integrals. The sum rule can be extended to as many functions as we need. Note that there are no properties of products and quotients. Just like the derivatives of the following will NOT work.

$$\int f(x)g(x)\mathrm{d}x \neq \int f(x)\mathrm{d}x\int g(x)\mathrm{d}x,\ \int \frac{f(x)}{g(x)}\mathrm{d}x \neq \frac{\int f(x)\mathrm{d}x}{\int g(x)\mathrm{d}x}.$$

Example 6.5 Evaluate the indefinite integral

$$\int \frac{2x^5-\sqrt{x}}{x}\mathrm{d}x.$$

Solution Rewrite the integrand as

$$f(x)=\frac{2x^5}{x}-\frac{\sqrt{x}}{x}=2x^4-\frac{1}{\sqrt{x}}=2x^4-x^{-1/2}.$$

Thus

$$\int f(x)\,dx = \int (2x^4 - x^{-1/2})\,dx\,.$$

We can integrate each of the two terms in the integrand separately. We obtain

$$\int f(x)\,dx = 2\,\frac{x^5}{5} - \frac{x^{1/2}}{1/2} + C = \frac{2}{5}x^5 - 2\sqrt{x} + C\,. \qquad\qquad \#$$

Your Practice 6.3   Evaluate the indefinite integral

$$\int \frac{x^2 + 4\sqrt{x}}{x}\,dx\,.$$

6.1.5   Differential Equation

In applications of calculus it is very common to have a situation as in Example 6.1, where it is required to find a function, given knowledge about its derivatives. This is related with the differential equation.

An equation that involves one or more of derivatives of an unknown function is called a *differential equation*. The equation

$$\frac{dy}{dx} = f(x)$$

is a simple example of a differential equation. Solving this equation means finding a function y with a derivative f. Therefore, the solutions of the differential equation are the antiderivatives of f. If F is one antiderivative of f, every function of the form $y = F(x) + C$ is a solution of that differential equation. The general solution of a differential equation involves an arbitrary constant (or constants). For example, the general solutions of

$$\frac{dy}{dx} = 9x^2$$

are given by

$$y = \int 9x^2\,dx = 3x^3 + C\,.$$

However, there may be some extra conditions given that will determine the constants and therefore uniquely specify the solution. For instance, if we are given the additional condition

$$y(1) = 0\,,$$

we can determine a particular solution curve passes through the point $(1, 0)$. Since the solutions of the differential equation are $y = 3x^3 + C$, we need to find C such that $y(1) = 3 \times 1^3 + C = 0$. From this equation, we see that $C = -3$, and we conclude that $y = 3x^3 - 3$ is the solution of this problem. Figure 6.2 shows the solution.

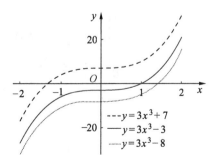

Figure 6. 2

Example 6. 6   Find the equation of the curve that passes through $(0, 4)$ and the slope of the curve is

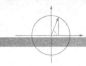

$12x^2 + 6x - 4$ at any point x.

Solution We want to find a function $y = f(x)$ such that
$$f'(x) = 12x^2 + 6x - 4,$$
and $y = 4$ when $x = 0$. Integrating $f'(x)$ we have
$$f(x) = \int f'(x) \, dx + C_1 = 12 \cdot \frac{1}{3}x^3 + 6 \cdot \frac{1}{2}x^2 - 4x + C = 4x^3 + 3x^2 - 4x + C.$$

To determine C we use the given condition $f(0) = 4$. Since $f(0) = C = 4$, the required function is
$$f(x) = 4x^3 + 3x^2 - 4x + 4. \qquad \qquad \#$$

If we are given the graph of a function f, it seems reasonable that we should be able to sketch the graph of an antiderivative F.

For instance, suppose that we are given that $F(0) = 1$. Then we have a place to start, the point $(0, 1)$, and the direction in which we move our pencil is given at each stage by the derivative $F'(x) = f(x)$.

In the next example we use the principles of this chapter to show how to graph F even when we don't have a formula for f. This would be the case, for instance, when $f(x)$ is determined by experimental data.

Example 6.7 The graph of a function f is given in Figure 6.3. Make a rough sketch of an antiderivative F, given that $F(0) = 2$.

Solution We are guided by the fact that the slope of $y = F(x)$ is $f(x)$. We start at the point $(0, 2)$ and draw F as an initially decreasing function since $f(x)$ is negative when $0 < x < 1$. Notice that $f(1) = f(3) = 0$, so F has horizontal tangents when $x = 1$ and $x = 3$. For $1 < x < 3$, $f(x)$ is positive and so F is increasing. We see that F has a local minimum when $x = 1$ and a local maximum when $x = 3$.

For $x > 3$, $f(x)$ is negative and so F is decreasing on $(3, +\infty)$. Since $f(x) \to 0$ as $x \to +\infty$, the graph of F becomes flatter as $x \to +\infty$. Also notice that $F''(x) = f'(x)$ changes from positive to negative at $x = 2$ and from negative to positive at $x = 4$, so F has inflection points when $x = 2$ and $x = 4$. We use this information to sketch the graph of the antiderivative in Figure 6.4. $\qquad \#$

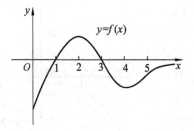

Figure 6.3

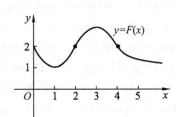

Figure 6.4

Example 6.8 Let $C(x)$ be the cost of producing x units of a commodity. If
$$C'(x) = 0.3x^2 + 2x$$

and the fixed cost is $2000, find $C(x)$ and the cost of producing 20 units.

Solution　We want to find $C(x)$, given $C'(x)=0.3x^2+2x$, $C(0)=2000$.

By antidifferentiation, we have

$$C(x) = \int C'(x)\mathrm{d}x + C_1 = \int (0.3x^2 + 2x)\mathrm{d}x + C_1 = 0.1x^3 + x^2 + C_1 .$$

Because $C(0)=2000$, then we get $C_1=2000$. Thus

$$C(x)=0.1x^3+x^2+2000.$$

The cost of producing 20 units is

$$C(20)=0.1\times20^3+20^2+2000=3200. \qquad\qquad \#$$

Your Practice 6.4　Find the cost function $C(x)$ when

$$C'(x)=40+0.4x$$

and 1000 Yuan at a zero production level. What is the cost at the production level of 100 units?

Example 6.9　Suppose that a falling body hits the ground with velocity -100 feet per second. What was the initial height of the body?

Solution　The motion is vertical and we choose the positive direction to be upward. We denote at time t the height above the ground is $h(t)$ and we know the velocity $v(t)$ is decreasing. It is known that, near the surface of the earth, a body falls with an acceleration about -32 feet for square second. We also know $v(0)=0$, $v(T)=-100$, $h(T)=0$ where T is the time at which the falling body hits the ground. Therefore, we have

$$a(t)=\frac{\mathrm{d}v}{\mathrm{d}t}=-32.$$

Integrating the equation above, we have

$$v(t)=-32t+C.$$

Because $v(0)=0$, then C to be zero. Thus $v(t)=-32t$.

Using $v(T)=-100$ we have $-100=-32T$ and $T=\dfrac{100}{32}=\dfrac{25}{8}$.

Since $h'(t)=v(t)$, we antidifferentiate again and obtain

$$h(t)=-16t^2+D.$$

Using the fact that $h(T)=0$ we have $0=-16\times\dfrac{25^2}{8}+D$, then $D=16\times\left(\dfrac{25}{8}\right)^2=\dfrac{625}{4}$,

and so

$$h(t)=-16t^2+\frac{625}{4}.$$

At time $t=0$ we have the initial height $h(0)=\dfrac{625}{4}=156.25$ (feet). $\qquad\qquad \#$

Example 6.10　In many cases, a tablet that is taken passes into the aqueous solution of the stomach where it slowly dissolves. The Noyes-Whitney is used to determine the dosage rates of varying dosage form:

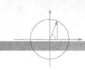
$$\frac{\mathrm{d}m}{\mathrm{d}t} = A\frac{D}{d}(C_s - C_b)$$

where m is the mass of dissolved material, A is the surface area of the solid, D is the diffusion coefficient, d is thickness of the concentration gradient, C_s is the particle surface (saturation) concentration, C_b is the concentration in the bulk solvent/solution (Figure 6.5).

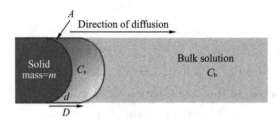

Figure 6.5

Then the mass of dissolved material is

$$m(t) = \int \frac{\mathrm{d}m}{\mathrm{d}t}\mathrm{d}t = \int A\frac{D}{d}(C_s - C_b)\mathrm{d}t = A\frac{D}{d}(C_s - C_b)t + K$$

where K is the constant of integration. To determine K, we suppose that the patient takes m_0 tablet. Then $m_0 = m(0) = 0 + K$ and $K = m_0$. Therefore,

$$m(t) = A\frac{D}{d}(C_s - C_b)t + m_0.$$

Exercise 6.1

1. Is $F(x) = (x+1)(x+2)$ an antiderivative of $f(x) = 2x + 3$? Explain.

2. Is $F(x) = e^{x^3/3}$ an antiderivative of $f(x) = e^{x^2}$? Explain.

3. Verify that $\int xe^x \mathrm{d}x = xe^x - e^x + C$.

4. Verify that $\int \ln x\mathrm{d}x = x\ln x - x + C$.

5. Find each indefinite integral.

(1) $\int 7\mathrm{d}x$;

(2) $\int \mathrm{d}t$;

(3) $\int 9x^2 \mathrm{d}x$;

(4) $\int (w^2 + 2e^w)\mathrm{d}w$;

(5) $\int \left(\frac{1}{x} - \frac{3}{x^2}\right)\mathrm{d}x$;

(6) $\int \frac{1}{x^4}\mathrm{d}x$;

(7) $\int \left(\frac{1}{e^{-x}} + \frac{1}{3x} + \frac{1}{x^5}\right)\mathrm{d}x$;

(8) $\int 5e^u \mathrm{d}u$;

(9) $\int e^{-u}(e^{2u} + e^u)\mathrm{d}u$;

(10) $\int (10x^9 - 12x^3 - 5)\mathrm{d}x$;

(11) $\int (10x^9 - 12x^3)\mathrm{d}x - 5$;

(12) $\int 10x^9 \mathrm{d}x - 12x^3 - 5$;

(13) $\int (6\sin t - 2\cos t)\mathrm{d}t$;

(14) $\int (6\sin t - 2\cos t)\mathrm{d}u$.

6. Find the function $y = y(t)$ such that

$\dfrac{dy}{dt}=\dfrac{20}{\sqrt{t}}$ and $y(1)=40$.

7. Find the function $x = x(t)$ such that $\dfrac{dx}{dt}=4e^t-2$ and $x(0)=1$.

8. Determine $f(x)$ given that $f''(x)= 8x^3-12x+3$.

9. Determine $h(t)$ given that $h''(t)= 6t-14+9e^t$, $h(0)=4$ and $h'(0)=8$.

10. Find the equation of the curve that passes through $(2, 3)$ if its slope is given by $\dfrac{dy}{dx}=4x-3$ for each x.

11. The area A of a healing wound changes at a rate given approximately by

$$\dfrac{dA}{dt}=-4t^{-3}, \ 1\leqslant t\leqslant 10,$$

where t is time in days and $A(1)=2$ square centimeters. What will the area of the wound be in 10 days?

12. A car is traveling at the rate of 88 feet per second when the brakes are applied. The car begins decelerating at a constant rate of 15 feet per square second.

(1) How many seconds elapse before the car stops?

(2) How far does the car travel during that time?

13. Suppose the car is in Problem 12 traveling at the rate of 44 feet per second. How long does it take for the car to stop? How far will the car travel?

6.2　The Definite Integral

6.2.1　Area Problem

The area problem is to definite integrals what the tangent and rate of change problems are to derivatives. It is probably easiest to see how we do this with an example. So, let us determine the area under the parabola $y = x^2$ from 0 to 1. In other words, we want to determine the area of the shaded region in Figure 6. 6.

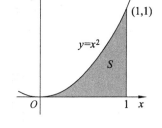

Figure 6. 6

Now, at this point, we cannot find the area of a region with curved sides exactly. However, we can estimate the area. We know how to compute areas of rectangles, so we approximate the area by rectangles.

Suppose we cut the region into n pieces with equal base (Figure 6. 7(a)). This is equivalent to divide the interval between 0 and 1 into n equal subintervals. Then in each interval we can form a rectangle whose height is given by the function value at a specific point in the interval. We add all rectangles up and the sum will be an estimate of the area. There are many ways we might do this, but let us take the height of the curve at the right endpoint of the subinterval as the height of the rectangle, as in Figure 6. 7(b).

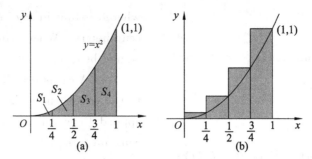

Figure 6. 7

Note that by choosing the height as we did each of the rectangles will overestimate the area since each rectangle takes in more area than the graph each time. Now let us estimate the area. First, the width of each of the rectangles is 1/4. The height of each rectangle is determined by the function value at the right endpoint and so the height of each rectangle is nothing more that the function value at the right endpoint. Let R_4 be the sum of the areas of these approximating rectangles. Here is the estimated area.

$$R_4 = \frac{1}{4}f\left(\frac{1}{4}\right) + \frac{1}{4}f\left(\frac{1}{2}\right) + \frac{1}{4}f\left(\frac{3}{4}\right) + \frac{1}{4}f(1)$$

$$= \frac{1}{4} \times \frac{1}{16} + \frac{1}{4} \times \frac{1}{4} + \frac{1}{4} \times \frac{9}{16} + \frac{1}{4}$$

$$= 0.234375.$$

Now, let us suppose that we want a better estimation. The easiest way to get a better approximation is to take more rectangles (i. e. increase n). Let us increase the number of rectangles that we used and see what happens. Here are the graphs showing the 10, 30 and 50 rectangles and the estimations in Figure 6. 8.

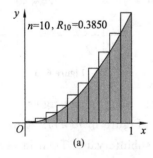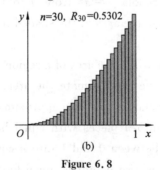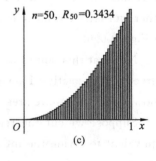

Figure 6. 8

We repeat this procedure with a larger number of strips and list the estimation in Table 6. 2.

Table 6. 2

n	R_n	n	R_n
10	0. 3850000	50	0. 3434000
20	0. 3587500	100	0. 3383500
30	0. 3501852	1000	0. 3338335

It looks as if R_n is approaching $\dfrac{1}{3}$ as n increases. Then we use this limit as the desired area.

Jumping straight to the general case (Figure 6. 9), assume that we have got a function $f(x)$ that is positive on some interval $[a, b]$. We want to determine the area of the region S that lies under the curve $y=f(x)$ from a to b. This means that S is bounded by the graph of a continuous function $y=f(x)$ (where $f(x) \geqslant 0$), the vertical lines $x=a$ and $x=b$, and the x-axis.

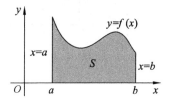

Figure 6. 9

We divide S into n strips $S_1, S_2, S_3, \cdots, S_n$ by drawing the vertical lines and as in Figure 6. 10. The interval $[a, b]$ is divided into n subintervals of equal length. These strips divide $[a, b]$ into n subintervals $[x_0, x_1], [x_1, x_2], [x_2, x_3], \cdots, [x_{n-1}, x_n]$ where $x_0 = a$ and $x_n = b$. The width of each of the n strips is

$$\Delta x = \frac{b-a}{n}.$$

Note that the subintervals do not have to be equal length, but it will make our work significantly easier. The right endpoints of each subintervals are

$$x_1 = a + \Delta x,$$
$$x_2 = a + 2\Delta x,$$
$$x_3 = a + 3\Delta x,$$
$$\cdots\cdots$$
$$x_n = a + n\Delta x = b.$$

Next in each interval, we approximate the ith strip S_i by a rectangle with width Δx and height $f(x_i)$, which is the value of f at the right endpoint (Figure 6. 11). Then the area of the ith rectangle is $f(x_i)\Delta x$.

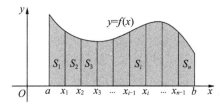

Figure 6. 10

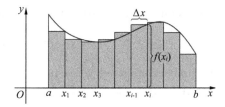

Figure 6. 11

Intuitively, the area of S is approximated by the sum of the areas of these rectangles, which is

$$A \approx R_n = f(x_1)\Delta x_1 + f(x_2)\Delta x_2 + \cdots + f(x_n)\Delta x_n.$$

We make approximation for different n as in Figure 6. 12.

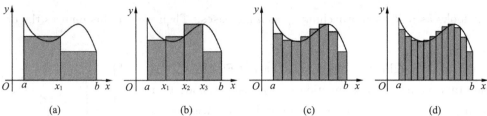

Figure 6.12

Notice that the rectangles approximate the area under the curve better and better as the number of strips increases, that is, as $n \to \infty$. Therefore we define the area of the region in the following way.

Definition 6.3

    The area A of the region S that lies under the graph of the continuous function f is the limit of the sum of the areas of approximating rectangles:

$$A = \lim_{n \to \infty} R_n$$

$$= \lim_{n \to \infty} [f(x_1)\Delta x_1 + f(x_2)\Delta x_2 + \cdots + f(x_n)\Delta x_n].$$

We will use summation notation or sigma notation at this point to simplify up our notation a little. The symbol $\sum\limits_{i=m}^{n}$ indicates a summation in which the letter i (called the index of summation) takes on consecutive integer values beginning with m and ending with n, that is, $m, m+1, \cdots$. For example,

$$\sum_{i=3}^{8} i^2 = 3^2 + 4^2 + 5^2 + 6^2 + 7^2 + 8^2,$$

$$\sum_{i=1}^{n} f(x_i)\Delta x = f(x_1)\Delta x + f(x_2)\Delta x + \cdots + f(x_n)\Delta x.$$

Using summation notation the area estimation is

$$A = \lim_{n \to \infty} \sum_{i=1}^{n} f(x_i)\Delta x.$$

The limit exists since f is continuous.

Note that the area is a defined quantity, which means that the height of rectangles makes no difference. We get the same value if we use left endpoints. We could take the height of the ith rectangle to be the value of f at any number x_i^* in the ith subinterval $[x_{i-1}, x_i]$ (see Figure 6.13). Such numbers $x_1^*, x_2^*, \cdots, x_n^*$ are called **sample points**. This gives us an estimate for the area of the form

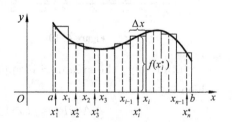

Figure 6.13

$$A = \lim_{n \to \infty} \sum_{i=1}^{n} f(x_i^*) \Delta x .$$

A sum of this form is called a **Riemann sum**, named for the 19th-century mathematician Bernhard Riemann, who developed the idea.

Some subtleties here are worth discussing. First, note that taking the limit of a sum is a little different from taking the limit of a function $f(x)$ as x goes to infinity. However, for now we assume that the computational techniques we used to compute limits of functions can also be used to calculate limits of sums. Second, we must consider what to do if the expression converges to different limits for different choices of sample point. Fortunately, this does not happen. Although the proof is beyond the scope of this text, it can be shown that if $f(x)$ is continuous on the closed interval $[a, b]$, then $\lim_{n \to \infty} \sum_{i=1}^{n} f(x_i^*) \Delta x$ exists and is unique (in other words, it does not depend on the choice of x_i^*).

6.2.2 Distance Problem

Find the distance traveled by an object during a certain time period if the velocity of the object is known at all times.

If the velocity remains constant, then the distance problem is easy to solve by means of the formula

distance＝velocity×time.

But if the velocity varies, it is not so easy to find the distance traveled.

Example 6.11   Suppose the odometer on our car is broken and we want to estimate the distance driven over a 30-second time interval. We take speedometer readings every five seconds and record them in Table 6.3 (Units: feet per second):

Table 6.3

t	0	5	10	15	20	25	30
$v(t)$	25	31	35	43	47	46	41

We consider how we might approximate a solution. During the first five seconds the velocity does not change very much, so we can estimate the distance traveled during that time by assuming that the velocity is constant. If we take the velocity during that time interval to be the velocity at the end of the interval(31 feet per second), then we obtain the approximate distance traveled during the first five seconds:

$$d_1 = 31 \text{ feet per second} \times 5 \text{ second} = 155 \text{ feet}.$$

Similarly, during the second time interval the velocity is approximately constant and we take it to be the velocity when $t = 10$ second. So our estimate for the distance traveled from $t = 5$ to $t = 10$ is

$$d_2 = 35 \text{ feet per second} \times 5 \text{ second} = 175 \text{ feet}.$$

If we add similar estimates for the other time intervals, we obtain an estimate for the total distance traveled:

$$(31\times5)+(35\times5)+(43\times5)+(47\times5)+(46\times5)+(41\times5)=1215(\text{feet}).$$

If we wanted a more accurate estimate, we could have taken velocity readings every two seconds, or even every second.

The General Case

In general, suppose an object moves with velocity $v=f(t)$, where $a\leqslant t\leqslant b$ and $f(t)\geqslant0$ (so the object always moves in the positive direction). We now want to approximate the change in position between time a and time b. We take the interval of time between a and b, divide it into n subintervals, and approximate the distance traveled during each of them. In detail, we take velocity readings at times

$$t_0(=a),\ t_1,\ t_2,\cdots,\ t_n(=b),$$

so that the velocity is approximately constant on each subinterval. If these times are equally spaced, then the time between consecutive readings is

$$\Delta t=\frac{b-a}{n}.$$

During the first time interval the velocity is approximately $f(t_1)$ and so the distance traveled is approximately $f(t_1)\Delta t$. Similarly, the distance traveled during the second time interval is about $f(t_2)\Delta t$ and the total distance traveled during the time interval is approximately

$$f(t_1)\Delta t+f(t_2)\Delta t+\cdots+f(t_n)\Delta t=\sum_{i=1}^{n}f(t_i)\Delta t.$$

The more frequently we measure the velocity, the more accurate our estimates become, so it seems plausible that the *exact* distance d traveled is the **limit** of such expressions:

$$d=\lim_{n\to\infty}\sum_{i=1}^{n}f(t_i)\Delta t.$$

Because the distance problem has the same form as our expressions for area, it follows that the distance traveled is equal to the area under the graph of the velocity function.

We will see that other quantities of interest in the natural and social sciences—such as the work done by a variable force or the cardiac output of the heart—can also be interpreted as the area under a curve. So when we compute areas in this chapter, bear in mind that they can be interpreted in a variety of practical ways.

6.2.3 The Definite Integral

> **Definition 6.4 (Definite Integral)**
>
> *If f is a continuous function defined on the interval $[a,b]$, we divide the interval $[a,b]$ into n subintervals of equal width $\Delta x=(b-a)/n$. We let $x_1,\ x_2,\cdots,\ x_n(x=b)$ be the endpoints of these subintervals. Then the definite integral of f from a to b is*
>
> $$\int_a^b f(x)\mathrm{d}x=\lim\sum_{i=1}^{n}f(x_i)\Delta x$$
>
> *provided that this limit exists. If it does exist, we say that f is integrable on $[a,b]$.*

Here we make some notes.

- The symbol $\int$ was introduced by Leibniz and is called an ***integral sign***. It is an elongated S and was chosen because an integral is a limit of sums.

- In the notation $\int_a^b f(x)\mathrm{d}x$, $f(x)$ is called the ***integrand*** and a and b are called the ***limits of integration***; a is the ***lower limit*** and b is the ***upper limit***.

- For now, the symbol $\mathrm{d}x$ has no meaning by itself; $\int_a^b f(x)\mathrm{d}x$ is a symbol. The $\mathrm{d}x$ simply indicates that the independent variable is x. The procedure of calculating an integral is called ***integration***.

- The definite integral $\int_a^b f(x)\mathrm{d}x$ is a number; it does not depend on x. In fact, we could use any letter in place of x without changing the value of the integral:

$$\int_a^b f(x)\mathrm{d}x = \int_a^b f(t)\mathrm{d}t = \int_a^b f(s)\mathrm{d}s .$$

- The definite integral of an integrable function can be approximated to within any desired degree of accuracy by a Riemann sum.

If $f(x)\geqslant 0$, the integral $\int_a^b f(x)\mathrm{d}x$ is the area under the curve $y=f(x)$ from a to b, and the Riemann sum $\sum_{i=1}^{n} f(x_i)\Delta x$ is the sum of areas of rectangles (Figure 6.11). If the function is below the x-axis we will get a negative area. If f takes on both positive and negative values (Figure 6.14), then the Riemann sum is the sum of the areas of the rectangles that lie above the x-axis and the ***negatives*** of the areas of the rectangles that lie below the x-axis. Then an definite integral can be interpreted as a net area:

$$\int_a^b f(x)\mathrm{d}x = A_1 - A_2$$

where A_1 is the area of the region above the x-axis and below the graph of f, and A_2 is the area of the region below the x-axis and above the graph of f (Figure 6.15).

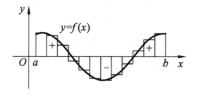

Figure 6.14

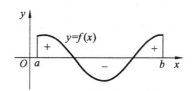

Figure 6.15

- Although we have defined $\int_a^b f(x)\mathrm{d}x$ by dividing $[a, b]$ into subintervals of equal width, there are situations in which it is advantageous to work with subintervals of unequal width. And there are methods for numerical integration that take advantage of unequal subintervals.

• If f is integrable on $[a, b]$, then the limit in Definition exists and gives the same value no matter how we choose the sample points. To simplify the calculation of the integral we often take the sample points to be right endpoints.

Now we can write the two problems in terms of definite integral. The area of the region S that lies under the curve $y = f(x)$ from a to b is

$$\text{area} = \int_a^b f(x)\mathrm{d}x .$$

The distance of an object traveled between a and b is

$$\text{distance} = \int_a^b f(t)\mathrm{d}t .$$

where $v = f(t)$ is the velocity the object moves.

We have defined the definite integral for an integrable function, but not all functions are integrable. The following theorem give the sufficient condition for the existence of definite integral.

Theorem 6.2

If f is continuous on $[a, b]$, or if f has only a finite number of jump discontinuities, then f is integrable on $[a, b]$; that is, the definite integral $\int_a^b f(x)\mathrm{d}x$ exists.

Exercise 6.2

1. Estimate the area of the region between the function $f(x) = x^2 - 4$ on $[0, 3]$ and the x-axis on the given interval using $n = 6$ and using

(1) the right end points of the subintervals for the height of the rectangles;

(2) the left end points of the subintervals for the height of the rectangles;

(3) the midpoints of the subintervals for the height of the rectangles.

2. Estimate the net area between $f(x) = 8x^2 - x^3 - 4$ and the x-axis on $[-2, 2]$ using $n = 8$ and the right end points of the subintervals for the height of the rectangles. Without looking at a graph of the function on the interval does it appear that more of the area is above or below the x-axis?

3. Estimate the net area between $f(x) = 5 + x - 2x^2$ on $[0, 4]$ and the x-axis using $n = 8$ and the right end points of the subintervals for the height of the rectangles. Without looking at a graph of the function on the interval does it appear that more of the area is above or below the x-axis?

4. Use the definition of the definite integral to evaluate the integral $\int_1^4 (2x + 3)\mathrm{d}x$.

5. Use the definition of the definite integral to evaluate the integral $\int_0^1 (6x - 1)\mathrm{d}x$.

6. The graph of g (Figure 6.16)

consists of two straight lines and a semicircle. Let $\pi=3.14$. Use it to evaluate the following integrals:

(1) $\int_0^2 g(x)\mathrm{d}x$;

(2) $\int_2^6 g(x)\mathrm{d}x$;

(3) $\int_6^7 g(x)\mathrm{d}x$;

(4) $\int_0^7 g(x)\mathrm{d}x$.

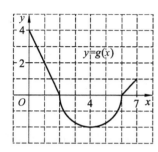

Figure 6.16

7. Calculate the definite integral by referring to Figure 6.17 with the indicated areas.

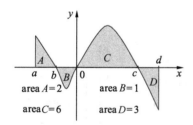

Figure 6.17

(1) $\int_b^0 f(x)\mathrm{d}x$;

(2) $\int_a^c f(x)\mathrm{d}x$;

(3) $\int_0^a f(x)\mathrm{d}x$;

(4) $\int_a^d f(x)\mathrm{d}x$.

8. Assume that $0<a<b<+\infty$. Use a geometric argument to show that

$$\int_a^b x\,\mathrm{d}x = \frac{b^2-a^2}{2} .$$

9. Use a graph to interpret the definite integral in terms of areas. Do not compute the integrals.

(1) $\int_{-2}^3 (x-3)\mathrm{d}x$;

(2) $\int_{-1}^2 (x^2-1)\mathrm{d}x$;

(3) $\int_{-\pi}^{\pi} \cos x\mathrm{d}x$;

(4) $\int_{0.5}^4 \ln x\mathrm{d}x$.

10. Find the value of integrals by interpreting it as the signed area under the graph of an appropriately chosen function.

(1) $\int_{-2}^3 |x|\,\mathrm{d}x$;

(2) $\int_{-3}^3 \sqrt{9-x^2}\mathrm{d}x$;

(3) $\int_2^5 (0.5x-4)\mathrm{d}x$;

(4) $\int_0^1 \sqrt{2-x^2}\mathrm{d}x$.

11. Verify each inequality without evaluating the integrals.

(1) $\int_0^1 x\mathrm{d}x \geqslant \int_0^1 x^2\,\mathrm{d}x$;

(2) $\int_1^2 x\mathrm{d}x \leqslant \int_1^2 x^2\,\mathrm{d}x$;

(3) $0 \leqslant \int_0^4 \sqrt{x}\mathrm{d}x \leqslant 8$;

(4) $\frac{1}{2} \leqslant \int_0^1 \sqrt{1-x^2}\mathrm{d}x \leqslant 1$.

12. Find the value of a $(a\geqslant 0)$ that maximizes $\int_0^a (4-x^2)\mathrm{d}x$.

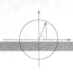

6.3   Properties of the Definite Integral

With the perspective that the definite integral of a function f over an interval $[a, b]$ measures the net signed area bounded by f and the x-axis over the interval, we naturally arrive at several different standard properties of the definite integral. In addition, it is helpful to remember that the definite integral is defined in terms of Riemann sums that fundamentally consist of the areas of rectangles.

If we consider the definite integral $\int_a^a f(x)\mathrm{d}x$ for any real number a, it is evident that no area is being bounded because the interval begins and ends with the same point. Hence,

$$\int_a^a f(x)\mathrm{d}x = 0.$$

When we defined the definite integral $\int_a^b f(x)\mathrm{d}x$, we implicitly assumed that $a < b$. But the definition as a limit of Riemann sums makes sense even if $a > b$. If we integrate from a to b, then in the defining Riemann sum $\Delta x = \dfrac{b-a}{n}$, while if we integrate from b to a, $\Delta x = \dfrac{a-b}{n} = -\dfrac{b-a}{n}$, and this is the only change in the sum used to define the integral. Therefore

$$\int_a^b f(x)\mathrm{d}x = -\int_b^a f(x)\mathrm{d}x.$$

Consider Figure 6.18. The area of the shaded rectangle is $c(b-a)$. It is then expected that the integral of a constant function $f(x) = c$ is the constant times the length of the interval

$$\int_a^b c\,\mathrm{d}x = c(b-a).$$

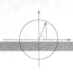

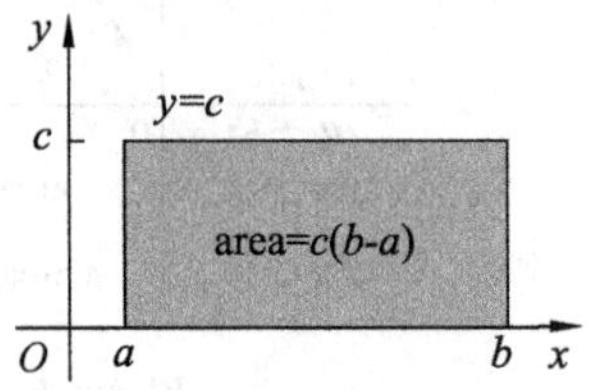

Figure 6.18

There are additional properties of the definite integral that we need to understand. Recall the Constant Multiple Rule and the Sum Rule for derivatives,

$$\frac{\mathrm{d}}{\mathrm{d}x}Cf(x) = C\frac{\mathrm{d}}{\mathrm{d}x}f(x),$$

$$\frac{\mathrm{d}}{\mathrm{d}x}[f(x)+g(x)] = \frac{\mathrm{d}}{\mathrm{d}x}f(x) + \frac{\mathrm{d}}{\mathrm{d}x}g(x).$$

These rules are useful because they enable us to deal individually with the simplest parts of certain functions and take advantage of the elementary operations of addition and multiplying by a constant. They also tell us that the process of taking the derivative respects addition and multiplying by constants in the simplest possible way.

It turns out that similar rules hold for the definite integral. First, let us consider the case of Constant Multiple Rule. We know that multiplying a function by a positive number C stretches or shrinks its graph vertically by a factor of C. So it stretches or shrinks each approximating rectangle by a factor C and therefore it has the effect of multiplying the area by C. Therefore the following principle holds:

Constant Multiple Rule

If f is a continuous function and C is any real number then

$$\int_a^b Cf(x)\mathrm{d}x = C\int_a^b f(x)\mathrm{d}x.$$

Finally, we see a similar situation geometrically with the sum of two functions f and g. As shown in Figure 6.19, if we take the sum of two functions f and g, at every point in the interval, the height of the function $f+g$ is given by $(f+g)(x)=f(x)+g(x)$, which is the sum of the individual function values of f and g. For each approximating rectangle, taking the same base and sample points (for instance, the right endpoints), the area of approximating rectangle in $\int [f(x)+g(x)]\mathrm{d}x$ is the sum of that in $\int f(x)\mathrm{d}x$ and in $\int g(x)\mathrm{d}x$.

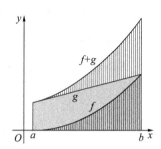

Figure 6.19

Stated in terms of definite integrals, we have the following general rule:

Sum Rule

If f and g are continuous functions, then

$$\int_a^b [f(x)+g(x)]\,\mathrm{d}x = \int_a^b f(x)\mathrm{d}x + \int_a^b g(x)\mathrm{d}x.$$

More generally, the Constant Multiple Rule and Sum Rule can be combined to make the observation that for any continuous functions f and g and any constants C and k,

$$\int_a^b [Cf(x)+kg(x)]\mathrm{d}x = C\int_a^b f(x)\mathrm{d}x + k\int_a^b g(x)\mathrm{d}x.$$

Example 6.12   If $\int_0^1 x^2\,\mathrm{d}x = \dfrac{1}{3}$, find $\int_0^1 (4+3x^2)\mathrm{d}x$.

Solution   We start by applying the Sum Rule and the Constant Multiple Rule,

$$\int_0^1 (4+3x^2)\mathrm{d}x = \int_0^1 4\mathrm{d}x + \int_0^1 3x^2\,\mathrm{d}x = \int_0^1 4\mathrm{d}x + 3\int_0^1 x^2\,\mathrm{d}x.$$

Since

$$\int_0^1 4\mathrm{d}x = 4(1-0) = 4,$$

$$\int_0^1 (4+3x^2)\mathrm{d}x = 4+3\times\frac{1}{3} = 5.$$

$\#$

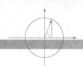

Next, we consider the results of subdividing a given interval. In Figure 6. 20, it can be seen: the area under $y=f(x)$ from a to c plus the area from c to b is equal to the total area from a to b. It is indicative of the following rule:

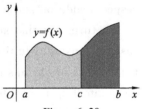

Figure 6. 20

Additive Interval Rule

If f is a continuous function and a, b, c are real numbers, then

$$\int_a^c f(x)\mathrm{d}x + \int_c^b f(x)\mathrm{d}x = \int_a^b f(x)\mathrm{d}x.$$

It turns out that the identity is true no matter what c is, but it is easiest to think about the meaning when $a \leqslant c \leqslant b$.

Example 6. 13 If we know $\int_0^{10} f(x)\mathrm{d}x = 17$ and $\int_0^8 f(x)\mathrm{d}x = 12$, find $\int_8^{10} f(x)\mathrm{d}x$.

Solution By Additive Interval Rule for integral interval we have

$$\int_0^8 f(x)\mathrm{d}x + \int_8^{10} f(x) = \int_0^{10} f(x)\mathrm{d}x.$$

So
$$\int_8^{10} f(x)\mathrm{d}x = \int_0^{10} f(x) - \int_0^8 f(x)\mathrm{d}x = 17 - 12 = 5.$$ #

Your Practice 6.5 If $\int_1^5 f(x)\mathrm{d}x = 7$ and $\int_3^5 f(x)\mathrm{d}x = 2$, find $\int_1^3 f(x)\mathrm{d}x$.

Exercise 6.3

1. Given that $\int_1^4 x\mathrm{d}x = 7.5$, $\int_1^4 x^2\mathrm{d}x = 21$, $\int_4^5 x^2\mathrm{d}x = \dfrac{61}{3}$, calculate the definite integral.

(1) $\int_1^4 (5x + x^2)\mathrm{d}x$;

(2) $\int_1^5 6x^2\mathrm{d}x$;

(3) $\int_4^4 (7x - 2)^2\mathrm{d}x$;

(4) $\int_4^1 x(1 - x)\mathrm{d}x$.

2. Suppose that the following information is known about the functions f, g, x^2 and x^3:

$\int_0^1 f(x)\mathrm{d}x = 2$, $\int_1^4 f(x)\mathrm{d}x = 3$,

$\int_0^1 g(x)\mathrm{d}x = -4$, $\int_1^4 f(x)\mathrm{d}x = 1$,

$\int_0^1 x^2\mathrm{d}x = \dfrac{1}{3}$, $\int_0^1 x^3\mathrm{d}x = \dfrac{1}{4}$,

$\int_1^4 x^2\mathrm{d}x = \dfrac{47}{3}$, $\int_1^4 x^3\mathrm{d}x = \dfrac{255}{4}$.

Use the provided information to evaluate each of the following definite integrals.

(1) $\int_4^1 f(x)\mathrm{d}x$;

(2) $\int_0^4 f(x)\mathrm{d}x$;

(3) $\int_0^1 [f(x) + g(x)]\mathrm{d}x$;

(4) $\int_1^4 [f(x) - 8x^3 + 3x^2]\mathrm{d}x$;

(5) $\displaystyle\int_{4}^{0}[4x^{3}+7g(x)]\mathrm{d}x$.

(6) $\displaystyle\int_{2}^{4}(x-2)^{2}\mathrm{d}x$.

3. Given that $\displaystyle\int_{0}^{a}x^{2}\mathrm{d}x=\frac{1}{3}a^{3}$. Evaluate:

4. Find $\displaystyle\int_{2}^{2}\cos 4x^{3}\mathrm{d}x$.

(1) $\displaystyle\int_{0}^{2}\frac{1}{2}x^{2}\mathrm{d}x$;

5. Find $\displaystyle\int_{-2}^{-2}e^{-x^{3}/4}\mathrm{d}x$.

(2) $\displaystyle\int_{-3}^{0}2x^{2}\mathrm{d}x$;

6. Find $a(a\geqslant 0)$ such that
$$\int_{1}^{a}(x-2)^{3}\mathrm{d}x=0.$$

(3) $\displaystyle\int_{1}^{3}\frac{1}{3}x^{2}\mathrm{d}x$;

7. Find $a(0\leqslant a\leqslant 2\pi)$ such that
$$\int_{0}^{a}\sin x\mathrm{d}x=0.$$

(4) $\displaystyle\int_{1}^{1}3x^{2}\mathrm{d}x$;

(5) $\displaystyle\int_{-2}^{3}\frac{3}{2}x^{2}\mathrm{d}x$;

6.4   Fundamental Theorem of Calculus

The fundamental theorem of calculus has two parts: the first part provides a method for computing definite integrals, and the second part links antiderivatives and integrals. Both Newton and Leibniz are to credited with the theorem.

Let us recall the physical example from the previous section. An object moves in a straight line with its speed function $v(t)=3t^{2}$ cm/sec. How far does the object travel between time $t=a$ and time $t=b$?

There are two reasonable ways to approach this problem. One way is to use antiderivatives. If $s(t)$ is the position of the object at time t, we know that $s(t)$ is an antiderivative of $v(t)$, i. e. ,$s'(t)=v(t)$ and $s(t)=t^{3}+C$. Therefore the distance the object travels is $s(b)-s(a)=b^{3}+C-(a^{3}+C)=b^{3}-a^{3}$. Notice that the C drops out; this means that it does not matter that what the exact value C is. In other words, to find the change in position between time a and time b we can use any antiderivative of the speed function $v(t)$—it need not be the one antiderivative that actually gives the location of the object.

The second approach to the problem is more difficult but also more general. By the definition of definite integral, the change in position between time a and time b is the definite integral of the speed on the integral $[a,b]$: $\displaystyle\int_{a}^{b}v(t)\mathrm{d}t$.

Combining the two quantities we have $\displaystyle\int_{a}^{b}v(t)\mathrm{d}t=s(b)-s(a)$ where $s'(t)=v(t)$. This means that the definite integral can be computed by finding any function with derivative $v(t)$, substituting a and b, and subtracting. We generalize this in a theorem.

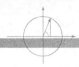

> **Theorem 6.3 (Fundamental Theorem of Calculus, Part Ⅰ)**
>
> *Suppose f is continuous on the interval* $[a, b]$, *then*
> $$\int_a^b f(x)\,dx = F(b) - F(a)$$
> *where F is any antiderivative of f, that is, a function such that* $F' = f$.

We rewrite this slightly:
$$\int_a^x f(t)\,dt = F(x) - F(a).$$

We have replaced the variable x by t and b by x. The substitution does not change the meaning because these are just different names for quantities.

We then take the two sides of the equation as functions. The expression $\int_a^x f(t)\,dt$ is a function: input a value for x, get out some other value. The expression $F(x) - F(a)$ is of course also a function, and its derivative is

$$\frac{\mathrm{d}}{\mathrm{d}x}[F(x) - F(a)] = F'(x) = f(x),$$

since $F(a)$ is a constant and has derivative zero. In other words, the odd looking function

$$G(x) = \int_a^x f(t)\,dt$$

has a derivative, and in fact $G'(x) = f(x)$. This is really just a restatement of the Fundamental Theorem of Calculus, and indeed is often called the Fundamental Theorem of Calculus, Part Ⅱ. To avoid confusion, some people call the two versions of the theorem "The Fundamental Theorem of Calculus, part Ⅰ" and "The Fundamental Theorem of Calculus, part Ⅱ", although unfortunately there is no universal agreement as to which is part Ⅰ and which part Ⅱ. Since it really is the same theorem, differently stated, some people simply call them both "Fundamental Theorem of Calculus (FTC)".

> **Theorem 6.4 (Fundamental Theorem of Calculus, Part Ⅱ)**
>
> *Suppose that f(x) is continuous on the interval* $[a, b]$ *and let*
> $$G(x) = \int_a^x f(t)\,dt,$$
> *then* $G'(x) = f(x)$.

Proof The integral $G(x) = \int_a^x f(t)\,dt$ may be interpreted as the signed area under $f(x)$, above the x-axis, and between a and x (Figure 6.21(a)).

To compute $G'(x)$, we start with the definition of the derivative in terms of a limit:

$$G'(x) = \lim_{h \to 0} \frac{G(x+h) - G(x)}{h}$$

$$= \lim_{h \to 0} \frac{1}{h}\left[\int_a^{x+h} f(t)\,dt - \int_a^x f(t)\,dt\right]$$

$$= \lim_{h \to 0} \frac{1}{h} \left[\int_a^x f(t) dt + \int_x^{x+h} f(t) dt - \int_a^x f(t) dt \right]$$

$$= \lim_{h \to 0} \frac{1}{h} \int_x^{x+h} f(t) dt .$$

To evaluate

$$\int_x^{x+h} f(t) dt ,$$

we interpret $\int_x^{x+h} f(t) dt$ as the signed area between x and $x+h$ (Figure 6.21(b)). When h is very small, this area will be very close to the area of the rectangle with base h and height $f(x)$. The signed area of this rectangle is $hf(x)$. Hence,

$$\lim_{h \to 0} \frac{1}{h} \int_x^{x+h} f(t) dt = \lim_{h \to 0} \frac{hf(x)}{h} = f(x)$$

which is what we wanted to show. In addition, we see that $G(x)$ is continuous, since it is differentiable. #

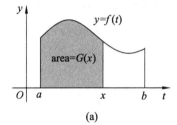 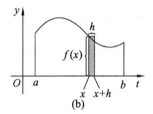

(a)   (b)

Figure 6.21

It is still true that we are depending on a geometric intuition to justify the argument, but we have isolated this part of the argument into two facts that are not too hard to prove. Once the last reference to interpretation has been removed from the proofs of these facts, we will have a real proof of the Fundamental Theorem. To show how one can make this argument mathematically rigourous, we present the complete proof of this result.

Proof of Theorem 6.3   We know from Theorem 6.4 that $G(x) = \int_a^x f(t) dt$ is an antiderivative of $f(x)$, and therefore any antiderivative $F(x)$ of $f(x)$ is of the form $F(x) = G(x) + C$. Then

$$F(b) - F(a) = G(b) + C - [G(a) + C] = G(b) - G(a) = \int_a^b f(t) dt - \int_a^a f(t) dt .$$

It is not hard to see that $\int_a^a f(t) dt = 0$, so this means that

$$F(b) - F(a) = \int_a^b f(t) dt,$$

which is exactly what Theorem 6.3 says. #

Note that the Fundamental Theorem does not define the definite integral; it is just provides a method for evaluating it. Also the Fundamental Theorem does not require $f(x) > 0$. When evaluating definite integrals, the symbol $F(x) \mid_a^b$ is used to denote the number $F(b)-F(a)$. The vertical line with subscript and superscript is used to indicate the operation "substitute and subtract" that is needed to finish the evaluation. For example, if $F(x)=x^4$, then $x^4 \mid_1^2$ means $F(2)-F(1)=2^4-1^4$. Some authors use other common notations such as $F(x)\mid_a^b$ and $[F(x)]_a^b$.

Example 6.14 Calculate $\int_1^3 e^x dx$.

Solution Note that $f(x)=e^x$ is continuous on $[1, 3]$. We need to find an antiderivative of $f(x)$. Note that FTC says we can use any antiderivative so we may use the simplest one $F(x)=e^x$, instead of $F(x)=e^x+2$ or $F(x)=e^x+C$. Then we must evaluate $F(3)-F(1)$:

$$F(3)=e^3, \ F(1)=e.$$

Therefore, the Fundamental Theorem gives

$$\int_1^3 e^x dx = F(3)-F(1)=e^3-e. \qquad \#$$

Example 6.15 Find the area under the parabola $y=x^2$ from 0 to 2.

Solution The required area A is the integral $\int_0^2 x^2 dx$. Since x^2 is continuous on $[0, 2]$ and $F(x)=\dfrac{1}{3}x^3$ is an antiderivative of x^2,

$$A = \int_0^2 x^2 dx = \left[\frac{x^3}{3}\right]_0^2 = \frac{2^3}{3} - \frac{0^3}{3} = \frac{8}{3}. \qquad \#$$

Always check that the integrand is continuous on the interval between the lower and the upper limit of integration. Errors may occur if you ignore the check step.

Example 6.16 What is wrong with the following calculation?

$$\int_{-1}^3 \frac{1}{x^2} dx = \left[\frac{x^{-1}}{-1}\right]_{-1}^3 = -\frac{1}{3} - 1 = -\frac{4}{3}.$$

Solution This calculation must be wrong because the answer is negative but $f(x)=\dfrac{1}{x^2}\geq 0$. The integral represents the area below the curve $y=f(x)$ and above the x-axis. The Fundamental Theorem of Calculus applies to continuous functions. It cannot be applied here because $f(x)=\dfrac{1}{x^2}$ is not continuous on $[-1, 3]$. In fact, f has an infinite discontinuity at 0, so $\int_{-1}^3 \dfrac{1}{x^2} dx$ does not exist. $\qquad \#$

Example 6.17 Evaluate $\int_3^6 \dfrac{dx}{x}$.

Solution Note that $\int_3^6 \dfrac{dx}{x} = \int_3^6 \dfrac{1}{x} dx$. An antiderivative of $f(x)=\dfrac{1}{x}$ is $F(x)=\ln|x|$, and because $3\leq x\leq 6$, we can write $F(x)=\ln x$. So

$$\int_3^6 \frac{1}{x} dx = [\ln x]_3^6 = \ln 6 - \ln 3 = \ln \frac{6}{3} = \ln 2. \qquad \#$$

Example 6.18 Given

$$f(x) = \begin{cases} 3x^2, & \text{if } x<1 \\ 2, & \text{if } x\geqslant 1 \end{cases}.$$

Evaluate each of the integral $\int_{-1}^{3} f(x)\mathrm{d}x$.

Solution   This function is not continuous at $x=1$ and $x=1$ is between the limits of integration. This means that the integrand is no longer continuous in the interval of integration and we simply cannot integrate functions that are not continuous in the interval of integration.

Also, even if the function was continuous at $x=1$ we would still have the problem that the function is actually two different equations depending where we are in the interval of integration.

Recalling the Additive Interval Rule, we can write the integral as follows,

$$\int_{-1}^{3} f(x)\mathrm{d}x = \int_{-1}^{1} f(x)\mathrm{d}x + \int_{1}^{3} f(x)\mathrm{d}x .$$

On each of these intervals the function is continuous. So, to integrate a piecewise function, all we need to do is to break up the integral at the break point(s) that happen to occur in the interval of integration and then integrate each piece. The integral in this case is then

$$\begin{aligned} \int_{-1}^{3} f(x)\mathrm{d}x &= \int_{-1}^{1} f(x)\mathrm{d}x + \int_{1}^{3} f(x)\mathrm{d}x \\ &= \int_{-1}^{1} 3x^2\,\mathrm{d}x + \int_{1}^{3} 2\mathrm{d}x \\ &= x^3\,|_{-1}^{1} + 2x\,|_{1}^{3} = 6. \end{aligned} \qquad \#$$

Your Practice 6.6   Evaluate $\int_{1}^{3}\left(4x - 2e^x + \dfrac{5}{x}\right)\mathrm{d}x$.

Example 6.19   The blood flux (volume of blood that passes through the blood vessel, Figure 6.22) is measured by

$$F = \int_{0}^{R} \frac{\pi P}{2\eta l} r(R^2 - r^2)\mathrm{d}r ,$$

where η is the viscosity of the blood, P is the pressure difference between the ends of the tube and l is the length. Integrate F.

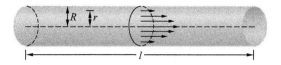

Figure 6.22   Blood vessel

Solution   The Fundamental Theorem gives

$$F = \frac{\pi P}{2\eta l}\int_{0}^{R}(R^2 r - r^3)\mathrm{d}r = \frac{\pi P}{2\eta l}\left[R^2\,\frac{r^2}{2} - \frac{r^4}{4}\right]_{0}^{R}$$

$$= \frac{\pi P}{2\eta l}\left[\frac{R^4}{2} - \frac{R^4}{4}\right] = \frac{\pi P R^4}{8\eta l}.$$

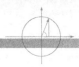

The final equation

$$F = \frac{\pi P R^4}{8\eta l}$$

is known as the Poiseuille's Law. It shows that the flux is proportional to the fourth power of the radius of the blood vessel.   #

There are a couple of nice facts about integrating even and odd functions over a symmetric interval $[a, b]$. For the graph of an odd function, the area between the curve and the horizontal axis to the left of $x=0$ is exactly the same as the area between the curve and the horizontal axis to the right of $x=0$, but opposite in sign.

> *If $f(x)$ is an odd function, then*
> $$\int_{-a}^{a} f(x)\,dx = 0.$$

However, for the graph of a typical even function, the area between the curve and the horizontal axis to the left of $x=0$ is again exactly the same as the area between the curve and the horizontal axis to the right of $x=0$, but unlike the case for odd functions, it has the same sign. Thus we have

> *If $f(x)$ is an even function, then*
> $$\int_{-a}^{a} f(x)\,dx = 2\int_{0}^{a} f(x)\,dx.$$

Note that in order to use these facts the limit of integration must be the same number, but opposite signs!

Example 6.20   Evaluate the following definite integrals.

(1) $\displaystyle\int_{-4}^{4} x^{2021}\,dx$;

(2) $\displaystyle\int_{-\frac{\pi}{2}}^{\frac{\pi}{2}} \cos x\,dx$.

Solution

(1) Since x^{2021} is odd and $[-4, 4]$ is symmetric, then $\displaystyle\int_{-4}^{4} x^{2021}\,dx = 0$.

(2) $\displaystyle\int_{-\frac{\pi}{2}}^{\frac{\pi}{2}} \cos x\,dx = 0$ because $\cos x$ is an even function and the integral interval is symmetric.   #

Example 6.21   Compute

$$\frac{d}{dx}\int_{1}^{x} (t^2 - e^t)\,dt$$

for $x > 1$.

Solution   First, note that $f(x) = x^2 - e^x$ is continuous for $x \geq 1$. If we set $G(x) = \int_{1}^{x} (t^2 - e^t)\,dt$ and apply the FTC, then

$$\frac{d}{dx} G(x) = \frac{d}{dx}\int_{1}^{x} (t^2 - e^t)\,dt = x^2 - e^x .$$ #

Example 6.22   Compute

$$\frac{\mathrm{d}}{\mathrm{d}x}\int_0^{x^2} (t^3 - 4)\,\mathrm{d}t .$$

Solution   Note that the upper limit of the integration is a function of x. We set $G(u) = \int_1^u (t^3 - 4)\,\mathrm{d}t$, $u > 0$. Then for $x > 0$,

$$G(x^2) = \int_0^{x^2} (t^3 - 4)\,\mathrm{d}t .$$

We wish to compute $\frac{\mathrm{d}}{\mathrm{d}x}G(x^2)$. To do so, we need to apply the Chain Rule. We set $u = x^2$, then

$$\frac{\mathrm{d}}{\mathrm{d}x} G(x^2) = \frac{\mathrm{d}G(u)}{\mathrm{d}u}\frac{\mathrm{d}u}{\mathrm{d}x}.$$

To compute $\dfrac{\mathrm{d}G(u)}{\mathrm{d}u} = \dfrac{\mathrm{d}}{\mathrm{d}u}\displaystyle\int_1^u (t^3 - 4)\,\mathrm{d}t$, we use the Fundamental Theorem of calculus:

$$\frac{\mathrm{d}}{\mathrm{d}u}\int_1^u (t^3 - 4)\,\mathrm{d}t = u^3 - 4 .$$

Since $\dfrac{\mathrm{d}u}{\mathrm{d}x} = \dfrac{\mathrm{d}x^2}{\mathrm{d}x} = 2x$, we find that

$$\frac{\mathrm{d}}{\mathrm{d}x} G(x^2) = (u^3 - 4) \cdot 2x$$

$$= 2x(x^6 - 4). \qquad\qquad \#$$

Exercise 6.4

1. Evaluate the integrals.

(1) $\displaystyle\int_1^4 (5x + 3)\,\mathrm{d}x$;

(2) $\displaystyle\int_0^1 e^x\,\mathrm{d}x$;

(3) $\displaystyle\int_1^5 \frac{2}{x}\,\mathrm{d}x$;

(4) $\displaystyle\int_5^2 (2x + 9)\,\mathrm{d}x$;

(5) $\displaystyle\int_1^4 3\sqrt{x}\,\mathrm{d}x$;

(6) $\displaystyle\int_4^{25} \frac{2}{\sqrt{x}}\,\mathrm{d}x$.

2. Find $\dfrac{\mathrm{d}y}{\mathrm{d}x}$.

(1) $y = \displaystyle\int_0^x \sqrt{3 + t}\,\mathrm{d}t$, $x > 0$;

(2) $y = \displaystyle\int_1^x u e^{u^2}\,\mathrm{d}u$;

(3) $y = \displaystyle\int_0^{x^2} \sqrt{u}\,\mathrm{d}u$, $x > 0$;

(4) $y = \displaystyle\int_2^{\ln x} e^{-t}\,\mathrm{d}t$, $x > 0$;

(5) $y = \displaystyle\int_x^5 \frac{1}{t^2}\,\mathrm{d}t$, $x > 0$;

(6) $y = \displaystyle\int_{x^2}^{x^3} \ln t\,\mathrm{d}t$, $x > 0$.

3. Compute

(1) $\displaystyle\lim_{x \to 0} \frac{1}{x^2}\int_0^x \sin t\,\mathrm{d}t$;

(2) $\displaystyle\lim_{h \to 0} \frac{1}{h}\int_0^h e^x\,\mathrm{d}x$.

4. Suppose that $\displaystyle\int_0^x f(t)\,\mathrm{d}t = 2x^2$, find $f(x)$.

5. Suppose that $\int_0^x f(t)\,\mathrm{d}t = \dfrac{1}{2}\tan(2x)$.

Find $f(x)$.

6.5 The Substitution Rule

To apply the Fundamental Theorem of Calculus we must find an antiderivative, and this is not always easy. It is not surprising that some integration techniques are closely related to differential rule because of the connection between differentiation and integration.

In this section we examine the Substitution Rule, which is the Chain Rule backwards, to help us find antiderivatives.

6.5.1 Substitution with Indefinite Integrals

Consider the Chain Rule

$$\{f\,[g(x)]\}' = f'[g(x)]\,g'(x).$$

Integrating both sides gives

$$\int f'[g(x)]\,g'(x)\mathrm{d}x = f\,[g(x)] + C.$$

The formula forms the basis for a method of integration called the ***substitution method***.

Theorem 6.5 (Substitution with Indefinite Integrals)

Let $u = g(x)$, where $g'(x)$ is continuous over an interval, let $f(x)$ be continuous over the corresponding range of g, and let $F(x)$ be an antiderivative of $f(x)$. Then

$$\int f\,[g(x)]\,g'(x)\mathrm{d}x = \int f(u)\,\mathrm{d}u$$
$$= F(u) + C$$
$$= F[g(x)] + C.$$

The method is called substitution because we substitute part of the integrand with the variable u and part of the integrand with $\mathrm{d}u$. It is also referred to as change of variables because we are changing variables to obtain an expression easier to work with for applying the integration rules.

Proof　Let f, g, u, and F be as specified in the theorem, then

$$\frac{\mathrm{d}}{\mathrm{d}x}F\,[g(x)] = F'[g(x)]g'(x) = f\,[g(x)]g'(x).$$

Integrating both sides with respect to x, we see that

$$\int f[g(x)]g'(x)\mathrm{d}x = F[g(x)] + C.$$

If we now substitute $u = g(x)$, and $\mathrm{d}u = g'(x)\mathrm{d}x$, we get

$$\int f[g(x)]\,g'(x)\mathrm{d}x = \int f(u)\mathrm{d}u = F(u) + C = F[g(x)] + C.$$

Example 6.23   Evaluate $\int (x^2 - 4)^3 x \mathrm{d}x$.

Solution   We let $u = x^2 - 4$ and then $\mathrm{d}u = 2x\mathrm{d}x$. We need to adjust the constants in our integral since they do not match up exactly with the expressions we are substituting. Rewrite the integral in terms of u:

$$\int (x^2 - 4)^3 x \mathrm{d}x = \frac{1}{2}\int (x^2 - 4)^3 (2x)\mathrm{d}x = \frac{1}{2}\int u^3 \mathrm{d}u.$$

Using the Power Rule for integrals, we have

$$\int u^3 \mathrm{d}u = \frac{u^4}{4} + C_1.$$

Substitute the original expression for x back into the solution, we have

$$\int (x^2 - 4)^3 x \mathrm{d}x = \frac{(x^2 - 3)^4}{8} + C.$$ #

> **Strategy for Integration by Substitution**
>
> (1) *Select an expression $g(x)$ within the integrand to be u such that $g'(x)$ is also part of the integrand.*
>
> (2) *Substitute $u = g(x)$ and $\mathrm{d}u = g'(x)\mathrm{d}x$ into the integral.*
>
> (3) *Evaluate the integral with respect to u.*
>
> (4) *Write the result in terms of x and the expression $g(x)$.*

Example 6.24   Use substitution to find the antiderivative of $\int 6x^2 (2x^3 - 4)^4 \mathrm{d}x$.

Solution   The first step is to choose an expression for u. We choose $u = 2x^3 - 4$ then $\mathrm{d}u = 6x^2 \mathrm{d}x$ and we already have $\mathrm{d}u$ in the integrand. Write the integral in terms of u:

$$\int 6x^2 (2x^3 - 4)^4 \mathrm{d}x = \int u^4 \mathrm{d}u.$$

Remember that $\mathrm{d}u$ is the derivative of the expression chosen for u, regardless of what is inside the integrand. Now we can evaluate the integral with respect to u:

$$\int u^4 \mathrm{d}u = \frac{u^5}{5} + C = \frac{(2x^3 - 4)^5}{5} + C.$$

We can check our answer by taking the derivative for the result of integration. We should obtain the integrand. Let $y = \dfrac{(2x^3 - 4)^5}{5}$ then we have

$$y' = \frac{1}{5} \cdot 5(2x^3 - 4)^4 \cdot 6x^2 = 6x^2 (2x^3 - 4)^4$$

which is exactly the expression we started with inside the integrand.   #

Your Practice 6.7   Use substitution to find the antiderivative of $\int 3x^2 (x^3 + 5)^6 \mathrm{d}x$.

Example 6.25   Use substitution to evaluate the integral $\int \dfrac{\sin t}{\cos^4 t} \mathrm{d}t$.

Solution   We know the derivative of $\cos t$ is $-\sin t$, so we set $u = \cos t$. Then $\mathrm{d}u = -\sin t \mathrm{d}t$. Substituting into the integral, we have

$$\int \frac{\sin t}{\cos^4 t}dt = -\int \frac{1}{u^4}du .$$

Evaluating the integral, we get

$$-\int \frac{1}{u^4}du = -\int u^{-4}du = -\left(-\frac{1}{3}\right)u^{-3} + C .$$

Putting the answer back in terms of t, we get

$$\int \frac{\sin t}{\cos^4 t}dt = \frac{1}{3\cos^3 t} + C . \qquad\qquad \#$$

Your Practice 6.8 Use substitution to evaluate the integral $\int \frac{\cos t}{\sin^3 t}dt$.

6.5.2 Substitution for Definite Integrals

Substitution can be used with definite integrals, too. However, using substitution to evaluate a definite integral requires a change to the limits of integration. If we change variables in the integrand, the limits of integration change as well.

Theorem 6.6 (Substitution for Definite Integrals)

Let $u = g(x)$, *where $g'(x)$ is continuous over an interval, let $f(x)$ be continuous over the corresponding range of g, and let $f(x)$ be an antiderivative of $f(x)$. Then*

$$\int_a^b f[g(x)]g'(x)dx = \int_{g(a)}^{g(b)} f(u)du.$$

We justify this theorem with some calculations here. From the substitution rule for indefinite integrals, if $F(x)$ is an antiderivative of $f(x)$, we have

$$\int f[g(x)]g'(x)dx = F[g(x)] + C .$$

Then

$$\int_a^b f[g(x)]g'(x)dx = F[g(x)]\Big|_a^b$$

$$= F[g(b)] - F[g(a)]$$

$$= F[g(u)]\Big|_{g(a)}^{g(b)}$$

$$= \int_{g(a)}^{g(b)} f(u)du$$

and we have the desired result.

Example 6.26 Use substitution to evaluate $\int_0^1 x^3 (5x^4 - 2)^3 dx$.

Solution Let $u = 5x^4 - 2$, so $du = 20x^3 dx$. Since the original function includes one factor of x^3 and $du = 20x^3 dx$, multiply both sides of the du equation by $1/20$. Then, $du = 20x^3 dx$ becomes $\frac{1}{20}du = x^3 dx$.

To adjust the limits of integration, note that when $x=0, u=-2$, and when $x=1, u=3$. Then

$$\int_0^1 x^3 (5x^4 - 2)^3 dx = \frac{1}{20}\int_{-2}^3 u^3 du .$$

Evaluating this expression, we get

$$\frac{1}{20}\int_{-2}^{3} u^3 \, du = \frac{1}{20} \cdot \frac{1}{4} u^4 \bigg|_{-2}^{3} = \frac{13}{16}.$$ #

Example 6.27   Use substitution to evaluate $\displaystyle\int_{0}^{1} x e^{x^2-1} \, dx$.

Solution   Let $u = x^2 - 1$. Then, $du = 2x \, dx$. To adjust the limits of integration, we note that when $x=0$, $u=-1$, and when $x=1$, $u=0$. So our substitution gives

$$\int_{0}^{1} x e^{x^2-1} \, dx = \frac{1}{2}\int_{-1}^{0} e^u \, du = \frac{1}{2} e^u \bigg|_{-1}^{0} = \frac{e-1}{2e}.$$ #

Substitution may be only one of the techniques needed to evaluate a definite integral. All of the properties and rules of integration apply independently, and trigonometric functions may need to be rewritten using a trigonometric identity before we can apply substitution. Also, we have the option of replacing the original expression for u after we find the antiderivative, which means that we do not have to change the limits of integration. These two approaches are shown in the following example.

Example 6.28   Use substitution to evaluate $\displaystyle\int_{0}^{\frac{\pi}{2}} \sin^2 \theta \, d\theta$.

Solution   First let us use a trigonometric identity to rewrite the integral. The Trig Identity $\sin^2\theta = \dfrac{1-\cos 2\theta}{2}$ allows us to rewrite the integral as

$$\int_{0}^{\frac{\pi}{2}} \frac{1-\cos 2\theta}{2} \, d\theta.$$

Then,

$$\int_{0}^{\frac{\pi}{2}} \frac{1-\cos 2\theta}{2} \, d\theta = \frac{1}{2}\int_{0}^{\frac{\pi}{2}} d\theta - \frac{1}{2}\int_{0}^{\frac{\pi}{2}} \cos 2\theta \, d\theta.$$

We can evaluate the first integral as it is, but we need to make a substitution to evaluate the second integral. Let $u = 2\theta$. Then, $du = 2 \, d\theta$, or $\dfrac{1}{2} du = d\theta$. Also, when $\theta = 0$, $u=0$, and when $\theta = \dfrac{\pi}{2}$, $u = \pi$. Expressing the second integral in terms of u, we have

$$\frac{1}{2}\int_{0}^{\frac{\pi}{2}} d\theta - \frac{1}{2}\int_{0}^{\frac{\pi}{2}} \cos 2\theta \, d\theta = \frac{1}{2}\int_{0}^{\frac{\pi}{2}} d\theta - \frac{1}{2} \cdot \frac{1}{2}\int_{0}^{\pi} \cos u \, du$$

$$= \frac{\theta}{2}\bigg|_{0}^{\pi/2} - \frac{1}{4}\sin u \bigg|_{0}^{\pi}$$

$$= \frac{\pi}{4}.$$ #

Your Practice 6.9   Evaluate $\displaystyle\int_{0}^{\frac{\pi}{2}} \cos^2 \theta \, d\theta$.

1. Write the functions in the brackets such that the identity holds.

(1) $x\mathrm{d}x=\mathrm{d}($);

(2) $\mathrm{e}^x\mathrm{d}x=\mathrm{d}($);

(3) $n\neq-1$, $x^n\mathrm{d}x=\mathrm{d}($);

(4) $k\neq0$, $\mathrm{e}^{kx+b}\mathrm{d}x=\mathrm{d}($);

(5) $\dfrac{1}{x}\mathrm{d}x=\mathrm{d}($);

(6) $\dfrac{1}{x-k}\mathrm{d}x=\mathrm{d}($).

2. Use substitution to evaluate the indefinite integral.

(1) $\displaystyle\int \cos^3 t \sin t\,\mathrm{d}t$;

(2) $\displaystyle\int_0^1 \dfrac{x^3}{x^4+2}\,\mathrm{d}x$;

(3) $\displaystyle\int_0^1 (2x+1)^4\,\mathrm{d}x$;

(4) $\displaystyle\int_{-2}^3 (3x-8)^9\,\mathrm{d}x$;

(5) $\displaystyle\int_0^1 (5x^3-1)^3 x^2\,\mathrm{d}x$;

(6) $\displaystyle\int_0^1 (x^2-1)^4 x\,\mathrm{d}x$;

(7) $\displaystyle\int_0^1 \dfrac{2x}{x^2+1}\,\mathrm{d}x$;

(8) $\displaystyle\int_0^1 x\mathrm{e}^{4x^2+3}\,\mathrm{d}x$.

3. Use the fact that $\cot x=\dfrac{\cos x}{\sin x}$ to evaluate

$$\int \cot x\,\mathrm{d}x.$$

6.6 Integration by Parts

Integration by parts is the Product Rule in integral form. We start with the Product Rule:

$$\frac{\mathrm{d}}{\mathrm{d}x}[f(x)g(x)]=f'(x)g(x)+f(x)g'(x).$$

We can apply integration to this equation and obtain

$$f(x)g(x)=\int f'(x)g(x)\mathrm{d}x+\int f(x)g'(x)\mathrm{d}x$$

and then rewrite this as

$$\int f(x)g'(x)\mathrm{d}x=f(x)g(x)-\int f'(x)g(x)\mathrm{d}x.$$

This may not seem particularly useful at first glance, but it turns out that in many cases we have an integral of the form $\int f(x)g'(x)\mathrm{d}x$ but that $\int f'(x)g(x)\mathrm{d}x$ is easier to integrate.

This technique for turning one integral into another is called ***Integration by Parts***, and is usually written in more compact form.

Theorem 6.7 (Integration by Parts)

Let u and v be differentiable functions, then

$$\int u\,dv = uv - \int v\,du$$

where $u = f(x)$ and $v = g(x)$ so that $du = f'(x)dx$ and $dv = g'(x)dx$.

To use this technique we need to identify likely candidates for $u = f(x)$ and $dv = g'(x)dx$. When choosing u and dv, keep in mind that we need to be able to readily find an antiderivative for dv and that du becomes simpler than u. Simpler could mean the power is reduced by one degree, or the original integral appears on the right side, etc.

After we have applied Integration by Parts, we then need to integrate $\int v\,du$. There is a danger to fall into a circular trap by choosing as the part to integrate (v) the term in the differential (du) from the first application of Integration by Parts. This does not provide us with any new information, instead brings us back to the original integral. For example, to evaluate $\int x^2 \sin x\,dx$, we choose

$$u = x^2 \text{ and } v = \sin x \text{ so that } du = 2x\,dx \text{ and } dv = -\cos x\,dx,$$

then

$$\int x^2 \sin x\,dx = -x^2\cos x + 2\int x\cos x\,dx.$$

If we ignore that the new integral is simpler than the original integral, which would tell us to continue in the same manner of selecting u and dv, we may fall into the circular trap of choosing

$$u = \cos x \text{ and } v = \frac{x^2}{2} \text{ so that } du = -\sin x\,dx \text{ and } dv = x\,dx,$$

so that

$$\int x^2 \sin x\,dx = -x^2\cos x + 2\int x\cos x\,dx$$

$$= -x^2\cos x + 2\left(\frac{x^2}{2}\cos x + \int \frac{x^2}{2}\sin x\,dx\right)$$

$$= \int x^2 \sin x\,dx.$$

This shows that with our carelessness we have wasted our time and are back at the beginning.

Example 6.29 Evaluate $\int x\ln x\,dx$.

Solution Let $u = \ln x$ so $du = \frac{1}{x}dx$. Then we must let $dv = x\,dx$ so $v = \frac{1}{2}x^2$ and

$$\int x\ln x\,dx = \frac{1}{2}x^2\ln x - \int \frac{1}{2}x^2 \cdot \frac{1}{x}dx = \frac{1}{2}x^2\ln x - \frac{1}{4}x^2 + C. \qquad \#$$

Your Practice 6.10 Evaluate $\int \ln x\,dx$.

Example 6.30 Evaluate $\int x^2 e^x dx$.

Solution Let $u = x^2$ so $du = 2x dx$. Then we must let $dv = e^x dx$ so $v = e^x$ and

$$\int x^2 e^x dx = x^2 e^x - \int 2x e^x dx .$$

To evaluate the integral $\int x e^x dx$, we must use Integration by Parts for a second time.

We set $u = x$ so $du = dx$. Then we must let $dv = e^x dx$ so $v = e^x$ and

$$\int x e^x dx = x e^x - \int e^x dx = x e^x - e^x + C_1 .$$

Combine these two equations above, we find

$$\int x^2 e^x dx = x^2 e^x - 2(x e^x - e^x + C_1) = x^2 e^x - 2x e^x + 2e^x + C$$

where $C = -2C_1$. #

Your Practice 6.11 Evaluate $\int x e^x dx$.

The following example shows using Integration by Parts repeatedly.

Example 6.31 Evaluate $\int e^x \cos x dx$.

Solution You can check that it does not matter which of the function you call u and v'. We set

$$u = \cos x \text{ and } dv = e^x dx,$$

then

$$u' = -\sin x \text{ and } v = e^x.$$

Therefore,

$$\int e^x \cos x dx = e^x \cos x + \int e^x \sin x dx. \tag{6.1}$$

We apply the Integration by Parts for a second time, with

$$u = \sin x \text{ and } dv = e^x dx.$$

Then

$$u' = \cos x \text{ and } v = e^x.$$

Therefore,

$$\int e^x \sin x dx = e^x \sin x - \int e^x \cos x dx. \tag{6.2}$$

Combining (6.1) and (6.2) yields

$$\int e^x \cos x dx = e^x \cos x + e^x \sin x - \int e^x \cos x dx.$$

We see that the integral $\int e^x \cos x dx$ appears on both sides. Rearranging the equation, we get

$$2\int e^x \cos x dx = e^x \cos x + e^x \sin x + C_1.$$

or

$$\int e^x \cos x \mathrm{d}x = \frac{1}{2} e^x (\cos x + \sin x) + C$$

with $C = \dfrac{C_1}{2}$. 　　　　　　　　　　　　　　　　　　　　　 #

We present a piece of practical advise: In integrals of the form $\int P(x) \sin ax \mathrm{d}x$, $\int P(x) \cos ax \mathrm{d}x$, and $\int P(x) e^{ax} \mathrm{d}x$, where $P(x)$ is a polynomial and a is a constant, the polynomial $P(x)$ should be considered as u and the expressions $\sin ax$, $\cos ax$, and e^{ax} as v'.

Your Practice 6.12 Evaluate $\int e^x \sin x \mathrm{d}x$.

Example 6.32 Evaluate $\int_0^1 x e^{-x} \mathrm{d}x$.

Solution We set
$$u = x \text{ and } \mathrm{d}v = e^{-x} \mathrm{d}x,$$
then
$$\mathrm{d}u = \mathrm{d}x \text{ and } v = -e^{-x}.$$
Therefore

$$
\begin{aligned}
\int_0^1 x e^{-x} \mathrm{d}x &= -x e^{-x} \Big|_0^1 - \int_0^1 (-e^{-x}) \mathrm{d}x \\
&= -1 \cdot e^{-1} - (-0 \cdot e^{-0}) + \int_0^1 e^{-x} \mathrm{d}x \\
&= -e^{-1} + [-e^{-x}]_0^1 = -e^{-1} + [-e^{-1} - (-e^{-0})] \\
&= -e^{-1} - e^{-1} + 1 = 1 - 2e^{-1}.
\end{aligned}
$$
　　　　　　　　　　　　　　　　　　　　　　　　　　　　 #

Exercise 6.6

Evaluate the integrals in Problems 1—10 by using Integration by Parts.

1. $\int x e^{x^2} \mathrm{d}x$.

2. $\int x \cos x \mathrm{d}x$.

3. $\int x \sec^2 x \mathrm{d}x$.

4. $\int x^2 \sin 2x \mathrm{d}x$.

5. $\int x^2 \cos x \mathrm{d}x$.

6. $\int x \sin 2x \mathrm{d}x$.

7. $\int_1^2 \ln x \mathrm{d}x$.

8. $\int_0^3 x^2 e^{-x} \mathrm{d}x$.

9. $\int_0^{\pi/3} x \sin x \mathrm{d}x$.

10. $\int_1^4 \sqrt{x} \ln \sqrt{x} \mathrm{d}x$.

11. Evaluating the integral $\int \cos^2 x \mathrm{d}x$ requires two steps. First, write $\cos^2 x$ as $\cos x \cdot \cos x$ and apply Integration by Parts to show that

$$\int \cos^2 x \mathrm{d}x = \sin x \cos x + \int \sin^2 x \mathrm{d}x.$$

Then, use $\sin^2 x + \cos^2 x = 1$ to replace $\sin^2 x$ in the integral on the right hand side, and complete the integration of $\int \cos^2 x \, dx$.

12. Evaluating the integral $\int \sin^2 x \, dx$ require two steps. First, write $\sin^2 x$ as $\sin x \cdot \sin x$ and apply Integration by Parts to show that

$$\int \sin^2 x \, dx = -\sin x \cos x + \int \cos^2 x \, dx.$$

Then, use $\sin^2 x + \cos^2 x = 1$ to replace $\cos^2 x$ in the integral on the right hand side, and complete the integration of $\int \sin^2 x \, dx$.

13. Use Integration by Parts to show that for $x > 0$,

$$\int \frac{1}{x} \ln x \, dx = (\ln x)^2 - \int \frac{1}{x} \ln x \, dx.$$

Then use this result to evaluate

$$\int \frac{1}{x} \ln x \, dx.$$

14. Use Integration by Parts to show that

$$\int x^n e^x \, dx = x^n e^x - n \int x^{n-1} e^x \, dx.$$

Such formulas are called reduction formula since they reduce the exponent of x by 1 each time they are applied. Then apply the reduction formula to compute

$$\int x^3 e^x \, dx.$$

15. Use Integration by Parts to show the reduction formula

$$\int x^n e^{ax} \, dx = \frac{1}{a} x^n e^{ax} - \frac{n}{a} \int x^{n-1} e^{ax} \, dx$$

where a $(a \neq 0)$ is a constant. Then compute

$$\int x^2 e^{-3x} \, dx.$$

16. Use Integration by Parts to show the reduction formula

$$\int (\ln x)^n \, dx = x(\ln x)^n - n \int (\ln x)^{n-1} \, dx.$$

Then compute

$$\int (\ln x)^3 \, dx.$$

Summary and Review

Key Concepts

- A function F is an antiderivative of the function f if $F'(x) = f(x)$ for all x in the domain of f.
- If F is an antiderivative of f, then every antiderivative of f is of the form $F(x) + C$ for some constant C.
- Solving the initial-value problem

$$\frac{dy}{dx} = f(x), \quad y(x_0) = y_0$$

requires us to find the set of antiderivatives of f and then to look for the particular antiderivative that also satisfies the initial condition.

- $\int_a^b f(x) \, dx$ denotes the definite integral of f over $[a, b]$, and this quantity is defined by the equation

$$\int_a^b f(x) \, dx = \lim_{n \to \infty} \sum_{i=1}^n f(x_i) \Delta x,$$

where $\Delta x = \dfrac{b-a}{n}$, $x_i = a + i\Delta x$ (for $i = 0, 1, \cdots, n$), and x_i satisfies $x_{i-1} \leqslant x_i \leqslant x_{i+1}$ (for $i = 1, \cdots, n$).

- The definite integral $\displaystyle\int_a^b f(x)\mathrm{d}x$ measures the exact net signed area bounded by f and the horizontal axis on $[a, b]$.

- For a velocity function v, $\displaystyle\int_a^b v(t)\mathrm{d}t$ measures the exact change in position of the moving object on $[a, b]$; when v is nonnegative, $\displaystyle\int_a^b v(t)\mathrm{d}t$ is the object's distance traveled on $[a, b]$.

- Substitution is a technique that simplifies the integration of functions that are the result of a Chain-Rule derivative. The term "substitution" refers to changing variables or substituting the variable u and $\mathrm{d}u$ for appropriate expressions in the integrand.

- When using substitution for a definite integral, we also have to change the limits of integration.

- Integration by Parts is the Product Rule in integral form.

Important Formulas

Differentiation Formulas

$$\frac{\mathrm{d}}{\mathrm{d}x}k = 0, \qquad \frac{\mathrm{d}}{\mathrm{d}x}x^n = nx^{n-1},$$

$$[cf(x)]' = cf'(x), \qquad [f(x) \pm g(x)]' = f'(x) \pm g'(x).$$

Properties of Indefinite Integrals

- $\displaystyle\int x^n \mathrm{d}x = \frac{1}{n+1}x^{n+1} + C,\ n \neq -1.$

- $\displaystyle\int \frac{1}{x}\mathrm{d}x = \ln|x| + C.$

- $\displaystyle\int e^x \mathrm{d}x = e^x + C.$

- $\displaystyle\int kf(x)\mathrm{d}x = k \int f(x)\mathrm{d}x.$

- $\displaystyle\int [f(x) \pm g(x)]\mathrm{d}x = \int f(x)\mathrm{d}x \pm \int g(x)\mathrm{d}x.$

Fundamental Theorem of Calculus

Suppose f is continuous on the interval $[a, b]$, then

$$\int_a^b f(x)\mathrm{d}x = F(b) - F(a)$$

where F is any antiderivative of f, that is, a function such that $F' = f$.

Fundamental Theorem of Calculus

Suppose that $f(x)$ is continuous on the interval $[a, b]$ and let

$$G(x) = \int_a^x f(t)\,dt,$$

then $G'(x) = f(x)$.

- Substitution with indefinite integrals:

$$\int f'[g(x)]g'(x)\,dx = \int f(u)\,du = F(u) + C = f[g(x)] + C.$$

- Integration by Parts:

$$\int u\,dv = uv - \int v\,du.$$

- Substitution for Definite integrals:

$$\int_a^b f[g(x)]g'(x)\,dx = \int_{g(a)}^{g(b)} f(u)\,du.$$

Glossary

- Antiderivative. A function F such that $F'(x) = f(x)$ for all x in the domain of f is an antiderivative of f.
- Indefinite integral. The most general antiderivative of $f(x)$ is the indefinite integral of f; we use the notation $\int f(x)\,dx$ to denote the indefinite integral of f.
- Initial-value problem. A problem that requires finding a function y that satisfies the differential equation $\dfrac{dy}{dx} = f(x)$ together with the initial condition $y(x_0) = y_0$.
- Change of variables. The substitution of a variable, such as u, for an expression in the integrand.
- Integration by substitution. A technique for integration that allows integration of functions that are the result of a Chain-Rule derivative.

Chapter 7　Applications of Integration

∷ Introduction

In this chapter, we will discuss a couple of applications of integrals. We will be focusing on areas, cumulative change, and average function values. There are many other applications, however many of them require advanced integration techniques that are not typically taught in this course.

7.1　Area between Curves

In this section we are going to find the area between two curves. We are already familiar with the interpretation of integrals as areas. If f is a nonnegative, continuous function in $[a, b]$, then

$$A = \int_a^b f(x)\,\mathrm{d}x$$

represents the area of the region bounded by the graph of $f(x)$, the x-axis, and the vertical lines $x=a$ and $x=b$. We will now discuss how to find the positive areas between two arbitrary curves, that is, the x-axis may not be a boundary of the region. Please note that we want to calculate positive areas; that is, the areas we compute in this section will always be positive.

Suppose that $f(x)$ and $g(x)$ are continuous functions in $[a, b]$. We want to find the area between the graphs of f and g.

We start with a simple case (Figure 7.1). We assume here that both f and g are nonnegative in $[a, b]$ and that $f(x) \geqslant g(x)$ in $[a, b]$. From Figure 7.1 we see that

$$A = \begin{bmatrix} \text{area between} \\ y = f(x) \text{ and } x\text{-axis} \end{bmatrix} - \begin{bmatrix} \text{area between} \\ y = g(x) \text{ and } x\text{-axis} \end{bmatrix}$$

$$= \int_a^b f(x)\,\mathrm{d}x - \int_a^b g(x)\,\mathrm{d}x$$

$$= \int_a^b [f(x) - g(x)]\,\mathrm{d}x .$$

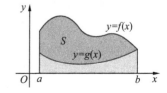

Figure 7.1

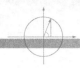

We now drop the assumption that both f and g are nonnegative in $[a, b]$. For this case (Figure 7.2), we can then obtain the same result. To derive the formula, we approximate the area by rectangles (Figure 7.3):

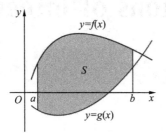

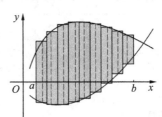

| Figure 7.2 | Figure 7.3 |

We split $[a, b]$ into n equal subin-tervals, each of length $\Delta x = \dfrac{b-a}{n}$. We choose an arbitrary point x in the subintervals to compute the heights of the approximating rectangles. From Figure 7.3, we see that the height of each rectangle is given by $f(x) - g(x)$ and the area of each rectangle is then $[f(x) - g(x)]\Delta x$. So, the area between the two curves is then approximated by

$$A \approx \sum_{i=1}^{n} [f(x) - g(x)]\Delta x .$$

The exact area is

$$A = \lim_{n \to \infty} \sum_{i=1}^{n} [f(x) - g(x)]\Delta x .$$

Now, recall the definition of the definite integral

$$A = \int_a^b [f(x) - g(x)]dx .$$

> *If f and g are continuous in $[a, b]$ and that $f(x) \geqslant g(x)$ for all $x \in [a, b]$, then the area of the region between the cures $y = f(x)$ and $y = g(x)$ from a to b is equal to*
> $$Area = \int_a^b [f(x) - g(x)]dx.$$

Example 7.1 Find the area between the curves $y = x^2 - 2$ and $y = -(x-1)^2 + 3$.

Solution We first sketch the boundary curves, as shown in Figure 7.4. The limits of integration for this will be the intersection points of the two curves. To find the points where the two curves intersect, we solve

$$x^2 - 2 = -(x-1)^2 + 3,$$
$$x^2 - 2 = -x^2 + 2x - 1 + 3,$$
$$2x^2 - 2x - 4 = 0,$$
$$2(x+1)(x-2) = 0.$$

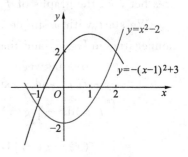

Figure 7.4

Therefore,

$$x = -1 \text{ and } x = 2$$

are the x-coordinates of the intersection points.

The area of the enclosed region is

$$\text{Area} = \int_{-1}^{2} [-(x-1)^2 + 3] - (x^2 - 2)\,dx$$

$$= \int_{-1}^{2} (-2x^2 + 2x + 4)\,dx$$

$$= \left[\frac{-2}{3}x^3 + x^2 + 4x\right]_{-1}^{2}$$

$$= \left(\frac{-16}{3} + 4 + 8\right) - \left(\frac{2}{3} + 1 - 4\right)$$

$$= 9. \qquad\qquad\#$$

When we compute the area of the region between two curves, we should always draw the bounding curves. This will help us to set up the appropriate integrals. Additional, we should note that the area formula always yields a nonnegative number, since it computes the positive area.

Your Practice 7.1   Find the area between the curves $y = x^2$ and $y = 3x + 4$.

Example 7.2   Determine the area of the region bounded by $y = 2x^2 + 10$, $y = 4x + 16$, $x = -2$ and $x = 5$.

Solution   In this case the last two pieces of information, $x = -2$ and $x = 5$, tell us the right and left boundaries of the region. The graph of this region is shown in Figure 7.5.

To find the intersection points, we solve

$$2x^2 + 10 = 4x + 16,$$

$$2x^2 - 4x - 6 = 0,$$

$$2(x+1)(x-3) = 0.$$

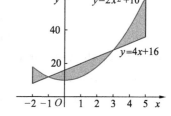

Figure 7.5

Therefore, the two curves exchange relative position at

$$x = -1 \text{ and } x = 3.$$

There are three regions in which one function is always the upper function and the other is always the lower function. So, all that we need to do is find to the area of each of the three regions, and then to add them up. Thus the area wanted is

$$\text{Area} = \int_{-2}^{-1} [2x^2 + 10 - (4x + 16)]\,dx + \int_{-1}^{3} [4x + 16 - (2x^2 + 10)]\,dx + \int_{3}^{5} [2x + 10 - (4x + 16)]\,dx$$

$$= \int_{-2}^{-1} (2x^2 - 4x - 6)\,dx + \int_{-1}^{3} (-2x^2 + 4x + 6)\,dx + \int_{3}^{5} (2x^2 - 4x - 6)\,dx$$

$$= \left[\frac{2}{3}x^3 - 2x^2 - 6x\right]_{-2}^{-1} + \left[-\frac{2}{3}x^3 + 2x^2 + 6x\right]_{-1}^{3} + \left[\frac{2}{3}x^3 - 2x^2 - 6x\right]_{3}^{5}$$

$$= \frac{14}{3} + \frac{64}{3} + \frac{64}{3} = \frac{142}{3}. \qquad\qquad\#$$

Sometimes we will be forced to work with functions in the form between $x = f(y)$ and

$x = g(y)$ on the interval $[c, d]$ (an interval of y values). When this happens, the derivation is identical. First we will start by assuming that $f(y) \geqslant g(y)$ on $[c, d]$. We can then divide up the interval into equal subintervals and build rectangles on each of these intervals (Figure 7.6).

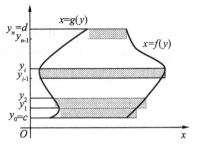

Following the work from above, we will arrive at the following formula for the area,

Figure 7.6

$$\text{Area} = \int_c^d [f(y) - g(y)] \, dy.$$

So, regardless of which form we use, the functions are in the same formula.

Example 7.3　Determine the area of the region enclosed by $x = \frac{1}{2} y^2 - 3$ and $y = x - 1$.

Solution　Firstly, we draw the bounding curves in Figure 7.7.

To have the intersection points, we solve the second equation for x and then setting them equal.

$$\frac{1}{2} y^2 - 3 = y + 1,$$

$$y^2 - 6 = 2y + 2,$$

$$y^2 - 2y - 8 = 0,$$

$$(y - 4)(y + 2) = 0.$$

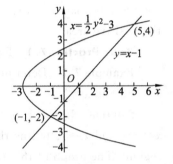

Figure 7.7

Therefore, the two curves intersect at $y = -2$ and $y = 4$ or in the full coordinates $(-1, -2)$ and $(5, 4)$.

Notice that there are two portions of the region that will have different lower function (Figure 7.8). When x is in the range $[-3, -1]$, the parabola is actually both the upper and the lower function. To use the formula referring to x, we need to solve the parabola for y. This gives

$$y = \pm \sqrt{2x + 6}$$

where the "$+$" sign gives the upper portion of the parabola and the "$-$" sign gives the lower portion.

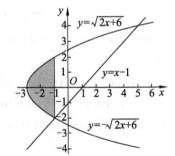

Figure 7.8

To compute the area, we need to split the integral into two parts:

$$A = \int_{-3}^{-1} [\sqrt{2x + 6} - (-\sqrt{2x + 6})] \, dx + \int_{-1}^{5} [\sqrt{2x + 6} - (x - 1)] \, dx.$$

While these integrals are more difficult than they should be. In this case the right boundary is always one function and the left boundary is the other. So we choose the vertical coordinate y to be the integration variable. We must rewrite the equation of the line in the form of $x = f(y)$. The area is then

$$A = \int_{-2}^{4} \left[(y+1) - \left(\frac{1}{2} y^2 - 3 \right) \right] dy$$

$$= \int_{-2}^{4} \left(-\frac{1}{2} y^2 + y + 4 \right) dy$$

$$= \left[-\frac{1}{6} y^3 + \frac{1}{2} y^2 + 4y \right]_{-2}^{4} = 18 .$$

♯

Exercise 7.1

1. Refer to Figure 7.9. Set up definite integrals that represent the indicated shaded areas over the given intervals.

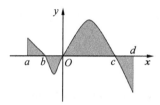

Figure 7.9

(1) Over interval $[a, b]$;

(2) Over interval $[0, c]$;

(3) Over interval $[c, d]$;

(4) Over interval $[a, d]$.

2. Find the area bounded by the graphs of the indicated equations over the given interval. Compute answers to three decimal places.

(1) $y = x^2 - 4$, $y = 0$, $0 \leqslant x \leqslant 3$;

(2) $y = x(1-x)$, $y = 0$, $-1 \leqslant x \leqslant 1$;

(3) $y = -e^x$, $y = 0$, $-1 \leqslant x \leqslant 1$.

3. Refer to Figure 7.10. Set up definite integrals that represent the indicated shaded areas over the given intervals.

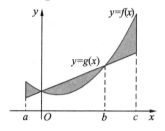

Figure 7.10

(1) Over interval $[a, 0]$;

(2) Over interval $[0, b]$;

(3) Over interval $[b, c]$;

(4) Over interval $[a, c]$.

4. Find the area bounded by the graphs of the indicated equations over the given interval. Compute answers to three decimal places.

(1) $y = x^2 + 1$, $y = 2x + 9$;

(2) $y = e^x$, $y = e^{-x}$, $x = -1$, $x = 4$.

5. A yeast culture is growing at a rate of $W'(t) = 0.3e^{0.1t}$ grams per hour. Find the area between the graph of W' and the t-axis over the interval $[0, 10]$ and interpret the results.

7.2　Average Values

7.2.1　Cumulative Change

We call $F(x) \big|_a^b = F(b) - F(a)$ the ***cumulative change*** or net change in $F(x)$ from $x = a$ to $x = b$. The cumulative change in a function is the definite integral of its derivative. To see why this is so, consider

$$\int_a^b F'(x)\mathrm{d}x = F(b) - F(a) .$$

On the right hand side, $F(b) - F(a)$ is the cumulative change in $F(x)$, while the integral $\int_a^b F'(x)\mathrm{d}x$ is a "sum" of instantaneous changes accumulated over $[a, b]$. Thus, the definite integral can be interpreted as the **cumulative** or net change in $F(x)$ between a and b. That is

$$\left[\begin{matrix}\text{cumulative} \\ \text{change in } [a, b]\end{matrix}\right] = \int_a^b \left[\begin{matrix}\text{instantaneous rate of} \\ \text{change at time } x\end{matrix}\right]\mathrm{d}x.$$

In particular,

$$\int_0^t v(t)\mathrm{d}t = s(t) - s(0)$$

means that $s(t) - s(0)$, the net distance traveled (final position minus initial position) is the integral of velocity.

If $V(t)$ is the volume of water in a reservoir at time t, then its derivative $V'(t)$ is the rate at which water flows into the reservoir at time t. So

$$\int_{t_1}^{t_2} V'(t)\mathrm{d}t = V(t_2) - V(t_1)$$

is the change in the amount of water in the reservoir between time t_1 and time t_2.

If the growth rate of a population is $\dfrac{\mathrm{d}P}{\mathrm{d}t}$, then

$$\int_a^b \frac{\mathrm{d}P}{\mathrm{d}t} = P(b) - P(a)$$

is the net change in population during the time period from a to b.

Example 7.4　If the birth rate of population is $b(t) = 2200\mathrm{e}^{0.024t}$ people per year and the death rate is $d(t) = 1460\mathrm{e}^{0.018t}$ people per year, find the area between these curves for $0 \leqslant t \leqslant 10$. What does this area represent?

Solution　We first determine which one is greater, the birth rate or the death rate. We see that

$$\frac{b(t)}{d(t)} = \frac{2200\mathrm{e}^{0.024t}}{1460\mathrm{e}^{0.018t}} > \frac{1460\mathrm{e}^{0.024t}}{1460\mathrm{e}^{0.018t}} = \frac{\mathrm{e}^{0.024t}}{\mathrm{e}^{0.018t}} = \mathrm{e}^{0.024t-0.018t} = \mathrm{e}^{0.006t} > 1.$$

Therefore, the birth rate is greater. Then the area between these curves is

$$A = \int_0^{10} (2200\mathrm{e}^{0.024t} - 1460\mathrm{e}^{0.018t})\mathrm{d}t$$

$$= \left[2200 \cdot \frac{1}{0.024}\mathrm{e}^{0.024t} - 1460 \cdot \frac{1}{0.018}\mathrm{e}^{0.018t}\right]_0^{10}$$

$$\approx 8868 .$$

Since the birth rate is greater than the death rate, we conclude that the area between these curves represents the increase of population between year $t = 0$ and $t = 10$.　　#

7.2.2　Definition of Average Value

The average of some finite set of values is a familiar concept. In the finite case, "average" refers to the arithmetic mean, the sum of the numbers divided by how many numbers are being averaged.

Suppose that the temperature (in ℃) recorded during a day followed the rule $f(x) = 0.001x^4 - 0.28x^2 + 25$, $-12 \leqslant x \leqslant 12$, where x is the number of hours from noon. How would you find the average temperature during the day? We cannot merely add up some number of temperatures and divide, since the temperature is changing continuously over the time interval. One approach is to get an approximation of the average temperature. Hence we take temperature readings every hour, then the arithmetic average temperature

$$\frac{f(x_1) + f(x_2) + \cdots + f(x_{24})}{24}$$

serves as an approximation.

Of course, if we compute more temperatures at more times, the average of these temperatures should be closer to the "real" average. We divide up the interval $[-12, 12]$ into n subintervals of equal length $\Delta x = \dfrac{b-a}{n}$, and use the function value at the right endpoint of each subinterval.

If we take the average of n temperatures at evenly spaced times, that is, we divide up the interval $[-12, 12]$ into n subintervals of equal length and use the function value at the right endpoint of each subinterval, we get

$$\frac{1}{n} \sum_{i=1}^{n} f(x_i) .$$

This is almost the sort of sum that we know turns into an integral; what is apparently missing is Δx. But in fact, the length of each subinterval is $\Delta x = \dfrac{24}{n}$, so rewriting slightly we have

$$\frac{1}{24} \sum_{i=1}^{n} f(x_i) \Delta x = \frac{1}{12 - (-12)} \sum_{i=1}^{n} f(x_i) \Delta x .$$

Now this has exactly the right form, so that in the limit we get average temperature $=$

$$\frac{1}{12 - (-12)} \int_{-12}^{12} f(x) \mathrm{d}x = \frac{1}{24} \int_{-12}^{12} (0.001x^4 - 0.28x^2 + 25) \mathrm{d}x \approx 15.7 .$$

We can expand this idea to any general function. The average values of f on $[a, b]$ can be expressed as an integral over $f(x)$ between a and b, divided by the length of the interval.

> *Suppose that $f(x)$ is continuous in $[a, b]$. The average values of f on the interval $[a, b]$ is*
> $$f_{\text{avg}} = \frac{\int_a^b f(x) \mathrm{d}x}{b - a} .$$

One way to think about the average value formula is to rewrite it as

$$f_{\text{avg}} \cdot (b - a) = \int_a^b f(x) \mathrm{d}x .$$

Think of $(b-a)$ as the width of a rectangle, and average as the height. Then the average value of a function on an interval is the height of a rectangle that has the same width as the interval and has the same area as the function on that interval.

Example 7.5　Find the average value of the cubic function $f(x)=x^3$ on the interval $[0, 1]$.

Solution　We use the integration formula

$$f_{avg} = \frac{1}{b-a}\int_a^b f(x)\,dx.$$

Hence,

$$f_{avg} = \frac{1}{1-0}\int_0^1 x^3\,dx = \int_0^1 x^3\,dx = \frac{x^4}{4}\Big|_0^1 = \frac{1}{4}.$$ #

Example 7.6　The average value of a function $y=f(x)$ over the interval $x\in[1, 5]$ is 2. What is the value of $\int_1^5 f(x)\,dx$?

Solution　By definition,

$$f_{avg} = \frac{1}{b-a}\int_a^b f(x)\,dx,$$

$$\int_a^b f(x)\,dx = f_{avg}\cdot(b-a).$$

Substituting the given values, we obtain

$$\int_1^5 f(x)\,dx = 2\cdot(5-1) = 8.$$ #

Example 7.7　The number of children in a large city was found to increase and then decrease rather drastically. If the number of children (in millions) over the 6-year period was given by

$$N(t)=-\frac{1}{4}t^2+t+4,\ 0\leqslant t\leqslant 6,$$

what was the average number of children in the city over the 6-year period? (Assume that $N=N(t)$ is continuous)

Solution　The average number of children in the city over the 6-year period is

$$\frac{1}{6-0}\int_0^6 N(t)\,dt = \frac{1}{6}\int_0^6\left(-\frac{1}{4}t^2+t+4\right)dt = \frac{1}{6}\left[-\frac{1}{12}t^3+\frac{1}{2}t^2+4t\right]_0^6 = 4\ (\text{millions}).$$ #

The Mean Value Theorem for Definite Integrals says a bit more about the value of the average value of a function.

Theorem 7.1 (the Mean Value Theorem for Definite Integrals)

　　Let $f(x)$ *be a continuous function on the closed interval* $[a, b]$. *Then there exists a point* c *in that interval such that*

$$f(c)=\frac{1}{b-a}\int_a^b f(x)\,dx.$$

In other words, the Mean Value Theorem for Definite Integrals states that there is at least one point c in the interval $[a, b]$ where $f(x)$ attains its average value f_{avg},

$$f(c) = f_{avg} = \frac{1}{b-a}\int_a^b f(x) \, dx .$$

The Mean Value Theorem for Definite Integrals should be fairly obvious when you look at the graph of function f and f_{avg}. For simplicity, we assume that $f(x)$ is positive. Geometrically, $\int_a^b f(x)dx$ represents the area between the graph of $f(x)$ and the x-axis, and $f_{avg} \cdot (b-a)$ is then equal to the area of the rectangle with height f_{avg} and width $b-a$

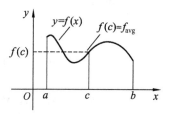

Figure 7. 11

(Figure 7. 11). Since the two rectangles are equal, the horizontal line $y = f_{avg}$ must intersect the graph of $f(x)$ at some point in the interval $[a, b]$. The x-coordinate of this intersection point is then the value of c in the Mean Value Theorem for Definite Integrals. A similar argument can be made when we do not assume that $f(x)$ is positive. In this general case, "area" is replaced by "signed area". The proof of this theorem is given in the following.

Proof   Since $f(x)$ is continuous on a closed interval, we conclude that f has an absolute maximum M and an absolute minimum m in $[a, b]$ by applying the Extreme Value Theorem, that is

$$m \leqslant f(x) \leqslant M \text{ for all } x \in [a, b]$$

and f attains both m and M for some values in $[a, b]$. Integralling on the interval, we therefore obtain

$$m(b-a) \leqslant \int_a^b f(x)dx \leqslant M(b-a) ,$$

or

$$m \leqslant \frac{1}{b-a}\int_a^b f(x)dx \leqslant M .$$

We set $I = \frac{1}{b-a}\int_a^b f(x)dx$ then $m \leqslant I \leqslant M$.

Applying the facts that $f(x)$ takes on all values between m and M on the interval $[a, b]$, and that I is a number between m and M, it follows from the Intermediate Value Theorem that there must be a number $c \in [a, b]$ such that $f(c)=I$, that is

$$f(c) = \frac{1}{b-a}\int_a^b f(x)dx . \qquad \#$$

Example 7. 8   Given the rational function $f(x)=\dfrac{2}{(x+1)^2}$. Find the values of c that satisfy the Mean Value Theorem for Definite Integrals for the function on the interval $[0, 3]$.

Solution   First we calculate the average value of the function $f(x)$ on the interval $[0, 3]$.

$$f_{avg} = \frac{1}{b-a}\int_a^b f(x)dx = \frac{1}{3}\int_0^3 \frac{2dx}{(x+1)^2} = \frac{2}{3}\left[-\frac{1}{x+1}\right]_0^3 = \frac{2}{3}\left(1-\frac{1}{4}\right) = \frac{1}{2} .$$

To determine the values of c, we solve the equation

$$f(c) = f_{avg}.$$

Hence,

$$\frac{2}{(c+1)^2} = \frac{1}{2}, \ (c+1)^2 = 4, \ c+1 = \pm 2, \ c_1 = 1, \ c_2 = -1.$$

We see that only the positive root $c_1 = 1$ lies in the interval $[0, 3]$, so the answer is $c = 1$.   #

Root Mean Square Value of a Function

The Root Mean Square (RMS) value is defined as the square root of the average (mean) value of the squared function $[f(x)]^2$ over the interval $[a, b]$. The corresponding integration formula is written in the form of

$$RMS = \sqrt{\frac{1}{b-a} \int_a^b [f(x)]^2 \, dx}.$$

The RMS value has many applications in mathematics, physics and engineering. For example, in physics, the RMS value of an alternating current (AC) is equal to the value of the direct current (DC) that dissipates the same power in a resistor.

Example 7.9 Find the RMS value of the sine function $f(t) = A \sin t$ over the interval $[0, 2\pi]$.

Solution   The RMS value is given by the integration formula

$$RMS = \sqrt{\frac{1}{2\pi} \int_0^{2\pi} (A \sin t)^2 \, dt}.$$

Applying the trig identity

$$\sin^2 t = \frac{1}{2}(1 - \cos 2t),$$

we have

$$RMS = \sqrt{\frac{1}{2\pi} \int_0^{2\pi} (A \sin t)^2 \, dt} = \sqrt{\frac{1}{2\pi} \int_0^{2\pi} \frac{A^2}{2}(1 - \cos 2t) \, dt}$$

$$= \sqrt{\frac{A^2}{4\pi} \int_0^{2\pi} (1 - \cos 2t) \, dt} = \sqrt{\frac{A^2}{4\pi} \left[t - \frac{\sin 2t}{2} \right]_0^{2\pi}}$$

$$= \sqrt{\frac{A^2}{4\pi} \cdot 2\pi} = \frac{A}{\sqrt{2}}.$$ #

Exercise 7.2

1. In 2016, the world consumption of natural gas was approximately 3528 bcm $(10^9 \, m^3)$ and was growing exponentially at about 1.6% per year. If the demand continues to grow at this rate, how many bcm of natural gas will be used from 2016 to 2030?

2. Find the average value of the function

$f(x)=1+x^2$ on the interval $[-1, 2]$.

3. Find the average value of the square root function $f(x)=\sqrt{x}$ on the interval $[0, 25]$.

4. Find the average value of the function $f(x)=\cos x$ on the interval $[0, \pi]$.

5. If the temperature in an aquarium (in degrees Celsius) is given by

$$C(t)=t^3-2t+10, \quad 0 \leqslant t \leqslant 2$$

over a 2-hour period, what is the average temperature over this period?

6. The daily temperature of the outside air is given by the equation

$$T(t)=20-5 \cos \frac{\pi t}{12},$$

where t is measured in hours ($0 \leqslant t \leqslant 24$) and T is measured in ℃. Find the average temperature between $t_0 = 6$ and $t_1 = 12$ hours.

7. Find the RMS value of the function $f(t)=A\cos t$ over the interval $[0, 2\pi]$.

8. Given the quadratic function $f(x)=(x+2)^2$. Find the values of c that satisfy the Mean Value Theorem for Definite Integrals for the function on the interval $[0, 9]$.

7.3   Improper Integrals

Recall that when we use the Fundamental Theorem of Calculus, the integrand must be continuous and the interval must be closed. There are two ways to extend the Fundamental Theorem of Calculus. One is to use an infinite interval, the other one is to allow the integrand containing a discontinuity on the interval. In either case, the integral is called an *improper integral*. One of the most important applications of this concept is probability distributions because determining quantities like the cumulative distribution or expected value typically require integrals on infinite intervals.

7.3.1   Integrating over an Infinite Interval

Is the area between the graph of $f(x)=e^{-x}$ and the x-axis over the interval $[0,+\infty)$ finite or infinite (Figure 7.12)? We know how to find the area of a region between 0 and t, namely,

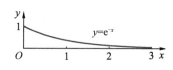

Figure 7.12

$$A(t) = \int_0^t e^{-x}\mathrm{d}x =-e^{-x} \mid_0^t = 1-e^{-t}.$$

We now let t tend to infinity and find

$$A=\lim_{t \to \infty} A(t)=\lim_{t \to \infty}(1-e^{-t})=1.$$

Since the limiting value exists, we can conclude that the area between the graph of $f(x)=e^{-x}$ and the x-axis over $[0,+\infty)$ is finite.

We therefore define an improper integral as a limit, taken as one of the limits of integration increases or decreases without bound.

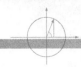

Definition 7.1(Improper Integral)

(1) Let $f(x)$ be continuous over an interval of the form $[0,+\infty)$. Then

$$\int_a^{+\infty} f(x)\,dx = \lim_{t \to +\infty} \int_a^t f(x)\,dx$$

provided this limit exists.

(2) Let $f(x)$ be continuous over an interval of the form $(-\infty, b]$. Then

$$\int_{-\infty}^b f(x)\,dx = \lim_{t \to -\infty} \int_t^b f(x)\,dx$$

provided this limit exists. In each case, if the limit exists, then the improper integral is said to converge. If the limit does not exist, then the improper integral is said to diverge.

(3) Let $f(x)$ be continuous over $(-\infty,+\infty)$. Then

$$\int_{-\infty}^{+\infty} f(x)\,dx = \int_{-\infty}^0 f(x)\,dx + \int_0^{+\infty} f(x)\,dx$$

provided that $\int_{-\infty}^0 f(x)\,dx$ and $\int_0^{+\infty} f(x)\,dx$ both converge. If either of these two integrals diverge, then $\int_{-\infty}^{+\infty} f(x)\,dx$ diverges.

Example 7.10 Determine whether the area between the graph of $f(x)=\dfrac{1}{x^2}$ and the x-axis over the interval $[1,+\infty)$ is finite or infinite.

Solution First we compute

$$A(t) = \int_1^t \frac{1}{x^2}\,dx = -\frac{1}{x}\Big|_1^t = 1 - \frac{1}{t}$$

and then let $t \to +\infty$. We find

$$\lim_{t \to +\infty} A(t) = \lim_{t \to +\infty}\left(1 - \frac{1}{t}\right) = 1.$$

Hence, the improper integral converges to 1,

$$\int_1^{+\infty} \frac{1}{x^2}\,dx = 1.$$

Therefore, the area between the graph of $f(x)=\dfrac{1}{x^2}$ and the x-axis over the interval $[1,+\infty)$ is finite.   #

Your Practice 7.2 Determine whether the area between the graph of $f(x)=\dfrac{1}{x^3}$ and the x-axis over the interval $[1,+\infty)$ is finite or infinite.

Example 7.11 Show that $\int_{-\infty}^0 \dfrac{1}{(x-1)^2}\,dx$ converges.

Solution Begin by rewriting $\int_{-\infty}^0 \dfrac{1}{(x-1)^2}\,dx$ as a limit from the definition. Thus,

$$\int_{-\infty}^0 \frac{1}{(x-1)^2}\,dx = \lim_{t \to -\infty}\int_t^0 \frac{1}{(x-1)^2}\,dx = \lim_{t \to -\infty}\left[-(x-1)^{-1}\big|_t^0\right]$$

$$= \lim_{t \to -\infty} \left(-\frac{1}{x-1} \Big|_t^0 \right) = \lim_{t \to -\infty} \left(1 + \frac{1}{t-1} \right) = 1.$$

We conclude that the improper integral converges to 1.　　　　　#

Example 7. 12　Compute $\displaystyle\int_{-\infty}^{+\infty} \frac{x}{1+x^2} \mathrm{d}x$.

Solution　Start by splitting up the integral:

$$\int_{-\infty}^{+\infty} \frac{x}{1+x^2} \mathrm{d}x = \int_{-\infty}^{0} \frac{x}{1+x^2} \mathrm{d}x + \int_{0}^{+\infty} \frac{x}{1+x^2} \mathrm{d}x .$$

If either $\displaystyle\int_{-\infty}^{0} \frac{x}{1+x^2} \mathrm{d}x$ or $\displaystyle\int_{0}^{+\infty} \frac{x}{1+x^2} \mathrm{d}x$ diverges, then $\displaystyle\int_{-\infty}^{+\infty} \frac{x}{1+x^2} \mathrm{d}x$ diverges. Compute each integral separately. We begin by computing

$$\int_{0}^{t} \frac{x}{1+x^2} \mathrm{d}x .$$

Using the substitution $u = 1 + x^2$ and $\mathrm{d}u = 2x\mathrm{d}x$, we find

$$\int_{0}^{t} \frac{x}{1+x^2} \mathrm{d}x = \int_{1}^{1+t^2} \frac{1}{2u} \mathrm{d}u = \frac{1}{2} \left[\ln|u| \right]_{1}^{1+t^2}$$

$$= \frac{1}{2} [\ln(1+t^2) - \ln 1] = \frac{1}{2} \ln(1+t^2).$$

Taking the limit $t \to +\infty$, we find

$$\int_{0}^{+\infty} \frac{x}{1+x^2} \mathrm{d}x = \lim_{t \to +\infty} \frac{1}{2} \ln(1+t^2) = +\infty.$$

Since one of the integrals is already divergent, we conclude that $\displaystyle\int_{-\infty}^{+\infty} \frac{x}{1+x^2} \mathrm{d}x$ diverges as well.　　　　　#

7.3.2　Discontinuous Integrand

Now let us examine integrals of functions containing an infinite discontinuity in the interval over which the integration occurs.

Consider an integral of the form $\displaystyle\int_{a}^{b} f(x)\mathrm{d}x$, where $f(x)$ is continuous over $[a, b)$ and discontinuous at b. Since the function $f(x)$ is continuous over $[a, t]$ for all values of t satisfying $a \leqslant t < b$, the integral $\displaystyle\int_{a}^{t} f(x)\mathrm{d}x$ is defined for all such values of t. Thus, it makes sense to consider the values of $a \leqslant t < b$ as t approaches b for $a \leqslant t < b$. That is, we define $\displaystyle\int_{a}^{b} f(x)\mathrm{d}x = \lim_{t \to b^-} \int_{a}^{t} f(x)\mathrm{d}x$, provided this limit exists (Figure 7. 13).

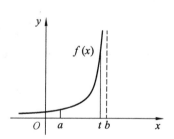

Figure 7. 13

We use a similar approach to define $\displaystyle\int_{a}^{b} f(x)\mathrm{d}x$, where $f(x)$ is continuous over $(a, b]$ and discontinuous at a. Now we proceed with a formal definition.

Definition 7.2 (Improper Integral for Discontinuous Integrand)

(1) Let $f(x)$ be continuous over $[a, b)$. Then,

$$\int_a^b f(x)\,dx = \lim_{t \to b^-} \int_a^t f(x)\,dx.$$

(2) Let $f(x)$ be continuous over $(a, b]$. Then,

$$\int_a^b f(x)\,dx = \lim_{t \to a^+} \int_t^b f(x)\,dx.$$

In each case, if the limit exists, then the improper integral is said to converge. If the limit does not exist, then the improper integral is said to diverge.

(3) If $f(x)$ is continuous over $[a, b]$ except at a point c in (a, b), then

$$\int_a^b f(x)\,dx = \int_a^c f(x)\,dx + \int_c^b f(x)\,dx$$

provided both $\int_a^c f(x)\,dx$ and $\int_c^b f(x)\,dx$ converge. If either of these integrals diverges, then $\int_a^b f(x)\,dx$ diverges.

Example 7.13　Evaluate $\int_0^4 \dfrac{1}{\sqrt{4-x}}\,dx$, if possible. State whether the integral converges or diverges.

Solution　The function $f(x) = \dfrac{1}{\sqrt{4-x}}$ is continuous over $[0, 4)$ and discontinuous at 4. By the definition, rewrite $\int_0^4 \dfrac{1}{\sqrt{4-x}}\,dx$ as limit form:

$$\int_0^4 \frac{1}{\sqrt{4-x}}\,dx = \lim_{t \to 4^-} \int_0^t \frac{1}{\sqrt{4-x}}\,dx.$$

We first compute the integral

$$\int_0^t \frac{1}{\sqrt{4-x}}\,dx = [-2\sqrt{4-x}]_0^t = -2\sqrt{4-t} + 4.$$

Taking the limit $t \to 4^-$, we find

$$\int_0^4 \frac{1}{\sqrt{4-x}}\,dx = \lim_{t \to 4^-} (-2\sqrt{4-t} + 4) = 4.$$

The improper integral converges.　　　　　　　　　　　　　　　　　　　　　#

Example 7.14　Evaluate $\int_0^1 \dfrac{1}{\sqrt{x}}\,dx$, if possible. State whether the integral converges or diverges.

Solution　The function $f(x) = \dfrac{1}{\sqrt{x}}$ is continuous over $(0, 1]$ and discontinuous at zero. By the definition, rewrite $\int_0^1 \dfrac{1}{\sqrt{x}}\,dx$ as limit form:

$$\int_0^1 \frac{1}{\sqrt{x}}\,dx = \lim_{t \to 0^+} \int_t^1 \frac{1}{\sqrt{x}}\,dx.$$

We compute the integral

$$\int_t^1 \frac{1}{\sqrt{x}} dx = [2\sqrt{x}]_t^1 = 2(1-\sqrt{t}).$$

Taking the limit $t \to 0^+$, we find

$$\int_0^1 \frac{1}{\sqrt{x}} dx = \lim_{t \to 0^+} 2(1-\sqrt{t}) = 2.$$

The improper integral converges.   #

Example 7.15   Evaluate $\int_{-1}^1 \frac{1}{x^2} dx$, if possible. State whether the integral converges

or diverges.

Solution   The function $f(x) = \frac{1}{x^2}$ is discontinuous at zero. We write

$$\int_{-1}^1 \frac{1}{x^2} dx = \int_{-1}^0 \frac{1}{x^2} dx + \int_0^1 \frac{1}{x^2} dx.$$

If either of the two integrals diverges, then the original integral diverges.

We compute the integral

$$\int_{-1}^t \frac{1}{x^2} dx = \left[-\frac{1}{x}\right]_{-1}^t = -\frac{1}{t} + 1.$$

As

$$\lim_{t \to 0^-} \left(-\frac{1}{t} + 1\right) = +\infty,$$

then $\int_{-1}^0 \frac{1}{x^2} dx$ diverges. Therefore, the improper integral $\int_{-1}^1 \frac{1}{x^2} dx$ diverges.   #

Your Practice 7.3   Evaluate $\int_{-1}^1 \frac{1}{x^3} dx$, if possible. State whether the integral

converges or diverges.

Exercise 7.3

1. Evaluate $\int_{-3}^{+\infty} e^{-x} dx$. State whether the improper integral converges or diverges.

2. Evaluate $\int_1^{+\infty} \frac{1}{x^{3/2}} dx$. State whether the improper integral converges or diverges.

3. Evaluate $\int_{-\infty}^{-1} \frac{1}{1+x^2} dx$. State whether the improper integral converges or diverges.

4. Evaluate $\int_{-\infty}^{+\infty} x^3 e^{-x^4} dx$. State whether the improper integral converges or diverges.

5. Evaluate $\int_0^2 \frac{1}{(x-1)^{2/5}} dx$. State whether the integral converges or diverges.

6. Evaluate $\int_{-2}^0 \frac{1}{(x+1)^{1/3}} dx$. State whether the integral converges or diverges.

7. Evaluate $\int_0^2 \frac{1}{x} dx$. State whether the integral converges or diverges.

Summary and Review

Key Concepts

- If f and g are continuous in $[a, b]$ and $f(x) \geqslant g(x)$ for all $x \in [a, b]$, then the area of the region between the curves $y = f(x)$ and $y = g(x)$ from a to b is equal to

$$\text{Area} = \int_a^b [f(x) - g(x)] \mathrm{d}x.$$

- The net change formula

$$\int_a^b f'(x) \mathrm{d}x = f(b) - f(a)$$

states that the cumulative change in a function is the definite integral of its derivative. When a quantity changes, the final value equals the initial value plus the integral of the rate of change.

- Suppose that $f(x)$ is continuous in $[a, b]$. The average values of f on the interval $[a, b]$ is

$$f_{\text{avg}} = \frac{1}{b-a} \int_a^b f(x) \mathrm{d}x.$$

- The Mean Value Theorem for Definite Integrals says that there exists a point c in the integrating interval such that

$$f(c) = \frac{1}{b-a} \int_a^b f(x) \mathrm{d}x$$

provided $f(x)$ is a continuous function.

- Integrals of functions over infinite intervals are defined in terms of limits.
- Integrals of functions over an interval for which the function has a discontinuity at an endpoint may be defined in terms of limits.

Glossary

Net Change Theorem. If we know change rate of a quantity, the Net Change Theorem says the future quantity is equal to the initial quantity plus the integral of the change rate of the quantity.

Key Equations

- Net Change Theorem.

$$F(b) = F(a) + \int_a^b F'(x) \mathrm{d}x$$

or

$$\int_a^b F'(x) \mathrm{d}x = F(b) - F(a).$$

- The average value

$$f_{\text{avg}} = \frac{1}{b-a} \int_a^b f(x) \mathrm{d}x$$

- Improper integral $\int_a^{+\infty} f(x) \mathrm{d}x = \lim\limits_{t \to +\infty} \int_a^t f(x) \mathrm{d}x$.

- Improper integral $\int_{-\infty}^b f(x) \mathrm{d}x = \lim\limits_{t \to -\infty} \int_t^b f(x) \mathrm{d}x$.

- Improper integrals $\int_{-\infty}^{+\infty} f(x) \mathrm{d}x = \int_{-\infty}^0 f(x) \mathrm{d}x + \int_0^{+\infty} f(x) \mathrm{d}x$.

Chapter 8 Probability and Statistics

⁚ Introduction

- ○ *The probability of events*
- ○ *The conditional probability and Independent Events*

- ○ *Random variables and distributions*
- ○ *Means and variances*
- ○ *Statistic Tools*

There are normally two kinds of phenomena in nature and human society. One is deterministic phenomenon, which is bound to take place under a certain condition. For instance, the sun rises in the east. The other one is nondeterministic or random phenomenon, in which outcomes are not sure to take place. Examples including tossing coins, rolling dice, forecasting the weather and so on.

The term probability refers to the study of randomness and uncertainty, and probability is a numerical measure of randomness and uncertainty.

8.1 The Probability of Events

8.1.1 Counting Techniques

The calculation of probability mainly depends on the knowledge of counting techniques. We need some counting rules.

If an experiment is performed in two stages, with n_1 ways to accomplish the first stage and n_2 ways to accomplish the second stage, then there are $n_1 \times n_2$ ways to accomplish the experiment. This rule can be extended to k stages easily. We call it ***the multiplication principle*** and express it in the following.

8.1.1.1 Permutations

A ***permutation*** is an ordered arrangement of a set of objects. For example, consider three letters a, b, and c. The possible permutations are abc, acb, bac, bca, cab, and cba. Thus we find that there are 6 distinct arrangements, because there are $n_1 = 3$ choices for the first position, then $n_2 = 2$ for the second, leaving only $n_3 = 1$ choice for the last position. So, by the multiplication principle, there are $n_1 \times n_2 \times n_3 = 3 \times 2 \times 1 = 6$ possible arrangements.

In general, n distinct objects can be arranged in $n \cdot (n-1) \cdot (n-2) \cdot \cdots \cdot 3 \cdot 2 \cdot 1$

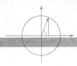

ways. We represent this product by the symbol $n!$, which is read "n factorial". Hence, the number of permutations (different ways of ordering/selecting) of n distinct objects is $n!$.

Note We define $0! = 1$.

Any ordered sequence of k objects taken from a set of n distinct objects is called a **permutation of size k objects**. A permutation is essentially different ways of ordering k of n objects, where the specific ordering is important. Different orderings of the same k objects are considered as different permutations. The number of permutations (different ways of selecting) k out of n objects is denoted by $P_{k,n}$. We have

$$P_{k,n} = \frac{n!}{(n-k)!}.$$

The outcome can be obtained from the multiplication principle: The 1st object can be selected in n different ways, the 2nd object can be selected in $n-1$ different ways, the 3rd object can be selected in $n-2$ different ways, $\cdots$, and the kth object can be selected in $n-k+1$ different ways. Therefore, the total number of possible selections is

$$P_{k,n} = n(n-1)(n-2)\cdots(n-k+1) = \frac{n!}{(n-k)!}.$$

For example, the number of three-letter code words using the letters in LOVE is just the number of permutations three out of four objects $P_{3,4} = 4 \times 3 \times 2 = 24$.

8.1.1.2 Combinations

In many problems we are interested in the number of ways of selecting k objects from n regardless of order.

Given a set of n distinct objects, any unordered subset of size k of the n objects is called a **combination**. The number of combinations of size k taken from the n distinct objects is denoted by $C_{k,n}$ or $\binom{n}{k}$. We have

$$C_{k,n} = \frac{P_{k,n}}{k!}.$$

Example 8.1 A committee of 4 people is to be formed from a group of 15 people. How many different committees are possible?

Solution Members are chosen regardless of order. Thus this is a combination problem of choosing k out n of objects. We know that there are $C_{4,15} = \frac{P_{4,15}}{4!} = 1365$ possible outcomes.   #

8.1.2 Sample Space and Events

8.1.2.1 Sample space

A **random experiment** is an experiment which can be performed over and over again under the same condition, and in which outcomes are more than ones, known, but is not predicted with certainty in each individual experiment. Tossing a coin and rolling a dice are examples of random experiments. The set of all possible outcomes of a random experiment is called the *sample space*, denoted by Ω. Each outcome in the sample space is called an element or a member of the sample space, or simply a sample point, denoted by ω.

In some experiments, it is helpful to list the elements of the sample space systematical by means of a tree diagram.

If we toss two fair coins, to list the elements of the sample space providing the most information, we construct a diagram of Figure 8.1, which is called a tree diagram. Now the various paths along the branches of the tree give the distinct sample points. Starting with the top left branch and moving to the right along the

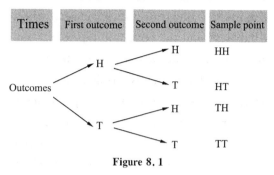

Figure 8.1

first path, we get the sample point HH, indicating the possibility that heads occur on two successive flips of the coin. Thus the sample space is $\Omega = \{HH, HT, TH, TT\}$.

8.1.2.2 Events

An *event* is a subset of a sample space, denoted by $A, B, C, \cdots$. An event is said to be simple if it consists of exactly one outcome and compound if it consists of more than one outcomes. Suppose that A is an event. We say that "the event A occurs" if the outcomes of the experiment are contained in the set A.

If an event always occurs in an experiment, we call it a *certain event*. The sample space Ω itself, is a certain event. An event never occurs in an experiment is called an *impossible event*. The empty set, denoted by $\varnothing$, which is also an event, an impossible event.

Example 8.2 Considering the experiment of tossing a dice. If we are interested in the number that shows on the top face, the sample space would be $\Omega = \{1, 2, 3, 4, 5, 6\}$.

The event A is that an odd number is obtained, and it can be represented as the subset $A = \{1, 3, 5\}$.

The event B is that the number smaller than 3 is obtained, and it can be represented as the subset $B = \{1, 2\}$.   ♯

Example 8.3 Suppose that two successive vehicles taking a particular freeway exit can turn right (R), turn left (L), or go straight (S). The sample space would be

$$\Omega = \{RR, RL, RS, LR, LS, LL, SR, SL, SS\}.$$

The event C is that two vehicles take different directions, and it can be represented as the subset $C = \{RL, RS, LR, LS, SR, SL\}$.

The event D is that two vehicles go in the same direction, and it can be represented as the subset $D = \{RR, LL, SS\}$.   ♯

8.1.2.3 Relations of events

An event is nothing but a set, so relationships and results from elementary set theory can be used to study events. The following operations will be used to construct new events from given events.

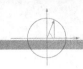

For events A and B, if every outcome in A belongs to B, which means that if A occurs and so does B, then we say that "A is a *subset event* of B", and denote $A \subset B$. If $A \subset B$ and $B \subset A$, then $A = B$. Figure 8.2 illustrates such subset, where events are visualized as "bubbles" and the rectangle represents the sample space. From this definition, we know that $A \subset \Omega$, for any event A.

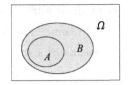

Figure 8.2

Considering the experiment of tossing a dice. If we are interested in the number that shows on the top face, the sample space would be $\Omega = \{1, 2, 3, 4, 5, 6\}$. Let x be the number that shows on the top face. The event $E = \{x \in \Omega, x \leqslant 8\}$ is the certain event, i. e. $E = \Omega$. The event $F = \{x \in \Omega, x \leqslant 0\}$ is the impossible event, i. e $F = \varnothing$. If event $A = \{x \in \Omega, x \leqslant 3\}$, and event $B = \{x \in \Omega, x \leqslant 4\}$, then $A \subset B$.

Suppose that A and B are events of the sample space Ω. The **union of two events** A and B, denoted by $A \cup B$ and read as "A union B", is the event consisting of all outcomes that are either in A alone or in B alone or in both events. In other words, $A \cup B$ means that A occurs, or B occurs, or both occur. The **intersection of two events** A and B, denoted by $A \cap B$ or AB, and read as "A intersected with B", is the event consisting of all outcomes that are in both A and B. Figures 8.3 and 8.4 show these event operations.

The operations of union and intersection can be extended to more than two events. Let $A_i (i = 1, 2, \cdots,)$ be events. Then **the union of an finite sequence events**

$$\bigcup_{i=1}^{n} A_i = A_1 \cup A_2 \cup \cdots \cup A_n$$

is the event consisting of all outcomes that belong to at least one of these n events. The *intersection*

$$\bigcap_{i=1}^{n} A_i = A_1 \cap A_2 \cap \cdots \cap A_n$$

is the event consisting of all outcomes that are common to all these n events. We use $\bigcup_{i=1}^{+\infty} A_i$ and $\bigcap_{i=1}^{+\infty} A_i$ when there are infinite events.

When A and B have no outcomes in common, namely, $A \cap B = \varnothing$, they are said to be **mutually exclusive** or **disjoint events**. In this situation, $A \cup B$ is often written as $A + B$. Figure 8.5 shows this situation.

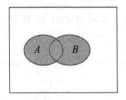

Figure 8.3

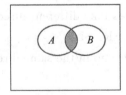

Figure 8.4

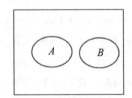

Figure 8.5

Note For n events $A_1, A_2, \cdots, A_n$, if any two of them are disjoint, then they are called the **pairwise disjoint events**.

The complement of event A with respect to Ω is the set of all outcomes in Ω that are not contained in A, denoted by $\overline{A}$ or A^c.

When we take complements of unions or intersections, the De Morgan's Laws are useful.

De Morgan's Laws

$$\overline{A \cup B} = \overline{A} \cap \overline{B},$$
$$\overline{A \cap B} = \overline{A} \cup \overline{B}.$$

Example 8.4   Toss a coin 10 times and the number of heads is observed. Let $A=\{0, 2, 6, 8, 9\}$, $B=\{1, 3, 4, 9\}$, and $C=\{1, 2, 4, 5\}$. Find $A \cup B$, $A \cap C$, $\overline{C}$, and $B \cup (A \cap C)$.

Solution $A \cup B$ is the set of all outcomes that belong to either A or B (or both). Thus $A \cup B=\{0, 1, 2, 3, 4, 6, 8, 9\}$. $A \cap C$ is the set of all outcomes that belong to both A and C. Therefore, $A \cap C=\{2\}$. We know $\Omega=\{0, 1, 2, 3, 4, 5, 6, 7, 8, 9, 10\}$ and then $\overline{C}=\{0, 3, 6, 7, 8, 9, 10\}$. Finally we get $B \cup (A \cap C)=\{1, 2, 3, 4, 9\}$.   #

Your Practice 8.1   An engineering construction firm is currently working on power plants at three different sites. Let $A_i(i=1, 2, 3)$ denote the event that the plant at site i is completed by the contract date. Use event operation to present the following event.

(1) At least one plant is completed by the contract date.

(2) All plants are completed by the contract date.

(3) Only the plant at site 1 is completed by the contract date.

(4) Exactly one plant is completed by the contract date.

We should learn to translate operations of events in the terms of sets and learn to use operations of events to decompose complicated events into simple ones.

Example 8.5   Suppose that A, B, and C are three events, then

(1) A, B and C all come up can be represented by $A \cap B \cap C$.

(2) Both A and B come up while C does not can be represented by $A \cap B \cap \overline{C}$.

(3) At least one of A, B and C comes up can be represented by $A \cup B \cup C$.

(4) Exactly two of A, B and C comes up can be represented by $A \cap B \cap \overline{C}+A \cap \overline{B} \cap C+\overline{A} \cap B \cap C$.

(5) At most two of A, B and C comes up can be represented by $\overline{A \cup B \cup C}$.   #

8.1.3 The Definition of Probability

What is probability? We begin with the mathematical definition of probability. The discipline of probability provides methods for quantifying the chances, or likelihoods, associated with the various outcomes of an experiment.

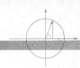

> **Definition 8.1 (Probability)**
>
> *Probability is a real-valued set function P that assigns, to each event A in the sample space Ω, a number $P(A)$, called the probability of the event A, which should satisfy the following properties:*
>
> (1) $P(A) \geqslant 0$.
>
> (2) $P(\Omega) = 1$.
>
> (3) *If A_1, A_2, $\cdots$, A_n, $\cdots$ is an infinite collection of disjoint events, then*
>
> $$P\left(\bigcup_{n=1}^{+\infty} A_n\right) = \sum_{n=1}^{+\infty} P(A_n).$$

Note that a probability is a number that is always between 0 and 1. We also get
$$P(\varnothing) = 0$$
since $\varnothing = \varnothing \cup \varnothing \cup \cdots$ and $P(\varnothing) = \sum_{n=1}^{+\infty} P(\varnothing)$.

Property (3) also holds for n disjoint events A_1, A_2, $\cdots$, A_n, that is
$$P\left(\bigcup_{i=1}^{n} A_i\right) = \sum_{i=1}^{n} P(A_i).$$
Particularly, for any event A, we have the complementary property
$$P(A) + P(\overline{A}) = 1 \text{ or } P(A) = 1 - P(\overline{A}).$$

The following theorem allows us to compute probability of unions of two sets (which are not necessary disjoint).

> **Theorem 8.1 (Additional Property)**
>
> *For any two events A and B, the probability of their union is*
> $$P(A \cup B) = P(A) + P(B) - P(A \cap B).$$

This can be illustrated in Figure 8.3. To compute $P(A \cup B)$, we add $P(A)$ and $P(B)$, but since we count $A \cap B$ twice, we need to subtract $P(A \cap B)$.

Example 8.6 Let A denote the event that the selected individual has a Visa credit card and B be the analogous event for a MasterCard. When $P(A) = 0.5$, $P(B) = 0.4$ and $P(AB) = 0.25$,

(1) compute the probability that the selected individual has at least one of the two types of cards;

(2) what is the probability that the selected individual has neither type of card?

(3) describe, in terms of A and B, the event that the selected student has a Visa card but not a MasterCard, and then calculate the probability of this event.

Solution (1) The event "the selected individual has at least one of the two types of cards" can be presented by $A \cup B$. Using the additional property, we obtain $P(A \cup B) = P(A) + P(B) - P(AB) = 0.5 + 0.4 - 0.25 = 0.65$.

(2) The event "the selected individual has neither type of card" can be represented by

$\overline{A} \cap \overline{B}$. Using De Morgan's Laws, we have $\overline{A} \cap \overline{B} = \overline{A \cup B}$. Applying the complementary property, we have $P(\overline{A} \cap \overline{B}) = P(\overline{A \cup B}) = 1 - P(A \cup B) = 1 - 0.65 = 0.35$.

(3) The event that the selected student has a Visa card but not a MasterCard can be represented by $A \cap \overline{B}$. Then $P(A \cap \overline{B}) = P(A) - P(AB) = 0.5 - 0.25 = 0.25$. #

Your Practice 8.2 Show that for any three events A, B, and C,

$$P(A \cup B \cup C) = P(A) + P(B) + P(C) - P(AB) - P(AC) - P(BC) + P(ABC).$$

8.1.4 Equally Likely Outcomes Model

In many experiments, the outcomes of a great deal of repeated experiments under a certain condition turn out to have some statistical regularity. For example, tossing a fair coin or fair dice once or twice (or any fixed number of times), each side has the same chance to be selected.

It is reasonable to assign equal probabilities to all possible outcomes. In this part, we consider the equally likely outcomes model.

> **Definition 8.2 (the Classical Probability)**
>
> When the various outcomes of an experiment are equally likely (the same probability is assigned to each simple event), letting N denote the number of outcomes in a sample space and N_A represent the number of outcomes contained in an event A, then the probability that A occurs is
>
> $$P(A) = \frac{\text{The number of outcomes contained in an event } A}{\text{The number of outcomes in the sample space}} = \frac{N_A}{N}.$$

Example 8.7 A ball is drawn at random from a bag containing seven black balls, four white balls and nine red balls. What is the probability that it is white?

Solution The sample space consists of 20 sample points, that is $N = 20$. Let A be the event that the ball is white. Then A consists of four sample points and $N_A = 4$. Thus the probability wanted is

$$P(A) = \frac{4}{20} = 0.2.$$ #

Example 8.8 In a single throw of two dice, what is the probability of getting a total of seven? How about a total smaller than four?

Solution The sample space is $\Omega = \{(i, j) \mid i, j = 1, 2, 3, 4, 5, 6\}$. Thus Ω consists of 36 sample points and $N = 36$.

Let $A = $ "getting a total of seven" and $B = $ "getting a total smaller than four". Then we have

$$A = \{(1, 6), (2, 5), (3, 4), (4, 3), (5, 2), (6, 1)\},$$

and

$$B = \{(1, 1), (1, 2), (2, 1)\}.$$

Thus $N_A = 6$ and $N_B = 3$. Therefore,

$$P(A) = \frac{N_A}{N} = \frac{6}{36} = \frac{1}{6},$$

$$P(B) = \frac{N_B}{N} = \frac{3}{36} = \frac{1}{12}. \qquad\qquad \#$$

Your Practice 8.3 A box contains six different balls, four red and two green. A child selects two balls at random. What is the probability that exactly one is red?

Exercise 8.1

1. How many 3-digit code numbers can we make from the numbers 1, 2, 3, 4 and 5, if

    (1) digits can be repeated;

    (2) digits can not be repeated.

2. How many 4-letter code words are possible using the letters in WRSTY, if

    (1) the letters can be repeated;

    (2) the letters can not be repeated.

3. An urn contains five blue and six green balls. We draw two balls from the urn. Find the sample space.

4. List all the possible outcomes of the experiment.

    (1) A coin is tossed two times, and the sequence of heads and tails is observed;

    (2) A coin is tossed three times, and the sequence of heads and tails is observed.

5. Select randomly one student from a school. Let A = "the student selected is female", B = "the student selected does not like to run", C = "the student selected is an athlete".

    (1) What do $AB\overline{C}$ and $A\overline{B}C$ mean respectively?

    (2) Under what condition $ABC = A$ holds?

6. If the sample space $\Omega = \{0, 1, \cdots, 9\}$. Let $A = \{1, 2, 3\}$, $B = \{2, 3, 4\}$, and $C = \{1, 4, 5, 7\}$. Find

    (1) $\overline{B}$;

    (2) $A \cap \overline{B}$;

    (3) $A \cap B \cap C$;

    (4) $B \cup (A \cap C)$.

7. Suppose that $P(A \cup B) = 0.6$ and $P(A \cup \overline{B}) = 0.7$. Find $P(A)$.

8. Suppose that $P(A) = 0.3$ and $P(B) = 0.5$, and $P(AB) = 0.2$. Find

    (1) $P(A \cup B)$;

    (2) $P(A \cap \overline{B})$;

    (3) $P(\overline{A} \cup \overline{B})$;

    (4) $P(\overline{A} \cap \overline{B})$.

9. Three balls are drawn in succession without replacement from a bag with five blue balls and six red ones. Find the probability that the first and the third are red, and the second is blue.

10. An elevator starts at the bottom floor with seven passengers and stopped at the 10th floor. Assume that each passenger leaves at each floor equally likely. Find the probability that no two passengers leave at a same floor.

11. Select at random 13 cards from a deck of 52 cards. Find the probability that it consists of 5 spades, 3 hearts, 3 diamonds and 2 clubs.

12. In a set of 40 randomly chosen people, what is the probability that no two have the same birthday, that is, have been born on the same day of the same month but not necessarily in the same year?

8.2   The Conditional Probability and Independent Events

8.2.1   The Conditional Probability

The probability of an event is frequently influenced by other events. In this section, we examine how the information "the event B has occurred" affects the probability assigned to the event A. We denote it as the conditional probability $P(A|B)$. The vertical bar "|" is read as "given", so the expression $P(A|B)$ is short for "the conditional probability of A given B".

Show you an example. Consider a statistic class consisting of 150 students, among whom 100 major in engineering. In the final exam, 36 students get the grade A, including 26 major in engineering. Let $A=$ "get the grade A" and $B=$ "major in engineering". So, for the whole class, the probability of getting the grade A is $P(A)=36/150=0.24$. But for the students majoring in engineering, we condition on the prior knowledge "majoring in engineering". Therefore it is the conditional probability $P(A|B)$ and $P(A|B)=26/100=0.26$.

Note that in this example, we have two sample spaces. One is the whole class, and the other is the students major in engineering. Thus, in a real world problem, we often need to discuss several sample space altogether, you should be careful not to confuse them. When computing $P(A|B)$, the sample space is reduced to B. In the reduced sample space B, the subset of students getting the grade A is exactly the event AB. Thus, $P(A|B)=26/100=0.26$. On the other hand, we also can write $P(A|B)=\dfrac{26/150}{100/150}=\dfrac{P(AB)}{P(B)}$. This give the definition of conditional probability.

Definition 8.3 (Conditional Probability)

For any two events A and B with $P(B)>0$, the conditional probability of A given that B has occurred, is defined by

$$P(A|B)=\frac{P(AB)}{P(B)}. \tag{8.1}$$

Note   We point out that the sample spaces on the left and right sides of Equation (8.1) are different (Figure 8.6). For $P(AB)$, the sample space is Ω. While for $P(A|B)$, the relevant sample space is no longer Ω but consists of outcomes in B.

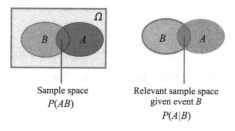

Sample space
$P(AB)$

Relevant sample space
given event B
$P(A|B)$

Figure 8.6

Example 8. 9 Suppose that of all individuals buying a certain digital camera, 0. 6 include an optional memory card in their purchase, 0. 4 include an extra battery, and 0. 3 include both a card and battery. Consider randomly selecting a buyer and let $A=$"memory card purchased " and $B=$"battery purchased". Then $P(A)=0.6$, $P(B)=0.4$ and $P($both purchased$)=P(AB)=0.3$. Given that the selected individual purchased an extra battery, the probability that an optional card was also purchased is

$$P(A\mid B)=\frac{P(AB)}{P(B)}=\frac{0.3}{0.4}=0.75.$$

That is, of all those purchasing an extra battery, 0. 75 purchased an optional memory card. Note that $P(A\mid B)\neq P(A)$ which means that the conditional probability is usually not equal to the unconditional probability.

From the definition of conditional probability, we obtain the following result:

Theorem 8. 2 (The Multiplication Rule)

For any two events A and B, the probability of their intersection is

$$P(AB)=P(A\mid B)P(B) \ (P(B)>0) \tag{8.2}$$

or

$$P(AB)=P(B\mid A)P(A) \ (P(A)>0). \tag{8.3}$$

Formulas (8. 2) and (8. 3) are particular useful for computing probabilities in two-stage experiments. The following example illustrates the use of these identities. We will see that there is a natural choice for which of the two events to condition on.

Example 8. 10 A card is withdrawn at random and not replaced from a deck of 52 cards. A second card is then drawn. Find the probability that the first card is an ace and the second a king.

Solution This is a two-stage experiment. We first draw a card and then another. Let $A=$"the first card is an ace" and $B=$"the second card is a king". Then $AB=$ "the first card is an ace and the second a king". Since the first card is drawn first, it will be easier to condition on the outcome of the first draw than on the second draw; that is, we will compute $P(B\mid A)$ rather than $P(A\mid B)$.

We have $P(A)=\frac{4}{52}=\frac{1}{13}$ since 4 out of 52 cards are aces and each card has the same probability of drawn. When an ace has been withdrawn, there are 51 cards left with 4 kings inside. Therefore we have $P(B\mid A)=\frac{4}{51}$.

Applying the Multiplication Rule we obtain

$$P(AB)=P(B\mid A)P(A)=\frac{1}{13}\times\frac{4}{51}=\frac{4}{663}. \qquad \#$$

8.2.2 The Law of Total Probability and the Bayes Formula

The law of total probability and Bayes formula are two important formulas in probability and statistics. They decompose the complex and comprehensive random events into several mutual exclusive simple events. The whole problem is transformed into local problems. One kind of problem is to obtain the desired result by calculating the probability of these simple events, and it is called the law of total probability. Another type of problem is to discuss the probability of the occurrence of each simple event under the condition that the result is given, which is known as the Bayes formula.

We say that events A_1, A_2, $\cdots$, A_n constitute a **_partition_** of the sample space Ω, if Ω is written as a union of those disjoint sets, that is,

$$A_1 \bigcup A_2 \bigcup \cdots \bigcup A_n = \Omega \text{ and } A_i \bigcap A_j = \varnothing \ (i \neq j).$$

We also say that events A_1, A_2, $\cdots$, A_n are mutually exclusive and exhaustive events.

We point out that a sample space has many partitions. As shown in Figure 8.7, the five events A_1, A_2, A_3, A_4, A_5 form a partition of the sample space Ω; the three events $A_1 A_2$, $A_3 A_4$, A_5 also make a partition of Ω.

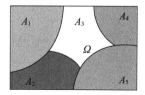

Figure 8.7

Theorem 8.3 (Law of Total Probability)

Let A_1, A_2, $\cdots$, A_n _be a partition of the sample space_ Ω _and_ $P(A_i) > 0$, _then for any other event_ B,

$$P(B) = \sum_{i=1}^{n} P(B \mid A) P(A_i). \tag{8.4}$$

Proof Because A_1, A_2, $\cdots$, A_n are mutually exclusive and exhaustive events, we have

$$A_1 \bigcup A_2 \bigcup \cdots \bigcup A_n = \Omega \text{ and } A_i \bigcap A_j = \varnothing \ (i \neq j).$$

We can write B as a union of disjoint sets using this partition of Ω:

$$B = B \bigcap \Omega = B \bigcap (\bigcup_{i=1}^{n} A_i) = \bigcup_{i=1}^{n} (BA_i)$$

as illustrated in Figure 8.8.

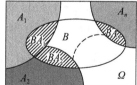

Figure 8.8

Applying the additional property and $BA_i \bigcap BA_j = \varnothing \ (i \neq j)$, we get

$$P(B) = P[\bigcup_{i=1}^{n} (BA_i)] = \sum_{i=1}^{n} P(BA_i) = \sum_{i=1}^{n} P(B \mid A_i) P(A_i). \qquad \#$$

Formula (8.4) is called **_the law of total probability_**.

Note If events A and $\overline{A}$ are a partition of the sample space Ω (Figure 8.9), then for any other event B,

$$P(B) = P(B \mid A) P(A) + P(B \mid \overline{A}) P(\overline{A}).$$

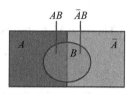

Figure 8.9

Example 8.11 A test for the HIV virus shows a positive result in 99% of all cases when the virus is actually present, and in 5% of all cases when the virus is not present (a false positive result). If such a test is administered to a randomly chosen individual, what is the probability that the test result is positive? We assume that the prevalence of the virus in the population is 1/200.

Solution We set $B=$ "the test result is positive". Individuals in this population fall into two groups, those who are infected with the HIV virus and those who are not. These two sets form a partition of the population. If we pick an individual at random from the population, then the person belongs to one of these two groups. We define

$$A=\text{"person is infected"},$$
$$\overline{A}=\text{"person is not infected"}.$$

Using the Law of Total Probability, we can write

$$P(B)=P(B|A)P(A)+P(B|\overline{A})P(\overline{A}).$$

Now, $P(A)=1/200$ and $P(\overline{A})=199/200$. Furthermore, $P(B|A)=0.99$ and $P(B|\overline{A})=0.05$. Hence

$$P(B)=0.99\times\frac{1}{200}+0.05\times\frac{199}{200}=0.0547. \qquad \#$$

Example 8.12 In a pharmaceutical factory, three machines, M_1, M_2 and M_3, make 70%, 20%, and 10%, respectively, of the tablets. It is known from past experience that 1%, 2% and 5% of the tablets made by each machine, respectively, are defective. Now, suppose that a finished tablet is randomly selected. What is the probability that it is defective?

Solution Let $A_i=$ "a tablet is made by machine M_i", $i=1, 2, 3$ and $B=$ "the tablet is defective". Then we have

$$P(A_1)=0.7, \ P(A_2)=0.2, \text{ and } P(A_3)=0.1.$$

We also have $P(B|A_1)=0.01$, $P(B|A_2)=0.02$, and $P(B|A_3)=0.05$.

Because events A_1, A_2, A_3 are a partition (Figure 8.10), now we use the Law of Total Probability to get

$$P(B) = \sum_{i=1}^{3}P(B|A_i)P(A_i)$$

$$=0.7\times0.01+0.2\times0.02+0.1\times0.05=0.016.$$

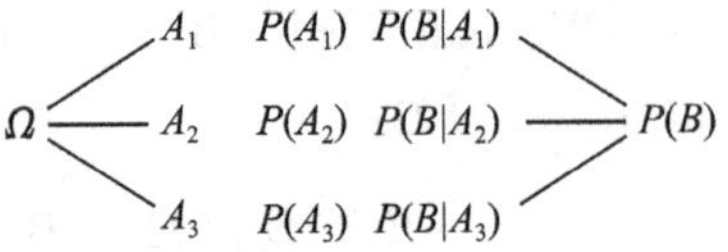

$$\#$$

Figure 8.10

We call $P(A_i|B)$ as the posterior probability of event A_i, that is, the probability of A_i after event B is observed. $P(A_i)$ by itself is then the prior probability, the belief we have in the likelihood of A_i in the absence of any additional information.

In real world problems, it is important to calculate a posterior probability from given a prior probability. Such a formula is called Bayes formula.

Theorem 8.4 (Bayes Formula)

Let A_1, A_2, A_3, $\cdots$, A_n be a collection of mutually exclusive and exhaustive events with prior probabilities $P(A_i)$, $i=1, 2, 3,\cdots$, n. Then for any other event B ($P(B)>0$), the posterior probability of A_j given that B has occurred is

$$P(A_j|B)=\frac{P(A_jB)}{P(B)}=\frac{P(B|A_j)P(A_j)}{\displaystyle\sum_{i=1}^{n}P(B|A_i)P(A_i)}. \tag{8.5}$$

Formula (8. 5) is called the **Bayes formula**.

Example 8. 13   In a mask factory, three workshops, W_1, W_2 and W_3, make 0. 3, 0. 45 and 0. 25, respectively, of the masks. It is known from past experience that 0. 02, 0. 03 and 0. 02 of the masks made by each machine, respectively, are defective. Now, if a product was chosen randomly and found to be defective, what is the probability that it was made by workshop W_3?

Solution   Let B_i = "the product is from workshop W_i" ($i = 1, 2, 3$), and $D =$ "the mask is defective". Then we have $P(B_1) = 0. 3$, $P(B_2) = 0. 45$, and $P(B_3) = 0. 25$.

We also have $P(D|B_1) = 0. 02$, $P(D|B_2) = 0. 03$, and $P(D|B_3) = 0. 02$.

First we use the Law of Total Probability to get

$$P(D) = \sum_{i=1}^{3} P(D|B_i)P(B_i) = 0. 3 \times 0. 02 + 0. 45 \times 0. 03 + 0. 25 \times 0. 02 = 0. 0245.$$

So we use Bayes formula to get the posterior probability

$$P(B_3|D) = \frac{P(DB_3)}{P(D)} = \frac{P(D|B_3)P(B_3)}{P(D)} = \frac{0. 25 \times 0. 02}{0. 0245} = 0. 204. \qquad \#$$

Example 8. 14   Approximately 1% of women aged $40 \sim 50$ have breast cancer. A woman with breast cancer has a 90% chance of a positive test from a mammogram, while a woman without breast cancer has a 10% chance of a false positive result. What is the probability a woman has breast cancer given that she just had a positive test?

Solution   Let $B =$ "a woman has breast cancer", and $A =$ "the test is positive", then we know $P(B) = 0. 01$, $P(A|B) = 0. 9$, and $P(A|\overline{B}) = 0. 1$.

We need to find the posterior probability $P(B|A)$. First we use the Law of Total Probability to get

$$P(A) = P(A|B)P(B) + P(A|\overline{B})P(\overline{B}) = 0. 9 \times 0. 01 + 0. 1 \times 0. 99 = 0. 108.$$

So we use the Bayes formula to get the posterior probability

$$P(B|A) = \frac{P(AB)}{P(A)} = \frac{P(A|B)P(B)}{P(A|B)P(B) + P(A|\overline{B})P(\overline{B})} = \frac{0. 9 \times 0. 01}{0. 108} = \frac{1}{12}. \qquad \#$$

Note   This answer is somewhat surprising and interesting. A positive test only means the woman has a $\frac{1}{12} \approx 8. 3\%$ chance of breast cancer, rather than 90%. But it makes sense: the test gives a false positive 10% of the time, so there will be a lot of false positives if the population size is large enough. Most of the positive test results will be incorrect.

Your Practice 8. 4   The population of a particular country consists of three ethnic groups. Each individual belongs to one of the four major blood groups. The accompanying joint probability (Table 8. 1) gives the proportions of individuals in the various ethnic group-blood group combinations. Suppose that an individual is randomly selected from the population, and define events by $A =$ "type A selected" and $C =$ "ethnic group 3 selected".

(1) Calculate $P(A)$, $P(C)$, and $P(A \cap C)$;

(2) Calculate both $P(A|C)$ and $P(C|A)$.

Table 8.1

Ethnic Group	Blood Group			
	O	A	B	AB
1	0.056	0.102	0.008	0.004
2	0.098	0.218	0.01	0.004
3	0.113	0.08	0.062	0.245

8.2.3 Independent Events

If events A and B are completely unrelated, then knowing that B has happened should not provide us any information about A. We can express this using conditional probabilities. Namely,

$$P(A|B)=P(A)$$

and we say that B and A are independent. We will not use this formula as the definition of independence; rather we will use the definition of condition probabilities to rewrite it. We find

$$\frac{P(AB)}{P(B)}=P(A).$$

Multiplying both sides by $P(B)$, we find $P(AB)=P(A)P(B)$. We use this as our definition.

Definition 8.4 (Independence)

Two events A and B are independent if and only if
$$P(AB)=P(A)P(B).$$

This means that, if events A and B are independent, then the probability of A is unchanged whether B occurs or not, that is the reason that the word "independent" is used.

Theorem 8.5

If events A and B are independent, so are the following pairs of events:

(1) $\overline{A}$ *and* B;

(2) A *and* $\overline{B}$;

(3) $\overline{A}$ *and* $\overline{B}$.

The proof of the formula is left to the readers.

Example 8.15 Tossing a fair six-sided dice once and we define events
$$A=\{2, 4, 6\}, B=\{1, 2, 3\}, \text{ and } C=\{1, 2, 3, 4\}.$$
So
$$AB=\{2\}, \text{ and } AC=\{2, 4\}.$$
We have
$$P(A)=\frac{1}{2}, P(B)=\frac{1}{2}, \text{ and } P(AB)=\frac{1}{6}\neq P(A)P(B),$$

$$P(C) = \frac{4}{6}, \text{ and } P(AC) = \frac{2}{6} = P(A)P(C).$$

Therefore, events A and B are dependent, whereas events A and C are independent. ♯

Example 8.16　Given that 5% of men and 0.25% of women are color-blind. One woman and one man are selected randomly, whether they are color-blind or not is independent. Find

(1) What is the probability that at most one of the two persons is color-blind?

(2) What is the probability that at least one of the two persons is color-blind?

Solution　Let $W =$ "the woman is color-blind", and $M =$ "the man is color-blind". The event that at most one of the two persons is color-blind is $\overline{W} \cup \overline{M}$, and the event that at least one of the two persons is color-blind is $W \cup M$.

Because whether two persons are color-blind or not is independent, we have that W and M are independent and $\overline{W}$ and $\overline{M}$ are also independent. We also know that $P(W) = 0.0025$, and $P(M) = 0.05$.

(1) Using De Morgan's Laws and independence of events W and M, we can get the probability that at most one of the two persons is color-blind:

$$P(\overline{W} \cup \overline{M}) = P(\overline{WM}) = 1 - P(WM) = 1 - P(W)P(M) = 0.000125.$$

(2) Using De Morgan's Laws yields

$$P(W \cup M) = 1 - P(\overline{W \cup M}) = 1 - P(\overline{W} \cap \overline{M}).$$

Using independence of events $\overline{W}$ and $\overline{M}$, we get

$$P(W \cup M) = 1 - P(\overline{W})P(\overline{M}) = 1 - [1 - P(W)][1 - P(M)] = 0.052375. \quad ♯$$

We can extend independence to more than two events. Events $A_1, A_2, \cdots, A_n$ are independent if for any $1 \leqslant i_1 < i_2 < \cdots < i_k \leqslant n$,

$$P(A_{i_1} A_{i_2} \cdots A_{i_k}) = P(A_{i_1})P(A_{i_2}) \cdots P(A_{i_k}). \tag{8.6}$$

Your Practice 8.5　Seventy percent of all vehicles examined at a certain emissions inspection station pass the inspection. Assuming that successive vehicles pass or fail independently of one another, calculate the following probabilities:

(1) P(all of the next two vehicles inspected pass);

(2) P(at least one of the next two inspected fails);

(3) P(exactly one of the next two inspected passes).

Exercise 8.2

1. From a deck of 52 cards, a card is withdrawn at random and not replaced, a second card is then drawn. Find the probability that the first card is an ace and the second a king.

2. A family has 3 children, one of which is a girl. Find the probability that there is at least one boy in this family.

3. Two cards are drawn successively and without replacement from an ordinary

deck of playing cards. Compute the probability of drawing

(1) two hearts;

(2) a heart on the first draw and a club on the second draw;

(3) a heart on the first draw and an ace on the second draw.

4. Let $A_1 = $ "the person who is left-eye-dominant", $A_2 = $ "the person who is right-eye-dominant", $B_1 = $ "the person who can folds the left thumb", $B_2 = $ "the person who can folds the right thumb". Probabilities of those events are list in Table 8.2.

Table 8.2

	B_1	B_2	Total
A_1	14%	20%	34%
A_2	40%	26%	66%
Total	54%	46%	1

Compute the following probability:

(1) $P(A_2 \cap B_2)$;

(2) $P(A_2 \cup B_2)$;

(3) $P(A_1 | B_1)$;

(4) $P(B_2 | A_2)$.

5. In a pharmaceutical factory, three machines, M_1, M_2 and M_3, make 35%, 40%, and 25% of the tablets respectively. It is known from past experience that 5%, 3% and 2% of the tablets made by each machine, respectively, are defective. Now, suppose that a finished tablet is randomly selected.

(1) What is the probability that it is defective?

(2) If a tablet was chosen randomly and found to be defective, what is the probability that it was made by machine M_3?

6. Let A and B be independent events with $P(A) = 0.6$, and $P(B) = 0.3$. Compute:

(1) $P(A \cap B)$;

(2) $P(A \cup B)$;

(3) $P(\overline{A} \cap \overline{B})$.

7. Let $P(A) = 0.2$, and $P(B) = 0.6$. Compute:

(1) $P(A \cup B)$, when A and B are independent;

(2) $P(A | B)$, when A and B are mutually exclusive.

8. Let A and B be independent events with $P(A) = 0.3$, and $P(B) = 0.5$. Compute:

(1) $P(A \cap B)$;

(2) $P(A \cap \overline{B})$;

(3) $P(\overline{A} \cap \overline{B})$;

(4) $P(\overline{A} \cap B)$;

(5) $P(\overline{A \cup B})$.

8.3　Random Variables and Distributions

8.3.1　Random Variables

In general, each outcome of an experiment can be associated with a number by specifying a rule of association. Such a rule of association is called a random variable. A random variable is a function from the sample space into the set of real numbers. Random variables are typically denoted by X, Y or Z, or other capital letters chosen from the end of the alphabet. We will often use the abbreviation r. v. in place of random variable. For

instance,

$$X: \Omega \rightarrow \mathbf{R}$$

describe a random variable X, which is a map from the sample space Ω to the set of real numbers. For each outcome ω in the sample space, there is a number $X(\omega)$ associates with it (Figure 8.11).

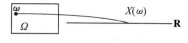

Figure 8.11

Example 8.17

(1) A fair dice is tossed. The number X shown on the top face is a random variable, which takes values in the set $\{1, 2, 3, 4, 5, 6\}$.

(2) The life of a bulb Y selected at random from bulbs produced by a company is a random variable, which takes values in the interval $(0, +\infty)$.　　　　　　♯

Note　The concept of a random variable allows us to pass from the experimental outcomes themselves to a numerical function of the outcomes.

Definition 8.5

A discrete random variable is a random variable that takes on a finite number of values $x_1, x_2, \cdots, x_n$ or an infinite number of values $x_1, x_2, \cdots, x_n, \cdots$.

Let Y be the number of students on a class list for a particular course who are absent on the first day of classes, then the possible values of Y are $0, 1, 2, \cdots, N$. So Y is a discrete random variable.

One type of the non-discrete random variable is the *continuous random variable* whose possible values consists of an entire interval on the number line. Experimental outcomes that are based on measurement scales such as time, weight, distance, and temperature can be described by continuous random variables.

8.3.2　The Probability Distribution of a Discrete Random Variable

Once a discrete random variable X is introduced, the sample space is no longer important. It suffices to list the possible values of X and their corresponding probabilities. This information is contained in the probability mass function of X.

Definition 8.6 (Probability Mass Function)

If the possible values of a discrete random variable X are $x_1, x_2, \cdots, x_n \cdots$, the probability distribution or probability mass function (pmf) is defined by

$$P(X=x_i)=p_i, \ i=1, 2, \cdots$$

or

X	x_1	x_2	$\cdots$	x_n	$\cdots$
P	p_1	p_2	$\cdots$	p_n	$\cdots$

Note If X is a discrete random variable, then we find that the probability mass function satisfy:

$$p_i \geqslant 0, \text{ and } \sum_{i=1}^{+\infty} p_i = 1.$$

Example 8.18 A fair coin is tossed for three times. Let X denote the number of head occurrence. Construct the distribution of X.

Solution We can find that the sample space is

$$\Omega = \{HHH, HHT, HTH, THH, HTT, THT, TTH, TTT\},$$

and the possible values of X are 0, 1, 2, 3.

We can find that $\{X=0\}$ means heads not appear in three times, hence applying the independence of events we get

$$P(X=0) = P(TTT) = P(T)P(T)P(T) = (1/2)^3 = 1/8.$$

We have

$$\{X=1\} = \{HTT\} \cup \{THT\} \cup \{TTH\},$$

and those three events are disjoint. Thus,

$$P(X=1) = P(\{HTT\} \cup \{THT\} \cup \{TTH\}) = P(HTT) + P(THT) + P(TTH).$$

Applying the independent of events we have

$$P(HTT) = P(THT) = P(TTH) = P(T)P(T)P(H) = (1/2)^3 = 1/8.$$

Therefore,

$$P(X=1) = 3/8.$$

A similar analysis leads to

$$P(X=2) = P(\{HHT\} \cup \{HTH\} \cup \{THH\}) = P(HHT) + P(HTH) + P(THH) = 3/8.$$
$$P(X=3) = P(HHH) = 1/8.$$

So the probability mass function of X is given by

X	0	1	2	3
P	1/8	3/8	3/8	1/8

\#

Example 8.19 If the probability mass function of random variable X is

X	-3	-1	1	10
P	0.14	$a/2$	0.55	$2a$

(1) Determine the parameter a.

(2) Find $P(X>0)$.

Solution (1) Apply the property of probability distribution, we get

$$\sum_{i=1}^{+\infty} p_i = 0.14 + \frac{a}{2} + 0.55 + 2a = 1,$$

$$a = 0.124.$$

Hence, the probability mass function of X is

X	-3	-1	1	10
P	0.14	0.062	0.55	0.248

(2) The possible values of random variable X are $-3, -1$, 1, 10, we have
$$\{X>0\} = \{X=1 \text{ or } 10\},$$
then $\qquad P(X>0) = P(X=1) + P(X=10) = 0.55 + 0.248 = 0.798.$ #

8.3.3 The Cumulative Distribution Function of a Random Variable

As we will see, so-called continuous random variables cannot be specified by giving a probability mass function. However, the cumulative distribution function of a random variable X (also known as the distribution function) allows us to treat discrete and continuous random variables in the same way.

Definition 8.7 (Cumulative Distribution Function)

The cumulative distribution function (cdf) $F(x)$ of a random variable X is the function defined by
$$F(x) = P(X \leqslant x), -\infty < x < +\infty.$$

Note (1) The cumulative distribution function $F(x)$ is defined on real numbers, not on sample space.

(2) Because $F(x)$ is the probability that the observed value of random variable X will be at most x, we have $0 \leqslant F(x) \leqslant 1$.

Example 8.20 If the random variable X has probability mass function

X	0	1	2
P	0.2	0.5	0.3

(1) Find $P(X \leqslant 0.5)$;

(2) Find the cumulative distribution function of X.

Solution (1) We know that X can take three possible values. The event $\{X \leqslant 0.5\}$ is equal to $\{X=0\}$. We have
$$P(X \leqslant 0.5) = P(X=0) = 0.2.$$

(2) Apply the definition of the cumulative distribution function, we have
$$F(x) = P(X \leqslant x) = \sum_{x_i \leqslant x} P(X=x_i), -\infty < x < +\infty.$$

We know that x should be discrete, because X can take three possible values. If $x<0$, then X can take no values. We have
$$F(x) = 0.$$

If $0 \leqslant x < 1$, then X can take only 0. We have
$$F(x) = P(X \leqslant x) = P(X=0) = 0.2.$$

If $1 \leqslant x < 2$, then X can take 0 and 1. We have
$$F(x) = P(X \leqslant x) = P(X=0) + P(X=1) = 0.7.$$

If $x \geqslant 2$, then X can take three possible values. We have
$$F(x) = P(X \leqslant x) = P(X=0) + P(X=1) + P(X=2) = 1.$$

Hence,

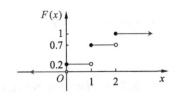

$$F(x) = \begin{cases} 0, & \text{if } x < 0; \\ 0.2, & \text{if } 0 \leqslant x < 1; \\ 0.7, & \text{if } 1 \leqslant x < 2; \\ 1, & \text{if } 2 \leqslant x. \end{cases}$$

We give the line graph for the cumulative distribution

Figure 8.12

function $F(x)$ in Figure 8.12.

#

We see that, for a discrete random variable X, the cumulative distribution function $F(x)$ jumps in each of the x_i, and is constant between successive x_i. The height of the jump at x_i is p_i.

Based on the above example, we list three properties of the cumulative distribution function $F(x)$ of a random variable X:

(1) For $a < b$ one has that $F(a) \leqslant F(b)$. This property is an immediate consequence of the fact that $a < b$ implies that the event $\{X \leqslant a\}$ is contained in the event $\{X \leqslant b\}$.

(2) Since $F(a)$ is a probability, the value of the cumulative distribution function is always between 0 and 1.

(3) $F(+\infty) = \lim\limits_{x \to +\infty} F(x) = 1$, and $F(-\infty) = \lim\limits_{x \to -\infty} F(x) = 0$.

In the following part, we will introduce some discrete random variable that models the number of successive amount of fixed number of trials.

8.3.3.1   the Bernoulli Distribution

The Bernoulli distribution is used to model an experiment with only two possible outcomes, often referred to as success and failure, usually encoded as 1 and 0. Such a experiment is called a ***Bernoulli trial***. Tossing a coin and buying a lottery are examples of Bernoulli trials.

Definition 8.8 (the Bernoulli Distribution)

A discrete random variable X is called a Bernoulli random variable or has a Bernoulli distribution with parameter p, if its probability mass function is given by
$$P(X=1) = p, \ P(X=0) = 1-p.$$
We denote this distribution by $X \sim B(1, p)$.

8.3.3.2   the Binomial Distribution

Suppose we toss the same coin successively and independently three times. Then there are eight possible outcomes for this experiment: HHH, HHT, HTH, TTH, HTT, THT, TTH, TTT. Let X be the number of H among the three trials, then the random variable X takes values 0, 1, 2, 3. For instance, $X(\text{HHH}) = 3$, $X(\text{HHT}) = 2$, $X(\text{TTT}) = 0$.

Using the independence of events we get

$$P(X=3)=P(\text{HHH})=p^3,$$

$$P(X=2)=P(\text{HHT})+P(\text{HTH})+P(\text{THH})=\binom{3}{2}p^2(1-p),$$

$$P(X=1)=P(\text{HTT})+P(\text{TTH})+P(\text{THT})=\binom{3}{2}p(1-p)^2,$$

$$P(X=0)=P(\text{TTT})=(1-p)^3.$$

The preceding random variable X is an example of a random variable with a binomial distribution with parameters $n=3$ and $p=1/2$.

Definition 8.9 (the Binomial Distribution)

A *discrete random variable* X *has a binomial distribution with parameters* n *and* p, *where* n *is an integer and* $0 \leqslant p \leqslant 1$, *if its probability mass function is given by*

$$b(x;\ n,\ p)=P(X=x)=\binom{n}{x}p^x(1-p)^{n-x},\ x=0,\ 1,\ 2,\cdots,\ n.$$

Note   We often write $X \sim B(n,\ p)$ or $X \sim Bin(n,\ p)$ to indicate that X is a binomial r. v. based on n trials with success probability p.

Example 8.21   Each of six randomly selected cola drinkers is given a glass containing cola S and one containing cola F. The glasses are identical in appearance except for a code on the bottom to identify the cola. Suppose there is actually no tendency among cola drinkers to prefer one cola to the other, then $p=P(\text{a selected individual prefers } S)=0.5$. Let X be the number among the six who prefer S, then $X \sim Bin(6,\ 0.5)$.   #

8.3.3.3   the Poisson Distribution

Definition 8.10 (the Poisson Distribution)

A *random variable* X *is said to have a Poisson random variable or Poisson distribution with parameter* $\lambda(\lambda>0)$, *if the probability mass function of* X *is*

$$p(x;\ \lambda)=P(X=x)=\frac{e^{-\lambda}\lambda^x}{x!},\ x=0,\ 1,\ 2,\cdots.$$

Note   We will often write $X \sim P(\lambda)$. The value of λ is frequency a rate per unit time or unit area. The constant e is the base of the natural logarithm system.

Example 8.22   Let X denote the number of arriving at the hospital during a given time period. Suppose that X has a Poisson distribution with $\lambda=4.5$, so the average number of arrivals is 4.5 patients. The probability of reaching five patients within the given time period is

$$P(X=5)=\frac{e^{-4.5}4.5^5}{5!}=0.1708.$$ #

8.3.4   Continuous Random Variables

Many experiments have outcomes that take values on a continuous scale. For example, we measure the pH value, the depth of a lake, and the length of life of a

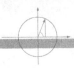

particular product. These experiments have continuous random variables naturally associated with them.

8.3.4.1 Probability density function

Continuous random variables take values in an entire interval. Thus the probabilities of the possible values of the outcomes approach zero. However, the probability that the possible values lie in some fixed interval $[a, b]$ will settle down. This motivates the following definition.

Definition 8.11 (Probability Density Function)

A random variable X is continuous if for a non-negative integrable function $f(x)$ and for any numbers a and b with $a \leqslant b$,

$$P(a < X \leqslant b) = \int_a^b f(x) \, \mathrm{d}x.$$

We call $f(x)$ the probability density function (or probability density)(pdf) of X.

The probability density function should satisfy:

(1) $f(x) \geqslant 0$, for every x;

(2) $\int_{-\infty}^{+\infty} f(x) \, \mathrm{d}x = 1$.

Property (1) says that $f(x)$ is non-negative. So we usually only write the positive part while the zero part is omitted. Property (2) tells that the area under the graph of the density function $f(x)$ is 1 (Figure 8.13).

Note that the probability that X lies in an interval $(a, b]$ is equal to the area under the probability density function $f(x)$ of X over the interval $(a, b]$ as shown in Figure 8.14. So if the interval gets smaller and smaller, the probability will go to zero. It follows that for any c,

$$P(X = c) = 0. \tag{8.7}$$

This implies that for continuous random variables you may be careless about the precise form of the intervals:

$$P(a \leqslant X \leqslant b) = P(a < X \leqslant b) = P(a < X < b) = P(a \leqslant X < b).$$

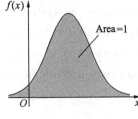

Figure 8.13

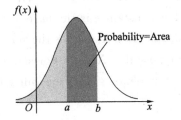

Figure 8.14

Example 8.23 If a random variable X has the probability density function

$$f(x) = \begin{cases} kx, & \text{if } 0 < x < 2; \\ 0, & \text{else.} \end{cases}$$

(1) Find the value of k;

(2) Calculate $P(0 \leqslant X \leqslant 1)$, $P(X > 1)$.

Solution　(1) We know

$$1 = \int_{-\infty}^{+\infty} f(x)\mathrm{d}x = \int_0^2 kx\,\mathrm{d}x = \left[\frac{kx^2}{2}\right]_0^2 = 2k.$$

Therefore, $k = \dfrac{1}{2}$ and

$$f(x) = \begin{cases} \dfrac{x}{2}, & \text{if } 0 < x < 2; \\ 0, & \text{else.} \end{cases}$$

(2) Using the definition, we get

$$P(0 \leqslant X \leqslant 1) = \int_0^1 f(x)\mathrm{d}x = \int_0^1 \frac{x}{2}\mathrm{d}x = \left[\frac{x^2}{4}\right]_0^1 = \frac{1}{4}.$$

$$P(X > 1) = \int_1^{+\infty} f(x)\mathrm{d}x = \int_1^2 \frac{x}{2}\mathrm{d}x = \left[\frac{x^2}{4}\right]_1^2 = \frac{3}{4}. \qquad \#$$

You should realize that discrete random variables do not have a probability density function $f(x)$ and continuous random variables do not have a probability mass function, but that both have a cumulative distribution function $F(x) = P(X \leqslant x)$.

There is a simple relation between the cumulative distribution function $F(x)$ and the probability density function $f(x)$ of a continuous random variable. It follows from integral calculus that

$$F(x) = P(X \leqslant x) = \int_{-\infty}^x f(t)\mathrm{d}t \text{ and } f(x) = \frac{\mathrm{d}}{\mathrm{d}x}F(x).$$

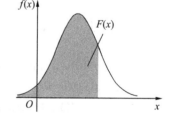

Hence, $F(x)$ is the area under the density curve to the left of x as shown in Figure 8.15.

Using the fact that for $a < b$ the event $X \leqslant b$ is a disjoint union of the events $X \leqslant a$ and $a < X \leqslant b$, we can express the probability that X lies in an interval $(a, b]$ directly in terms of either f or F:

Figure 8.15

$$P(a < X \leqslant b) = \int_a^b f(t)\mathrm{d}t = F(b) - F(a).$$

Example 8.24　If a random variable has the probability density function

$$f(x) = \begin{cases} \dfrac{1}{8} + \dfrac{3x}{8}, & \text{if } 0 < x < 2; \\ 0, & \text{else.} \end{cases}$$

(1) Find cumulative distribution function of X;

(2) Calculate $P(1 \leqslant X \leqslant 1.5)$.

Solution

(1) Apply the definition of the cumulative distribution function, we have

$$F(x) = P(X \leqslant x) = \int_{-\infty}^x f(t)\mathrm{d}t, \ -\infty < x < +\infty.$$

We know that x should be discussed, because the probability density function $f(x)$

Calculus for Medicine and Pharmacy

can take different expressions in different intervals.

If $x \leqslant 0$, then for every $t < x$, $f(t) = 0$. We have

$$F(x) = \int_{-\infty}^{x} f(t)\mathrm{d}t = 0 \,.$$

If $0 \leqslant x < 2$, then for every $t < x$, $f(t)$ can take two different expressions. We have

$$F(x) = \int_{-\infty}^{x} f(t)\mathrm{d}t = \int_{0}^{x} \left(\frac{1}{8} + \frac{3t}{8} \right)\mathrm{d}t = \frac{x}{8} + \frac{3x^2}{16} \,.$$

If $x \geqslant 2$, we can get

$$F(x) = \int_{-\infty}^{x} f(t)\mathrm{d}t = \int_{0}^{2} \left(\frac{1}{8} + \frac{3t}{8} \right)\mathrm{d}t = 1 \,.$$

So,

$$F(x) = \begin{cases} 0, & \text{if } x \leqslant 0; \\ \dfrac{x}{8} + \dfrac{3x^2}{16}, & \text{if } 0 \leqslant x < 2; \\ 1, & \text{if } x \geqslant 2. \end{cases}$$

(2) We can use two ways to get the probability. Method 1 uses the cdf:
$$P(1 \leqslant X \leqslant 1.5) = F(1.5) - F(1) = 0.297.$$

Method 2 uses the pdf:

$$P(1 \leqslant X \leqslant 1.5) = \int_{1}^{1.5} \left(\frac{1}{8} + \frac{3x}{8} \right)\mathrm{d}t = 0.297 \,. \qquad \#$$

Your Practice 8.6   A continuous random variable X has probability density function

$$f(x) = \begin{cases} \dfrac{3(1-x^2)}{2}, & \text{if } 0 < x < 1; \\ 0, & \text{else.} \end{cases}$$

(1) Find the cumulative distribution function of X;

(2) Calculate $P(-1 \leqslant X \leqslant 0.5)$.

8.3.4.2   The Uniform Distribution

We may encounter a continuous random variable that describes an experiment where the outcome is completely arbitrary outcome, except that we know that it lies between certain bounds. The arbitrary proposition means that subintervals of the same length should have the same probability. This motivates the following definition.

Definition 8.12 (the Uniform Distribution)

A continuous random variable X is said to have a uniform distribution or uniform random variable on the interval (a, b) if the probability density function of X is

$$f(x) = \begin{cases} \dfrac{1}{b-a}, & \text{if } a < x < b; \\ 0, & \text{else.} \end{cases}$$

We denote this distribution by $X \sim U(a, b)$.

The probability density function of the uniform distribution is shown in Figure 8.16.

Your Practice 8.7   Give the cumulative distribution function $F(x)$ of a random variable that has a $U(a, b)$ distribution.

8.3.4.3　The Exponential Distribution

The family of exponential distributions provides probability models that are very widely used in engineering and science disciplines.

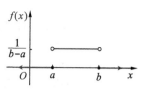

Figure 8.16

Definition 8.13 (the Exponential Distribution)

A continuous random variable X is said to have an exponential distribution or exponential random variable with parameter λ $(\lambda > 0)$, if the probability density function of $f(x)$ is

$$f(x) = \begin{cases} \lambda e^{-\lambda x}, & if\ x > 0; \\ 0, & else. \end{cases}$$

We denote this distribution by $X \sim E(\lambda)$.

The probability density function of the exponential distribution is shown in Figure 8.17.

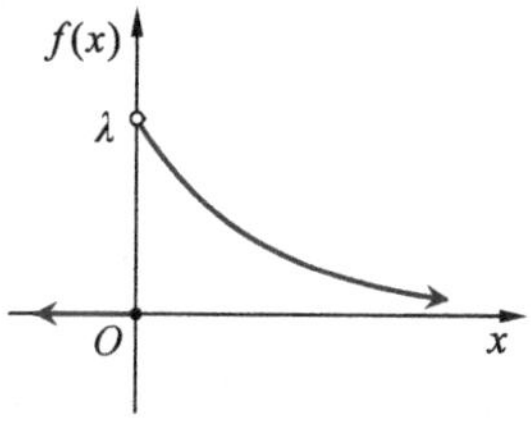

The cumulative distribution function of the exponential distribution is given by

$$F(x) = \begin{cases} 1 - e^{-\lambda x}, & if\ x > 0; \\ 0, & else. \end{cases}$$

Figure 8.17

The exponential distribution satisfies the memoryless property, i.e., if X has an exponential distribution, then for every s, $t > 0$,

$$P(X > s + t \mid X > s) = P(X > t).$$

Actually, this follows directly from

$$P(X > s + t \mid X > s) = \frac{P(X > s + t)}{P(X > s)} = \frac{e^{-\lambda(s+t)}}{e^{-\lambda s}} = e^{-\lambda t} = P(X > t).$$

Your Practice 8.8　A study of the response time of a certain computer system yields that the response time in seconds has an exponentially distributed time with parameter 0.25. What is the probability that the response time exceeds five seconds?

8.3.4.4　The Normal Distribution

The normal distribution is the most important one in all of probability and statistics. Many numerical populations have distributions that can be fit very closely by an appropriate normal curve. Examples include heights, weights, and other physical characteristics.

Definition 8.14 (the Normal Distribution)

A continuous random variable X is said to have a normal distribution or normal random variable with parameters μ and σ^2, where $-\infty < \mu < +\infty$ and $\sigma > 0$, if the probability density function of X is

$$f(x) = \frac{1}{\sqrt{2\pi}\sigma} \exp\left\{ -\frac{(x-\mu)^2}{2\sigma^2} \right\}, \quad -\infty < \mu < +\infty. \tag{8.8}$$

We denote this distribution by $X \sim N(\mu, \sigma^2)$.

The probability density function and the cumulative distribution function of the normal random variable are shown in Figures 8.18 and 8.19.

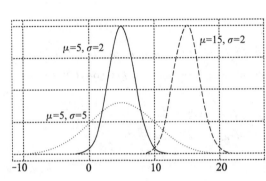

Figure 8.18

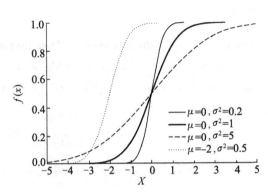

Figure 8.19

If X has an $N(\mu, \sigma^2)$ distribution, then its cumulative distribution function is given by

$$F(x) = \int_{-\infty}^{x} \frac{1}{\sqrt{2\pi}\sigma} \exp\left\{ -\frac{(t-\mu)^2}{2\sigma^2} \right\} dt, \quad -\infty < x < +\infty.$$

Unfortunately there is no explicit expression for $f(x)$; $f(x)$ has no antiderivative. However, any $N(\mu, \sigma^2)$ distributed random variable can be turned into an $N(0, 1)$ distributed random variable by a simple transformation. As a consequence, a table of the $N(0, 1)$ distribution suffices. The latter is called the standard normal distribution, and because of its special role the letter φ has been reserved for its probability density function

$$\varphi(z) = \frac{1}{\sqrt{2\pi}} e^{-\frac{z^2}{2}}, \quad -\infty < z < +\infty. \tag{8.9}$$

We denote this distribution by $Z \sim N(0, 1)$.

Theorem 8.6

If X has a normal distribution with parameters μ and σ^2 ($\sigma > 0$), then

$$Z = \frac{X - \mu}{\sigma}$$

has a standard normal distribution.

Proof We first determine the cumulative distribution function of Z and then the probability density by differentiating.

Let $F_X(x)$ be the distribution function of X, $F_Z(z)$ be the distribution function of Z. Since $\sigma > 0$, we have: for any z,

$$F_Z(z) = P(Z \leqslant z) = P\left(\frac{X - \mu}{\sigma} \leqslant z \right) = P(X \leqslant \mu + \sigma z) = F_X(\mu + \sigma z).$$

By differentiating $F_Z(z)$ (using the Chain Rule), we obtain the probability density

$$f_Z(z) = \frac{\mathrm{d}}{\mathrm{d}z}F_Z(z) = \frac{\mathrm{d}F_X(\mu+\sigma z)}{\mathrm{d}z}$$

$$= \frac{\mathrm{d}F_X(\mu+\sigma z)}{\mathrm{d}(\mu+\sigma z)}\frac{\mathrm{d}(\mu+\sigma z)}{\mathrm{d}x} = \sigma f_X(\mu+\sigma z).$$

Substituting x in Equation (8.8) with $\mu+\sigma z$, we get

$$f_Z(z) = \frac{1}{\sqrt{2\pi}}\mathrm{e}^{-\frac{z^2}{2}}.$$

Then $Z \sim N(0, 1)$.   #

The probability density function of the standard normal random variable is shown in Figure 8.20.

Note that φ is symmetric about zero: $\varphi(-z) = \varphi(z)$ for each z. The corresponding cumulative distribution function is denoted by Φ:

$$\Phi(z) = \int_{-\infty}^{z} \varphi(t)\mathrm{d}t = \int_{-\infty}^{z} \frac{1}{\sqrt{2\pi}}\mathrm{e}^{-\frac{t^2}{2}}\mathrm{d}t.$$

Thus the value of $\Phi(z)$ is the area under the pdf and to the left of z as shown in Figure 8.21. The table for the standard normal distribution is given in Appendix B. The table contain the values of $\Phi(z)$.

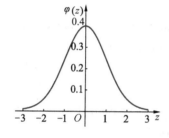

Figure 8.20

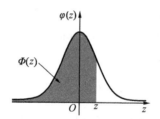

Figure 8.21

Proposition 8.1

If the standard normal random variable Z with the cumulative distribution function $\Phi(z)$, then we have

(1) $\Phi(0) = 0.5$;

(2) $\Phi(-z) = 1 - \Phi(z)$;

(3) $P(a \leqslant Z \leqslant b) = \int_{a}^{b} \varphi(z)\mathrm{d}z = \Phi(b) - \Phi(a)$.

Example 8.25 A random variable Z has a standard normal distribution. Using the cumulative distribution function $\Phi(z)$, we can obtain

(1) $P(-0.34 < Z \leqslant 0.62) = \Phi(0.62) - [1 - \Phi(0.34)] = 0.7324 - 1 + 0.6331 = 0.3655$.

(2) $P(Z > -0.65) = 1 - \Phi(-0.65) = \Phi(0.65) = 0.7422$.   #

Example 8.26 If $X \sim N(1.5, 4)$, calculate $P(|X| < 3)$.

Solution For $X \sim N(1.5, 4)$, using Theorem 8.6, we have

$$\frac{X-1.5}{2} \sim N(0, 1).$$

Hence, $P(|X|<3)=P(-3<X<3)=P\left(-2.25<\dfrac{X-1.5}{2}<0.75\right)$

$$=\Phi(0.75)-[1-\Phi(2.25)]=0.7734-1+0.9878=0.7612. \quad \#$$

This example leads to the following results.

If $X \sim N(\mu, \sigma^2)$, *then*

(1) $P(a \leqslant X \leqslant b)=P\left(\dfrac{a-\mu}{\sigma} \leqslant Z \leqslant \dfrac{b-\mu}{\sigma}\right)=\Phi\left(\dfrac{b-\mu}{\sigma}\right)-\Phi\left(\dfrac{a-\mu}{\sigma}\right);$

(2) $P(X \leqslant a)=\Phi\left(\dfrac{a-\mu}{\sigma}\right);$

(3) $P(b \leqslant X)=1-\Phi\left(\dfrac{b-\mu}{\sigma}\right).$

Exercise 8.3

1. What values can c be in order that the following sequences become a discrete random variable.

(1) $P(X=k)=\dfrac{c}{n}$, $k=1, 2, \cdots, n$;

(2) $P(X=k)=\dfrac{k}{c}$, $k=1, 2, 3, 4$;

(3) $P(X=k)=ck$, $k=1, 2, \cdots, 10$;

(4) $P(X=k)=\dfrac{c\lambda^k}{k!}$, $\lambda>0$, $k=1, 2, \cdots$.

2. Suppose that X has the probability mass function $P(X=k)=\dfrac{k}{15}$, $k=1, 2, 3, 4, 5$. Calculate

(1) $P(X=1 \text{ or } X=2)$;

(2) $P(1<X<3.5)$;

(3) $P(1 \leqslant X \leqslant 3.5)$.

3. The random variable X follows a Poisson distribution with $P(X=1)=P(X=2)$. Find $P(X=3)$.

4. Let a ball be taken at random from an urn that contains five blue, three white and six green balls. Let $X=1$ if the outcome is a blue ball, $X=5$ if the outcome is a white ball, $X=10$ if the outcome is a green ball.

(1) Find the probability mass function of X;

(2) Find the cdf of X.

5. We tossed a coin repeatedly until the first heads showed up. Assume that the probability of heads is p with $p \in (0, 1)$. Let Y be a random variable that counts the number of trials until the first heads shows up.

(1) Show that $P(Y=1)=p$, $P(Y=2)=(1-p)p$.

(2) Explain why $P(Y=j)=(1-p)^{j-1}p$, for $j=1, 2, \cdots$. This is called the **Geometric distribution**.

(3) Proof $\sum\limits_{j \geqslant 1} P(Y=j)=1$.

6. What values can c be in order that the following function become a pdf.

(1) $f(x)=cx^2$, $1\leqslant x\leqslant 2$;

(2) $f(x)=\dfrac{c}{x^2}$, $x\geqslant 1$;

(3) $f(x)=4x^c$, $0\leqslant x\leqslant 1$;

(4) $f(x)=ce^{-2x}$, $x\geqslant 0$.

7. The probability density function of X is given by $f(x)=2(1-x)$, $0\leqslant x\leqslant 1$.

(1) Calculate $P(0<X<0.5)$, $P(1/4<X<3/4)$, $P(X=0.5)$, $P(X\geqslant 0.5)$;

(2) Find the cumulative distribution function of X.

8. Suppose that $X\sim U(0, 10)$.

(1) Calculate $P(0<X<2)$, $P(X=5)$, $P(X\geqslant 8)$;

(2) Find the cumulative distribution function of X.

9. Let $Z\sim N(0, 1)$, compute the following probability:

(1) $P(0\leqslant Z<0.5)$;

(2) $P(Z>-0.5)$;

(3) $P(|Z|\geqslant 0.5)$.

10. Let $Z\sim N(0, 1)$, find values of c such that

(1) $P(Z\geqslant c)=0.025$;

(2) $P(Z<c)=0.05$;

(3) $P(|Z|<c)=0.95$;

(4) $P(|Z|\leqslant c)=0.9$.

11. If X has a normal distribution with parameters 6 and 25, find the following probability:

(1) $P(6<X\leqslant 12)$;

(2) $P(X>21)$;

(3) $P(|X-6|<5)$.

8.4   Means and Variances

Means and Variances summarize a random variable by numbers. The expected value, also called the expectation or mean, gives the center in the sense of average value of the distribution of the random variable. The variance measures the spread of the distribution of the random variable.

8.4.1   Means

8.4.1.1   The discrete case

Assume a player tosses a dice. He wins 8 Yuan when he gets six and lost 2 Yuan otherwise. If he tossed 12 times, how much would he get? What most people would do to answer this question is to take the weighted average

$$8\times\frac{1}{6}+(-2)\times\frac{5}{6}=-\frac{1}{3}$$

and conclude that the player would get $12\times\left(-\dfrac{1}{3}\right)=-4$ (Yuan). This weighted average is what we call the expected value or expectation of the random variable X whose distribution is given by

$$P(X=8)=\frac{1}{6}, \ P(X=-2)=\frac{5}{6}.$$

It might happen that the player is unlucky and that each time he lost, in which case he lost 24 Yuan. At the other extreme, he may be lucky and wins every time. However, it is a mathematical fact that the conclusion about 4 Yuan lost is correct in the following sense:

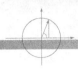

for a large number n of toss the total gain will be around n times $-\dfrac{1}{3}$ Yuan with high probability. This example illustrates the following definition.

> **Definition 8. 15**
>
> *If the probability mass function of a discrete variable X is*
> $$P(X=x_i)=p_i, \ i=1, 2,\cdots.$$
> *Then, the expectation of X is*
> $$E(X)= \sum_i x_i P(X=x_i)= \sum_i x_i p_i.$$

We also call $E(X)$ the expected value or the mean of X. Since the expectation is determined by the probability distribution of X only, we also speak of the expectation or mean of the distribution.

Example 8. 27 The probability mass function of the amount of memory X (GB) in a purchased flash drive was given as

X	0	1	2	3	4
P	0. 08	0. 15	0. 45	0. 27	0. 05

Compute the expectation of X.

Solution Using the definition of the mean, we have

$$E(X) = \sum_{i-1}^{5} x_i p_i = 0 \times 0.08 + 1 \times 0.15 + 2 \times 0.45 + 3 \times 0.27 + 4 \times 0.05 = 2.06 . \ \#$$

Your Practice 8.9 Let X be the discrete random variable that takes the values -2, 0, 2, 4, and 16, each with probability $1/5$. Compute the expectation of X.

When the range of X is finite, the sum in the definition is always defined. When the range of X is countably infinite, we must sum an infinite number of terms. Such sums can be infinite, depending on the distribution of X. We will not encounter any cases of discrete random variables where this sum is undefined.

We can easily extend the definition of the expected value of X to the expected value of a function of X. Let $g(x)$ be a function of x. Then

$$E[g(X)] = \sum_i g(x_i)P(X = x_i) = \sum_i g(x_i)p_i . \tag{8.10}$$

8.4.1.2 The continuous case

This point of view also leads the way to how one should define the expected value of a continuous random variable. For example, let X be a continuous random variable whose probability density function $f(x)$ is zero outside the interval $[0, 1]$. It seems reasonable to approximate X by the discrete random variable Y, taking the values

$$\frac{1}{n}, \frac{2}{n}, \cdots, \frac{n-1}{n}, 1.$$

Using area of rectangles to approximate the area of the curved region (Figure 8.22), we have a good idea of the size of the probability

$$P\left(Y=\frac{k}{n}\right)\approx\frac{1}{n}f\left(\frac{k}{n}\right).$$

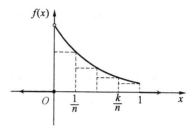

We have

$$E(Y) = \sum_{k=1}^{n}\frac{k}{n}P\left(Y=\frac{k}{n}\right)\approx\frac{k}{n}f\left(\frac{k}{n}\right)\cdot\frac{1}{n}.$$

It is reasonable that the expectation $E(Y)$ of Y should approximate the expectation $E(X)$ of X. By the

Figure 8. 22

definition of a definite integral, for large n the right-hand side is close to

$$\int_{0}^{1}xf(x)\mathrm{d}x.$$

This motivates the following definition.

Definition 8. 16

The expectation of a continuous random variable X with probability density function $f(x)$ is the number

$$E(X)=\int_{-\infty}^{+\infty}xf(x)\mathrm{d}x.$$

Example 8. 28 Suppose the probability density function of a random variable X is given by

$$f(x)=\begin{cases}2x, & \text{if } 0<x<1;\\ 0, & \text{else.}\end{cases}$$

Find $E(X)$.

Solution Using the definition of the mean, we have

$$E(X) = \int_{-\infty}^{+\infty}xf(x)\mathrm{d}x = \int_{0}^{1}x\cdot 2x\mathrm{d}x = \frac{2x^{3}}{3}\bigg|_{0}^{1} = \frac{2}{3}.$$ #

Your Practice 8. 10 Compute the expectation of a random variable U that is uniformly distributed over $[2, 5]$.

We can easily extend the definition of the expected value of X to the expected value of a function of X. Let $g(x)$ be a function of x. Then

$$E[g(X)] = \int_{-\infty}^{+\infty}g(x)f(x)\mathrm{d}x.\qquad(8.11)$$

8.4.2 Variances

The mean of X measures the fluctuation center of the random variable, whereas the variance of X measures the amount of variability or dispersion.

Definition 8. 17 Variance

Suppose a random variable X with mean $\mu=E(X)$. The variance of X, denoted by $V(X)$, σ_{X}^{2} (or σ^{2} for short), is denoted by

$$V(X)=E[(X-\mu)^{2}].$$

The standard deviation (SD) of X is $\sigma=\sqrt{V(X)}$.

If X is a discrete random variable with probability mass function p_i, then

$$V(X) = \sum_{i=1}^{+\infty} (x_i - \mu)^2 p_i .$$

If X is a continuous random variable with probability density function $f(x)$, then

$$V(X) = \int_{-\infty}^{+\infty} (x - \mu)^2 f(x) \mathrm{d}x .$$

Note　The quantity $h(X) = (X - \mu)^2$ is the squared deviation of X from its mean, and $E[h(X)]$ is the expected squared deviation. If most of the probability distribution is close to μ, then σ^2 will be relatively small. However, if there are x values far from μ that have large $p(x)$ (or $f(x)$), then σ^2 will be quite large.

Proposition 8.2

Let a and b be constant, for a random variable X, we have

(1) $E(aX+b) = aE(X) + b$;

(2) $V(aX+b) = a^2 V(X)$.

The first property says that the expected value of a linear function of X is the linear function evaluated at the expected value of X. The second property tells us what happens to the variance when we multiply a random variable by a constant factor; it is important to note that the constant factor is squared when we pull it out of the variance. Furthermore, we see that the variance is unchanged when we shift a random variable by a constant term. The proof of the formula is left to the readers.

We apply these formulas to do some calculations.

Example 8.29　The probability distribution of a random variable X is

X	-2	-1	0	1	3
P	0.3	0.1	0.2	0.1	0.3

Find $E(X)$, $V(X)$, $E(2X+3)$ and $V(2X+3)$.

Solution　Using the definition of the mean, we have

$$E(X) = \sum_{i=1}^{5} x_i p_i = (-2) \times 0.3 + (-1) \times 0.1 + 0 \times 0.2 + 1 \times 0.1 + 3 \times 0.3 = 0.3 .$$

Using the definition of the variance, we have

$$\begin{aligned}
V(X) &= \sum_{i=1}^{5} (x_i - \mu)^2 p_i \\
&= (-2 - 0.3)^2 \times 0.3 + (-1 - 0.3)^2 \times 0.1 + (0 - 0.3)^2 \times 0.2 + \\
&\quad (1 - 0.3)^2 \times 0.1 + (3 - 0.3)^2 \times 0.3 \\
&= 4.01.
\end{aligned}$$

Using the property of the mean, we obtain

$$E(2X+3) = 2E(X) + 3 = 2 \times 0.3 + 3 = 3.6.$$

Using the property of the variance, we obtain

$$V(2X+3)=4V(X)=4\times4.01=16.04. \qquad \#$$

It is often necessary to discuss sums of random variables. We collect some rules without proof. Let X and Y be two discrete random variables, then $X+Y$ is also a discrete random variable. We have

$$E(X+Y)=E(X)+E(Y).$$

We can use our rules to find an alternate formula for the variance

$$V(X)=E(X^2)-(EX)^2. \qquad (8.12)$$

This formula is often more convenient to use, since it leads to algebraically simpler expressions. Note that $E(X^2)\neq(EX)^2$ unless $V(X)=0$.

We give an example to calculate the variance by the two ways.

Example 8.30　Suppose the probability density function of X is

$$f(x)=\begin{cases} \dfrac{x}{2}, & \text{if } 0<x<2, \\ 0, & \text{else.} \end{cases}$$

Find the mean and variance of X.

Solution　$E(X) = \displaystyle\int_{-\infty}^{+\infty} xf(x)\mathrm{d}x = \int_0^2 x\cdot\frac{x}{2}\mathrm{d}x = \frac{x^3}{6}\Big|_0^2 = \frac{4}{3}$.

Method 1:

Because $E(X^2) = \displaystyle\int_{-\infty}^{+\infty} x^2 f(x)\mathrm{d}x = \int_0^2 x^2\cdot\frac{x}{2}\mathrm{d}x = \frac{x^4}{8}\Big|_0^2 = 2$.

So, $V(X)=E(X^2)-(EX)^2=2-\left(\dfrac{4}{3}\right)^2=\dfrac{2}{9}$.

Method 2:

$$V(X) = E\left[\left(X-\frac{4}{3}\right)^2\right] = \int_0^2\left(x-\frac{4}{3}\right)^2\cdot\frac{x}{2}\mathrm{d}x = \frac{2}{9}. \qquad \#$$

The rule for the expected value of a product of random variables is more complicated. Namely, we need the condition that the two random variables are independent. The definition of the independence of random variables is similar to that of the independence of events. Namely, when X and Y are discrete random variables, we say that X and Y are independent if

$$P(X=x, Y=y)=P(X=x)P(Y=y)$$

or $\qquad\qquad P(x\leqslant x, Y\leqslant y)=P(X\leqslant x)P(Y\leqslant y)$

for every x and y. We can now state how to deal with the expected value of a product of independent random variables.

Proposition 8.3

If X and Y are two independent random variables, then

$$E(XY)=[E(X)][E(Y)].$$

This rule allows us to compute the variance of the sum of two independent random variables.

Namely, suppose that X and Y are independent, then we have

$$V(X\pm Y)=V(X)+V(Y).$$

Exercise 8.4

1. The probability mass function of X is given by

X	-1	0	1	2
P	1/6	1/3	1/6	1/3

Find $E(X)$, $V(X)$, $E(3X+8)$, $V(3X+8)$, $E(X^4)$.

2. The probability mass function of X is given by

X	-2	-1	0	1	2	3
P	0.1	0.1	0.2	0.3	0.2	0.1

Find $E(X)$, $E(X^2)$, $V(X)$, $E(4X+5)$, $V(4X+5)$, $E(X^3)$.

3. If $X\sim U(0, 10)$. Calculate $E(X)$, $V(X)$, $E(3X+8)$, $V(3X+8)$, $E(X^3)$.

4. If $X\sim B(n, p)$, $E(X)=2.4$, $V(X)=1.44$. Find n and p.

5. If $X\sim U(a, b)$, $E(X)=3$, $V(X)=1/3$. Calculate $P(1<X<3)$.

6. The probability density function of X is given by $f(x)=a+bx^2$, $0\leqslant x\leqslant 1$, and $E(X)=3/5$. Find a and b.

7. The probability density function of X is given by $f(x)=30x(1-x)^4$, $0\leqslant x\leqslant 1$. Find $E(X)$, $E(7X+8)$, $V(X)$, $V(7X+8)$.

8. Let X be uniformly distributed on the set

$$S=\{1, 2,\cdots, n\}$$

where n is a positive integer; that is,

$$P(X=k)=\frac{1}{n}, \ k\in S.$$

Find $E(X)$, $V(X)$.

8.5 Statistics Tools

The purpose of statistics is to generalize from properties of a small body of data to statement concerning properties of similar data. The discipline of statistics teaches us how to make intelligent judgments and informed decisions in the presence of uncertainty and variation.

8.5.1 Random Samples and Statistics

A *population* is a set which contains all the observed values of the experiment. Every single value is called an *individual*. The number of individuals in the population is called a *sample size*. The population with a finite sample size is said to be a finite population, and the population with an infinite sample size is said to be an infinite population. For example, the set of all cars of a certain type is a population. The set of some people suffering from a certain disease is a population.

For any given population, there is a probability mass function or probability density function which describes the distribution of the values in the population. So, the population is a random variable that has the probability distribution or probability density function.

A common purpose of statistical inference is to generalize from properties of a small body of data to statements concerning properties of a population. Such small body is called a sample. More specifically, a *sample* is a subset of the population from which we can draw conclusions about the whole population. In many cases, such as the observation of the population is destructive or the number of the population is too large, we are not able to investigate a whole population, a subset of observation from the population can help us make inferences concerning the same population. For example, in attempting to determine the average length of life of a certain brand of light bulb, it would be impossible to testify all such bulbs. We are obliged to get conclusions regarding a population by its sample.

If our inferences from the sample to the population are valid, we must obtain samples that are representative for the population, and we call this sample a random sample. A *random sample* of size n of a population X, denoted by $(X_1, X_2, \cdots, X_n)$, is a collection of n random variables, where X_k is the kth observation. If $(X_1, X_2, \cdots, X_n)$ is a random sample from the population X, then random variables $X_1, X_2, \cdots, X_n$ are independently and identically distributed with the population X.

It is desirable to choose a random sample that the observation are made independently and randomly.

We often use capital letters for the random variable and lower-case letter for the value of the random variable, so $(x_1, x_2, \cdots, x_n)$ is an observed value of the particular random sample $(X_1, X_2, \cdots, X_n)$.

In the following part, we give some important statistics.

Definition 8.18

Let $(X_1, X_2, \cdots, X_n)$ be a random sample from the population X and $h(X_1, X_2, \cdots, X_n)$ be any function of $(X_1, X_2, \cdots, X_n)$, where h has not unknown parameters, then $h(X_1, X_2, \cdots, X_n)$ is said to be a statistic.

Example 8.31   Suppose (X_1, X_2) be a random sample drawn from the population $X \sim N(\mu, \sigma^2)$, where μ is known but σ^2 is unknown, then $\min\{X_1, X_2\}$, $\frac{X_1+X_2}{2}-\mu$ are statistics. But $\frac{X_1+X_2}{\sigma}$ is not a statistic.   #

The two most important statistics are the *sample mean* and the *sample variance*.

Let $(X_1, X_2, \cdots, X_n)$ be a random sample from the population X, and $(x_1, x_2, \cdots, x_n)$ are observed values of the sample. The sample mean and the sample variance are defined as follows,

$$\text{sample mean}: \overline{X} = \frac{1}{n} \sum_{i=1}^{n} X_i$$

$$\text{sample variance}: S^2 = \frac{1}{n-1} \sum_{i=1}^{n} (X_i - \overline{X})^2 .$$

The sample mean is thus the arithmetic average of the observations. The sample variance is the sum of the squared deviations from the sample mean, divided by $n-1$.

The definition of the sample variance is not very convenient for computation. We usually use an alternate form

$$S^2 = \frac{1}{n-1} \left(\sum_{i=1}^{n} X_i^2 - n\overline{X}^2 \right) .$$

The proof of the formula is left to the readers.

Example 8.32 Given the values 29.5, 49.3, 30.6, 28.2, 28.0, 26.3, 33.9, 29.4, 23.5, 31.6. We compute the sample mean to be

$$\overline{x} = \frac{1}{10} \sum_{i=1}^{10} x_i = \frac{310.3}{10} = 31.03$$

and the sample variance

$$S^2 = \frac{1}{10-1} \sum_{i=1}^{10} (x_i - \overline{x})^2 = \frac{1}{9} \sum_{i=1}^{10} (x_i - 31.03)^2 = 49.3 . \qquad \#$$

Your Practice 8.11 Compute the sample mean and the sample variance for the values 1.62, 3.31, 4.57, 5.42, 6.71.

Any statistic computed from a sample will vary from sample to sample, since the samples are random subsets of the population. Therefore statistics are random variables with their own probability distributions.

The probability distribution of a statistic is called a *sampling distribution*. If the sample size n is very large, one can show that

$$\frac{\overline{X} - \mu}{\sigma/\sqrt{n}}$$

is approximately standard normally distributed.

8.5.2　Estimating Means and Proportions

8.5.2.1　Estimating means

We saw in section 8.4 that the mean and the variance are useful parameters for describing the probability distribution of a population. If we wish to learn something about the distribution of some quantities from a random sample of the population, we might want to know what the mean and variance of the population distribution are. We will use the sample mean and the sample variance to estimate the mean and the variance of the population.

We assume that the population distribution has finite mean μ and finite variance σ^2. These two parameters are unknown to us, and we wish to estimate them by talking a random sample $(X_1, X_2, \cdots, X_n)$ of size n from the population X. The X_k are independent and identically distributed according to the distribution of the population with

$E(X_k) = \mu$ and $V(X_k) = \sigma^2$, $k=1, 2, \cdots, n$.

To estimate the mean and the variance of the population distribution, we will use the sample mean and the sample variance defined in the previous subsection. We know that the sample mean and the sample variance are also random variable. As such, we can compute their means and variance. The means of the sample mean is

$$E(\overline{X}) = E\left(\frac{1}{n}\sum_{i=1}^{n}X_i\right) = \frac{1}{n}\sum_{i=1}^{n}E(X_i) = \frac{1}{n}(n\mu) = \mu .$$

Using independence of the observations, the variance of the sample mean is

$$V(\overline{X}) = V\left(\frac{1}{n}\sum_{i=1}^{n}X_i\right) = \frac{1}{n^2}\sum_{i=1}^{n}V(X_i) = \frac{1}{n^2}(n\sigma^2) = \frac{\sigma^2}{n} .$$

We see from this that the expected value of the sample mean is equal to the population mean. The spread of the distribution of $\overline{X}$ is described by the variance of $\overline{X}$. Since the variance of $\overline{X}$ becomes smaller as the sample size increases, we conclude that the sample mean of large samples shows less variation about its mean than the sample mean of small samples. This implies that the larger the sample size, the more accurately the mean of the population can be estimated.

We also can compute and get the mean of the sample variance,

$$E(S^2) = E\left[\frac{1}{n-1}\left(\sum_{i=1}^{n}X_i^2 - n\overline{X}^2\right)\right] = \sigma^2 .$$

That is, the expected value of the sample variance is equal to the variance of the population. This is the reason that we divided by $n-1$ instead of n when computing the sample variance.

The proof of the formula is left to the readers.

Note If the population distribution has finite mean μ and finite variance σ^2, then we can use the sample mean X as an estimator of μ, and the sample variance S^2 as an estimator of σ^2.

Let us look at an example to illustrate how we would estimate the mean and the variance of a characteristic of a population.

Example 8.33 A machine produces pills. Suppose that the weights (in grams) of the following sample of independent observations from a population

3.1, 3.5, 3.3, 3.7, 4.5, 4.2, 2.8, 3.9, 3.5, 3.3.

Estimate the mean and the variance.

Solution To estimate the mean, we compute the sample mean $\overline{X}$. We sum the 10 numbers in the sample and divide the result by 10, which yields

$$\overline{x} = \frac{1}{10}\sum_{i=1}^{10}x_i = 3.58 .$$

Thus, the estimate for the mean is 3.58.

To estimate the variance, we compute the sample variance S^2. We square the difference between each sample point and the sample mean, and add the results. We then

divide this number by 9. We find

$$\sigma^2 = \frac{1}{9} \sum_{i=1}^{10} (x_i - 3.58)^2 = 0.262 .$$

Thus, our estimate for the variance is 0.262.   #

In the previous example, we estimated the population mean and the population variance from a sample of size 10. Since we do not know the population parameters we have no idea how good our estimates are. How can we assess the quality of our estimates?

8.5.2.2 Confidence interval

In scientific publications, one frequently finds the sample mean reported under a heading of the form "Mean $\pm$ S. E. ". What does "Mean $\pm$ S. E. " mean? When we write "Mean$\pm$S. E. ", we specify an interval, namely, [Mean $-$ S. E. , Mean $+$ S. E.]. The expression "Mean" stands for the sample mean $\overline{X}$. The expression "S. E. " stands for the standard error which serves as an estimate for the standard deviation of the sample mean. It is denoted by $S_{\overline{X}}$ and defined as

$$S_{\overline{X}} = \frac{S}{\sqrt{n}} ,$$

where S is the square root of the sample variance, called the **sample standard deviation**.

Since we use "Mean" ($\overline{X}$) as an estimate for the population mean μ, we would like this interval to contain μ. Surely, since $\overline{X}$ is a random variable, if we took repeated samples and computed such intervals for each sample, not all the intervals would contain μ. But maybe we can at least find out what fraction of these intervals (or similar intervals) contain the population mean μ. In other words, we might wish to know before taking the sample what the probability is that the interval [Mean $-$ S. E. , Mean $+$ S. E.] or more generally, [Mean$-a$S. E. , Mean$+a$S. E.], where a is a positive constant, will contain μ. To be concrete, we will try to determine a so that this probability is equal to 0.95.

If the sample size is very large, one can show that $\dfrac{\overline{X}-\mu}{\sigma/\sqrt{n}}$ is approximately standard normally distributed. If Z is standard normally distributed, then

$$P(-1.96 \leqslant Z \leqslant 1.96) = 0.95.$$

Hence, the event

$$-1.96 \leqslant \frac{\overline{X}-\mu}{\sigma/\sqrt{n}} \leqslant 1.96 \tag{8.13}$$

is probability approximately 0.95 for n sufficiently large.

Rearranging the terms in Equation (8.13), we find

$$-1.96 \frac{\sigma}{\sqrt{n}} < \overline{X} - \mu < 1.96 \frac{\sigma}{\sqrt{n}}$$

or

$$\overline{X} - 1.96 \frac{\sigma}{\sqrt{n}} < \mu < \overline{X} + 19.6 \frac{\sigma}{\sqrt{n}} .$$

We can thus write

$$P\left(\overline{X}-1.96\frac{\sigma}{\sqrt{n}}<\mu<\overline{X}+19.6\frac{\sigma}{\sqrt{n}}\right)\approx0.95,\text{ for large } n. \tag{8.14}$$

This means that if we repeatedly draw random samples of size n from a population with mean μ and standard deviation σ, then in about 95% of the samples, the interval $\left[\overline{X}-1.96\frac{\sigma}{\sqrt{n}},\ \overline{X}+19.6\frac{\sigma}{\sqrt{n}}\right]$ would contain the true mean μ. Such an interval is referred to as a 95% *confidence interval*.

Notice that this interval contains the parameter σ. If we do not know μ, we probably do not know σ either. We might then wish to replace σ by the square root of the sample variance, denoted by S. Fortunately, when n is large, S will be very close to σ and Equation (8.14) holds approximately when σ is replaced by S.

Thus we find that for large n,

$$P\left(\overline{X}-1.96\frac{S}{\sqrt{n}}<\mu<\overline{X}+19.6\frac{S}{\sqrt{n}}\right)\approx0.95.$$

Rewriting the event in interval notation, we obtain

$$P\left(\mu\in\left[\overline{X}-1.96\frac{S}{\sqrt{n}},\ \overline{X}+19.6\frac{S}{\sqrt{n}}\right]\right)\approx0.95.$$

The interval in this expression is of the form

$$[\text{Mean}-1.96\text{S. E.},\ \text{Mean}+1.96\text{S. E.}] \tag{8.15}$$

We succeeded in determining what fraction of intervals of the form (8.15) contain the mean. Namely, if n is large, and we take repeated samples each of size n, then 95% of the intervals $[\text{Mean}-1.96\text{S. E.},\ \text{Mean}+1.96\text{S. E.}]$ would contain the true mean. If we wanted 99% of such intervals to contain the true mean, we would need to replace the factor 1.96 by 2.58, since if Z is standard normally distributed, then $P(-2.58\leqslant Z\leqslant2.58)=0.99$ (95% and 99% are the most frequently used percentages for confidence intervals). Since $P(-1\leqslant Z\leqslant1)=0.68$, we conclude that if the sample size is large, approximately 68% of intervals of the form $[\text{Mean}-a\text{S. E.},\ \text{Mean}+a\text{S. E.}]$ contain the population mean μ.

We wish to emphasize that the preceding discussion requires that the sample size n is large. Whether or not a particular n can be considered large depends on the population distribution. If the samples X_k are normally distributed with mean μ and standard deviation σ, then one can show that $\dfrac{\overline{X}-\mu}{\sigma/\sqrt{n}}$ is standard normally distributed for all n. When we replace σ by S in Equation (8.13) in this case, then n is considered large for $n\geqslant40$. That is, for $n\geqslant40$, $\dfrac{\overline{X}-\mu}{S/\sqrt{n}}$ is then approximately standard normally distributed. The more the distribution of the X_k differs from the normal distribution, the larger n needs to be to use the normal distribution as an approximation.

Example 8.34 There are a large number of bagged pills, from which 16 bags are randomly taken, and the weight (unit: g) is as follows:

506, 508, 499, 503, 504, 510, 497, 512, 514, 505, 493, 496, 506, 502, 509, 496.
Assuming that the weight of bagged pills approximately obeys normal distribution, try to find out a 0.95 confidence interval of population mean μ.

Solution When $n=16$, the sample mean is

$$\overline{x} = \frac{1}{16} \sum_{i=1}^{16} x_i = 503.75 .$$

The sample standard deviation:

$$S = \sqrt{S^2} = \sqrt{\frac{1}{15} \sum_{i=1}^{16} (X_i - 503.75)^2} = 6.2022 .$$

Since the population approximately obeys normal distribution, we have a 95% confidence interval of population mean μ as

$$\left[\overline{X} - 1.96 \frac{S}{\sqrt{n}}, \ \overline{X} + 19.6 \frac{S}{\sqrt{n}} \right] = \left[503.75 - 1.96 \frac{6.2022}{\sqrt{16}}, \ 503.75 + 1.96 \frac{6.2022}{\sqrt{16}} \right]$$

$$= [500.7, 506.8].$$

So, $[500.7, 506.8]$ is a 0.95 confidence interval of μ. $\qquad\qquad$ #

8.5.2.3 Estimating proportions

Of particular interest is the case of estimating proportions. For instance, an experiment which has two possible outcomes that are generically called success and failure. Let p denote the probability of a success and $q = 1 - p$ denote the probability of a failure. The population distribution of this experiment is Bernoulli distribution with parameter p, where the unknown parameter p is a proportion.

Now we wish to estimate parameter p by talking a random sample $(X_1, X_2, \cdots, X_n)$ of size n from the population $X \sim B(1, p)$. Hence, X_k are independent and identically distributed according to the distribution of the population with $E(X_k) = p$, $V(X_k) = p(1-p)$.

We find

$$E(\overline{X}) = E\left(\frac{1}{n} \sum_{i=1}^{n} X_i \right) - \frac{1}{n} \sum_{i=1}^{n} E(X_i) = \frac{1}{n} (np) = p .$$

Using independence of the observations, the variance of the sample mean is

$$V(\overline{X}) = V\left(\frac{1}{n} \sum_{i=1}^{n} X_i \right) = \frac{1}{n^2} \sum_{i=1}^{n} V(X_i) = \frac{1}{n^2} [np(1-p)] = \frac{p(1-p)}{n} .$$

The sample mean $\overline{X}$ will serve as an estimate for the success probability p. We denote the estimate for p by $\hat{p}$ (read as "p hat"). That is, if we observe k successes in a sample of size n, then

$$\hat{p} = \frac{k}{n} .$$

To find the standard error in the case of k successes in a sample of size n, in the literature, you will typically find the standard error for proportion p as

$$S_{\hat{p}} = \sqrt{\frac{\hat{p}(1-\hat{p})}{n-1}}$$

or
$$S_{\hat{p}} = \sqrt{\frac{\hat{p}(1-\hat{p})}{n}}.$$

The proof of the formula is left to the readers. For large n, the two numbers are very close, so that it does not matter which you use.

Example 8.35　A pharmaceutical factory produced a batch of drugs. 100 pieces were selected, 22 pieces were found to be defective, give a 95% confidence interval of the defective proportion p.

Solution　The sample mean is $\overline{X} = \frac{22}{100} = 0.22$.

The estimate for the defective proportion is $\hat{p} = \overline{X} = 0.22$.

The standard error for proportion p is

$$S_{\hat{p}} = \sqrt{\frac{\hat{p}(1-\hat{p})}{n}} = \sqrt{\frac{0.22 \times 0.78}{100}} = 0.0414.$$

Since $n = 100$ is large, we find a 95% confidence interval as
$$[0.22 - 1.96 \times 0.0414, \ 0.22 + 1.96 \times 0.0414] = [0.1389, 0.3011]. \qquad \#$$

8.5.3　Linear Regression

Regression analysis is a useful tool to investigate how two or more variables are related. We often want to see how a certain variables of interest is affected by one or more variables. The simplest deterministic mathematical relationship between two variables is a linear relationship. In this section, we discuss the linear relationship between two quantitative variables, that is a simple linear regression.

In simple linear regression, we predict scores on one variable from the scores on a second variable. The variable we are predicting is called the **criterion variable** (or dependent variable) and is referred to as Y. The variable we are basing our predictions on is called the **predictor variable** (or deterministic variable) and is referred to as X. When there is only one predictor variable, the prediction method is called simple regression. In simple linear regression, the predictions of Y when plotted as a function of X form a straight line.

The example data in Table 8.3 are plotted in Figure 8.23. You can see that there is a positive relationship between X and Y. If you were going to predict Y from X, the larger the value of X, the larger your prediction of Y.

Table 8.3　Example data

X	Y
1	1
2	2
3	1.3
4	3.75
5	2.25

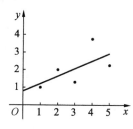

Figure 8.23

Linear regression consists of finding the best-fitting straight line through the points. The best-fitting line is called a ***regression line***. The black line in Figure 8. 23 is the regression line and consists of the predicted score on Y for each possible value of X. The vertical lines in Figure 8. 24 from the points to the regression line represent the deviations of the actual values from the predict ones, that is, the errors of prediction. The shorter the vertical line, the smaller its error of prediction.

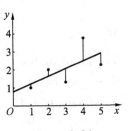

Figure 8. 24

Linear regression attempts to model the relationship between two variables by fitting a linear equation. A simple linear regression model has the following form:

$$Y = a + bX + \varepsilon, \ \varepsilon \sim N(0, \sigma^2),$$

where ε is the random error, X is a deterministic variable and Y is a dependent variable, and the actual observed value of y is associated, but not determined by the value of x.

Our goal is to estimate a and b from the data. The data consists of points (x_k, y_k), $k = 1, 2, \cdots, n$. Choose a and b so that the sum of the squared deviations

$$h(a, b) = \sum_{k=1}^{n} [y_k - (a + bx_k)]^2$$

is minimized. The deviation $y_k - (a + bx_k)$ are called ***residuals***. The procedure of finding a and b is called ***method of least squares***. The resulting straight line is called ***the least square line*** (or linear regression line.)

We will now derive the general formula for finding a and b. We first rewrite the residuals. We set

$$\overline{x} = \frac{1}{n} \sum_{k=1}^{n} x_k, \ \overline{y} = \frac{1}{n} \sum_{k=1}^{n} y_k$$

and
$$y_k - (a + bx_k) = (y_k - \overline{y}) + (\overline{y} - a - b\overline{x}) - b(x_k - \overline{x}).$$

In the following, we will simply write $\sum$ instead of $\sum_{k=1}^{n}$. If we square the expression and sum over k, we find

$$\sum [y_k - (a + bx_k)]^2 = \sum (y_k - \overline{y})^2 + n(\overline{y} - a - b\overline{x})^2 +$$
$$b^2 \sum (x_k - \overline{x})^2 - 2b \sum (x_k - \overline{x})(y_k - \overline{y}) +$$
$$2(\overline{y} - a - b\overline{x}) \sum (y_k - \overline{y}) -$$
$$2b(\overline{y} - a - b\overline{x}) \sum (x_k - \overline{x}). \tag{8.16}$$

The last two terms are equal to zero. We introduce notation to simplify our derivation:

$$SS_{xx} = \sum (x_k - \overline{x})^2 = \sum x_k^2 - n\overline{x}^2,$$
$$SS_{xy} = \sum (x_k - \overline{x})(y_k - \overline{y}) = \sum x_k y_k - n\overline{x}\,\overline{y},$$
$$SS_{yy} = \sum (y_k - \overline{y})^2 = \sum y_k^2 - n\overline{y}^2.$$

Using this notation, the right-hand side of Equation (8. 16) can be written as

$$SS_{yy} + n(\overline{y} - a - b\overline{x})^2 + b^2 SS_{xx} - 2b SS_{xy}.$$

The last two terms suggest that we should complete the square:

$$SS_{yy} + n(\overline{y} - a - b\overline{x}) + SS_{xx}\left[b^2 - 2b\frac{SS_{xy}}{SS_{xx}} + \left(\frac{SS_{xy}}{SS_{xx}}\right)^2\right] - \frac{(SS_{xy})^2}{SS_{xx}}$$

$$= n(\overline{y} - a - b\overline{x})^2 + SS_{xx}\left(b - \frac{SS_{xy}}{SS_{xx}}\right)^2 + SS_{yy} - \frac{(SS_{xy})^2}{SS_{xx}}.$$

Thus we have written the sum of the squared deviations as a sum of two squares plus an additional term. We can minimize the expression by setting each squared expression equal to zero:

$$\overline{y} - a - b\overline{x} = 0,$$

$$b - \frac{SS_{xy}}{SS_{xx}} = 0.$$

Solving for a and b yields

$$b = \frac{SS_{xy}}{SS_{xx}},$$

$$a = \overline{y} - b\overline{x}.$$

These expressions serve as estimates for a and b, denoted by $\hat{a}$ and $\hat{b}$. Summarizing our results, we have the following conclusion.

The linear regression line is given by

$$\hat{y} = \hat{a} + \hat{b}x$$

with

$$\hat{b} = \frac{\sum(x_k - \overline{x})(y_k - \overline{y})}{\sum(x_k - \overline{x})^2}, \tag{8.17}$$

$$\hat{a} = \overline{y} - \hat{b}\overline{x}. \tag{8.18}$$

Example 8.36　Fit a linear regression line $\hat{y} = \hat{a} + \hat{b}x$ about (x, y) through the points $(1, 1.62)$, $(2, 3.31)$, $(3, 4.57)$, $(4, 5.42)$, $(5, 6.71)$.

Solution　To facilitate the computation, we construct Table 8.4.

Table 8.4

x_k	y_k	$x_k - \overline{x}$	$y_k - \overline{y}$	$(x_k - \overline{x})(y_k - \overline{y})$	$(x_k - \overline{x})^2$
1	1.62	-2	-2.706	5.412	4
2	3.31	-1	-1.016	1.016	1
3	4.57	0	0.244	0	0
4	5.42	1	1.094	1.094	1
5	6.71	2	2.384	4.768	4
$\overline{x} = 3$	$\overline{y} = 4.326$		$\sum(y_k - \overline{y})^2 = 15.29$	$\sum(x_k - \overline{x})(y_k - \overline{y}) = 12.29$	$\sum(x_k - \overline{x})^2 = 10$

Now,

$$\hat{b} = \frac{12.29}{10} = 1.229,$$

$$\hat{a} = 4.326 - 1.229 \times 3 = 0.639.$$

Hence, the linear regression line is given by

$$\hat{y} = 1.23x + 0.64.$$

This line and the data points are shown in Figure 8.25.

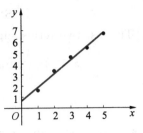

Figure 8.25

Exercise 8.5

1. Given a sample of ten data:

29.5, 49.3, 30.6, 28.2, 28.0, 26.3, 33.9, 29.4, 23.5, 31.6.

Compute:

(1) the sample mean;

(2) the sample variance s^2;

(3) the sample standard deviation s.

2. Given a sample of ten data:

3.1, 3.5, 3.3, 3.7, 4.5, 4.2, 2.8, 3.9, 3.5, 3.3.

Compute:

(1) the sample mean;

(2) the sample variance s^2;

(3) the sample standard deviation s.

3. A random sample of size 10 from the normal distribution $N(\mu, 4)$ yielded the following data:

55.9, 56.6, 57.6, 55.1, 57.5, 56.1, 60.0, 58.3, 52.6, 58.5.

Find an estimate for μ.

4. A random sample of size 5 from the normal distribution $N(\mu, \sigma^2)$ yielded $\bar{x} = 8.34$, $s = 0.03$.

Find an estimate for μ and σ^2.

5. A random sample of size 16 from the normal distribution $N(\mu, 25)$ yielded $\bar{x} = 73.8$. Find a 95% confidence interval for μ.

6. A random sample of size 12 from the normal distribution $N(\mu, \sigma^2)$ yielded $\bar{x} = 66.3$, $s = 8.4$. Find a 95% confidence interval for μ.

7. Fit a linear regression line $\hat{y} = \hat{a} + \hat{b}x$ through the points (70, 87), (67, 73), (74, 79), (70, 83), (80, 88), (64, 79), (84, 98), (74, 91), (80, 96), (82, 94).

8. Fit a linear regression line $\hat{y} = \hat{a} + \hat{b}x$ through the points (2, 1.8), (4, 1.5), (6, 1.4), (8, 1.1), (10, 1.1), (12, 0.9).

Summary and Review

Important Terms, Symbols, and Concepts

- Suppose that an experiment consists of k ordered tasks. Task 1 has n_1 possible outcomes, task 2 has n_2 possible outcomes, $\cdots$, and task k has n_k possible outcomes. The total number of possible outcomes of the experiment is $n_1 \times n_2 \times n_3 \times \cdots \times n_k$. This is called the multiplication principle.

- Any ordered sequence of k objects taken from a set of n distinct objects is called a permutation of size k objects. The number of permutations (different ways of ordering/selecting) k out of n objects is denoted by $P_{k,n}$.

- Given a set of n distinct objects, any unordered subset of size k of the objects is called a combination. The number of combinations of size k that can be formed from the n distinct objects is denoted by $C_{k,n}$ or $\binom{n}{k}$.

- The set of all possible outcomes of a statistical experiment is called a sample space, denoted by Ω or S.

- An event is a subset of a sample space, denoted by A, B, C, $\cdots$. An event is said to be simple if it consists of exactly one outcome and compound if it consists of more than one outcome.

- Probability is a real-valued set function P that assigns, to each event A in the sample space Ω, a number $P(A)$, called the probability of the event A, which should satisfy the following properties: (1) $P(A) \geqslant 0$; (2) $P(\Omega) = 1$; (3) If A_1, A_2, $\cdots$, A_n, $\cdots$ is an infinite collection of disjoint events, then $P(\bigcup_{n=1}^{+\infty} A_n) = \sum_{n=1}^{+\infty} P(A_n)$.

- When the various outcomes of an experiment are equally likely, letting N denote the number of outcomes in a sample space and N_A represent the number of outcomes contained in an event A, then $P(A) = \dfrac{N_A}{N}$.

- For any two events A and B, the conditional probability of A given that B has occurred, denoted by $P(A|B)$, is defined by $P(A|B) = \dfrac{P(AB)}{P(B)}$.

- Two events A and B are mutually independent if and only if $P(AB) = P(A)P(B)$. Otherwise, they are dependent.

- The cumulative distribution function, denoted by $F(x)$, is $F(x) = P(X \leqslant x)$, $-\infty < x < +\infty$.

- Any random variable X whose only possible values are 0 and 1 and $P(X=1) = p$, $P(X=0) = 1 - p$ is called a Bernoulli distribution. The Bernoulli distribution is denoted by $X \sim B(1, p)$.

- A random variable X is said to have a Binomial distribution, if the Probability mass function of X is $P(X=x) = \binom{n}{x} p^x (1-p)^{n-x}$, $x = 0$, 1, 2, $\cdots$, n. The Binomial distribution is denoted by $X \sim B(n, p)$.

- A random variable X is said to have a Poisson distribution with parameter $\lambda (\lambda > 0)$, if the probability function of X is $P(X=x) = \dfrac{e^{-\lambda} \lambda^x}{x!}$, $x = 0$, 1, 2, $\cdots$. The Poisson

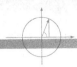
distribution is denoted by $X \sim P(\lambda)$.

- A continuous random variable X is said to have a uniform distribution on the interval (a, b), if the probability density function of X is $f(x) = \dfrac{1}{b-a}$, $a < x < b$. The uniform distribution is denoted by $X \sim U(a, b)$.

- A continuous random variable X is said to have an exponential distribution with parameter $\lambda(\lambda > 0)$, if the probability density function of $f(x)$ is $f(x) = \lambda e^{-\lambda x}$, $x > 0$. The exponential distribution is denoted by $X \sim E(\lambda)$.

- A continuous random variable X is said to have a normal distribution with parameters μ and σ^2, if the probability density function of X is $f(x; \mu, \sigma) = \dfrac{1}{\sqrt{2\pi}\sigma} \cdot \exp\left\{ -\dfrac{(x-\mu)^2}{2\sigma^2} \right\}$, $-\infty < \mu < +\infty$, $\sigma > 0$. The normal distribution is denoted by $X \sim N(\mu, \sigma^2)$.

- A random variable Z is called a standard normal distribution, if the probability density function of Z is $f(z) = \dfrac{1}{\sqrt{2\pi}} e^{-\frac{z^2}{2}}$ $(-\infty < z < +\infty)$. The standard normal distribution is denoted by $Z \sim N(0, 1)$.

- If the probability mass function of a discrete variable X is
$$P(X = x_i) = p_i, \quad i = 1, 2, \cdots,$$
then, the expectation X is
$$E(X) = \sum_i x_i P(X = x_i) = \sum_i x_i p_i.$$

- Suppose that X is a continuous random variable with probability density function $f(x)$, then $E(X) = \displaystyle\int_{-\infty}^{+\infty} x f(x) \, dx$.

- A random sample of size n of a random variable X is a collection of n random variables $(X_1, X_2, \cdots, X_n)$, which are independent and identically distributed with the population X, where X_k is the kth observation.

- The sample mean $\overline{X}$ is used as an estimate for the population mean μ. The sample variance S^2 serves as an estimate for the population variance σ^2.

- The simple linear regression model can be expressed as $Y = a + bx + \varepsilon$, $\varepsilon \sim N(0, \sigma^2)$, where a, b are unknown parameters. Based on the data $(x_1, y_1), \cdots, (x_n, y_n)$, the estimates $\hat{a}$, $\hat{b}$ of a, b can be obtained, and $\hat{y} = \hat{a} + \hat{b}x$ is called a linear regression line.

Important Formula

- The law of total probability: Let $A_1, A_2, \cdots, A_n$ be a partition of the sample space, then for any other event B, $P(B) = \displaystyle\sum_{i=1}^{n} P(B|A_i)P(A_i)$.

- Bayes formula: Let $A_1, A_2, \cdots, A_n$ be a partition of the sample space, then for any other event B for which $P(B) > 0$, we have $P(A_j \mid B) = \dfrac{P(A_j B)}{P(B)} = \dfrac{P(B \mid A_j) P(A_j)}{\displaystyle\sum_{i=1}^{n} P(B \mid A_i) P(A_i)}$.

- Let $(X_1, X_2, \cdots, X_n)$ be a random sample from the population X. The sample mean is $\overline{X} = \dfrac{1}{n} \displaystyle\sum_{i=1}^{n} X_i$. The sample variance is $S^2 = \dfrac{1}{n-1} \displaystyle\sum_{i=1}^{n} (X_i - \overline{X})^2$. The sample standard deviation is $S = \sqrt{S^2}$.

- For large n, a 95% confidence interval of the population mean μ is

$$\left[\overline{X} - 1.96 \, \frac{S}{\sqrt{n}}, \ \overline{X} + 1.96 \, \frac{S}{\sqrt{n}} \right].$$

- The linear regression line is given by

$$\hat{y} = \hat{a} + \hat{b} x$$

with

$$\hat{b} = \frac{\sum (x_k - \overline{x})(y_k - \overline{y})}{\sum (x_k - \overline{x})^2},$$

$$\hat{a} = \overline{y} - \hat{b} \overline{x}.$$

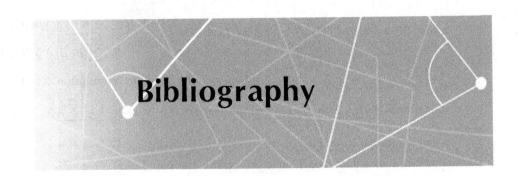

Bibliography

[1] BARNETT R A, ZIEGLER M R, BYLEEN K E. Calculus for business, economics, life sciences, and social sciences[M]. 14th ed. New York: Pearson, 2019.

[2] BITTINGER M L, ELLENBOGEN D J, SURGENT S A. Calculus and its applications[M]. 10th ed. New York: Pearson, 2019.

[3] Lial M L, GREENWELL R N, RITCHEY N P. Calculus with applications[M]. 11th ed. New York: Pearson, 2015.

[4] DONALD S L. Brief calculus for management and the life and social sciences[M]. Toronto: Irwin, 1997.

[5] STEWART J. Calculus[M]. 7th ed. Boston: Cengage Learning, 2012.

[6] LIAL M L, HUNGERFORD T W, HOLCOMB J P, et al. Mathematics with applications in the management, natural, and social sciences [M]. New York: Pearson, 2018.

[7] THOMAS G B, Jr WEIR M D, HASS J R. Thomas' calculus[M]. New York: Pearson, 2014.

[8] Neuhauser C. Calculus for biology and medicine[M]. Hoboken: Prentice Hall, 2000.

[9] THOMPSON S P, GARDNER M. Calculus made easy[M]. New York: St. Martin's Press, 1998.

[10] GOLDSTEIN L, LAY D, SCHNEIDER D, et al. Calculus and its applications [M]. 14th ed. New York: Pearson, 2017.

[11] GUICHARD D. Calculus: early transcendentals [M/OL]. Walla: Whitman College, 2009 [2021−02−01]. https://www. whitman. edu/mathematics/calculus_online/.

[12] LI X, HE D Q, JIANG W B. Medical advanced mathematics [M]. Chinese Edition. Beijing: Peking University Medical Press, 2013.

[13] MA J Z. Advanced mathematics for medicine higher mathematics[M]. Chinese Edition. Beijing: Science Press, 2019.

[14] WEI J, BIAN Q X. Advanced mathematics for medicine[M]. Chinese Edition. Hefei: University of Science and Technology of China Press, 2020.

[15] DEKKING F M, KRAAIKAMP C, LOPUHAA H P, et al. A modern introduction to probability and statistics[M]. Berlin: Springer, 2005.

[16] ROSS S. A first course in probability [M]. 6th ed. Hoboken: Prentice Hall, 1984.

[17] RIFFENBURGH R H, GILLEN D L. Statistics in medicine[M]. 4th ed. Cambridge: Academic Press, 2020.

Appendix A Differentiation and Integration Formulas

Basic Differentiation Formulas

1. $(cu)' = cu'$

2. $(u \pm v)' = u' \pm v'$

3. $(uv)' = u'v + uv'$

4. $\left(\dfrac{u}{v}\right)' = \dfrac{u'v - uv'}{v^2}$

5. $\dfrac{dy}{dx} = \dfrac{dy}{du} \cdot \dfrac{du}{dx}$

6. $(c)' = 0$

7. $(x^n)' = nx^{n-1}$

8. $(e^x)' = e^x$

9. $(\ln x)' = \dfrac{1}{x}$

10. $(\sin x)' = \cos x$

11. $(\cos x)' = -\sin x$

12. $(\tan x)' = \sec^2 x$

13. $(\cot x)' = -\csc^2 x$

14. $(\sec x)' = \sec x \tan x$

15. $(\csc x)' = -\csc x \cot x$

Basic Integration Formulas

1. $\displaystyle\int kf(x)\,dx = k\int f(x)\,dx$

2. $\displaystyle\int [f(x) \pm g(x)]\,dx = \int f(x)\,dx \pm \int g(x)\,dx$

3. $\displaystyle\int dx = x + C$

4. $\displaystyle\int x^n\,dx = \dfrac{n+1}{x^{n+1}} + C,\ n \neq -1$

5. $\displaystyle\int \dfrac{1}{x}\,dx = \ln|x| + C$

6. $\displaystyle\int e^x\,dx = e^x + C$

7. $\displaystyle\int \sin x\,dx = -\cos x + C$

8. $\displaystyle\int \cos x\,dx = \sin x + C$

9. $\displaystyle\int \tan x\,dx = -\ln|\cos x| + C$

10. $\displaystyle\int \cot x\,dx = \ln|\sin x| + C$

11. $\displaystyle\int \sec x\,dx = \ln|\sec x + \tan x| + C$

12. $\displaystyle\int \csc x\,dx = -\ln|\csc x + \cot x| + C$

13. $\displaystyle\int \sec^2 x\,dx = \tan x + C$

14. $\displaystyle\int \csc^2 x\,dx = -\cot x + C$

15. $\displaystyle\int \sec x \tan x\,dx = \sec x + C$

16. $\displaystyle\int \csc x \cot x\,dx = -\csc x + C$

Appendix B Table of the cdf of the Standard Normal Distribution

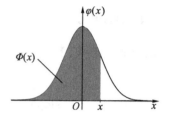

x	0.00	0.01	0.02	0.03	0.04	0.05	0.06	0.07	0.08	0.09
0.0	0.50000	0.50399	0.50798	0.51197	0.51595	0.51994	0.52392	0.52790	0.53188	0.53586
0.1	0.53983	0.54380	0.54776	0.55172	0.55567	0.55962	0.56360	0.56749	0.57142	0.57535
0.2	0.57926	0.58317	0.58706	0.59095	0.59483	0.59871	0.60257	0.60642	0.61026	0.61409
0.3	0.61791	0.62172	0.62552	0.62930	0.63307	0.63683	0.64058	0.64431	0.64803	0.65173
0.4	0.65542	0.65910	0.66276	0.66640	0.67003	0.67364	0.67724	0.68082	0.68439	0.68793
0.5	0.69146	0.69497	0.69847	0.70194	0.70540	0.70884	0.71226	0.71566	0.71904	0.72240
0.6	0.72575	0.72907	0.73237	0.73565	0.73891	0.74215	0.74537	0.74857	0.75175	0.75490
0.7	0.75804	0.76115	0.76424	0.76730	0.77035	0.77337	0.77637	0.77935	0.78230	0.78524
0.8	0.78814	0.79103	0.79389	0.79673	0.79955	0.80234	0.80511	0.80785	0.81057	0.81327
0.9	0.81594	0.81859	0.82121	0.82381	0.82639	0.82894	0.83147	0.83398	0.83646	0.83891
1.0	0.84134	0.84375	0.84614	0.84849	0.85083	0.85314	0.85543	0.85769	0.85993	0.86214
1.1	0.86433	0.86650	0.86864	0.87076	0.87286	0.87493	0.87698	0.87900	0.88100	0.88298
1.2	0.88493	0.88686	0.88877	0.89065	0.89251	0.89435	0.89617	0.89796	0.89973	0.90147
1.3	0.90320	0.90490	0.90658	0.90824	0.90988	0.91149	0.91308	0.91466	0.91621	0.91774
1.4	0.91924	0.92073	0.92220	0.92364	0.92507	0.92647	0.92785	0.92922	0.93056	0.93189
1.5	0.93319	0.93448	0.93574	0.93699	0.93822	0.93943	0.94062	0.94179	0.94295	0.94408
1.6	0.94520	0.94630	0.94738	0.94845	0.94950	0.95053	0.95154	0.95254	0.95352	0.95449
1.7	0.95543	0.95637	0.95728	0.95818	0.95907	0.95994	0.96080	0.96164	0.96246	0.96327
1.8	0.96407	0.96485	0.96562	0.96638	0.96712	0.96784	0.96856	0.96926	0.96995	0.97062
1.9	0.97128	0.97193	0.97257	0.97320	0.97381	0.97441	0.97500	0.97558	0.97615	0.97670
2.0	0.97725	0.97778	0.97831	0.97882	0.97932	0.97982	0.98030	0.98077	0.98124	0.98169
2.1	0.98214	0.98257	0.98300	0.98341	0.98382	0.98422	0.98461	0.98500	0.98537	0.98574
2.2	0.98610	0.98645	0.98679	0.98713	0.98745	0.98778	0.98809	0.98840	0.98870	0.98899
2.3	0.98928	0.98956	0.98983	0.99010	0.99036	0.99061	0.99086	0.99111	0.99134	0.99158
2.4	0.99180	0.99202	0.99224	0.99245	0.99266	0.99286	0.99305	0.99324	0.99343	0.99361
2.5	0.99379	0.99396	0.99413	0.99430	0.99446	0.99461	0.99477	0.99492	0.99506	0.99520
2.6	0.99534	0.99547	0.99560	0.99573	0.99585	0.99598	0.99609	0.99621	0.99632	0.99643
2.7	0.99653	0.99664	0.99674	0.99683	0.99693	0.99702	0.99711	0.99720	0.99728	0.99736
2.8	0.99744	0.99752	0.99760	0.99767	0.99774	0.99781	0.99788	0.99795	0.99801	0.99807
2.9	0.99813	0.99819	0.99825	0.99831	0.99836	0.99841	0.99846	0.99851	0.99856	0.99861
3.0	0.99865	0.99869	0.99874	0.99878	0.99882	0.99886	0.99889	0.99893	0.99896	0.99900

Answers to Even-numbered Problems

Chapter 1

Exercise 1.1

2. (2) $(-\infty, 0]$ and $[3, +\infty)$.

4. (2) The slope is 2, the y-intercept is $\dfrac{3}{2}$.

6. $\dfrac{6}{7}x - y = \dfrac{9}{2}$.

8. (2) $y = \dfrac{3}{2}x + \dfrac{1}{2}$.

10. (2) 0.53.

Exercise 1.2

2. (2) 1.

(4) Does not exist.

4. (2) For $x = 1$, we have $y = 1$ or $y = -1$, thus this equation can not define a function.

(4) For $x = 1$, we have $y = 1$ or $y = -1$, thus this equation can not define a function.

6. (2) $\left(-\infty, -\dfrac{4}{3}\right)$ and $\left(-\dfrac{4}{3}, +\infty\right)$.

8. Even; Neither odd nor even; Odd.

10. (2) Even.

12. Decreasing.

Exercise 1.3

2. (2)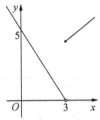

(4)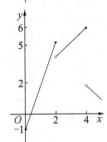

4. Horizontal asymptote at $y = 1$; Vertical asymptote at $x = -1$ and $x = 1$.

6. (2) 10000.

8. (2) $y = -0.0006x + 7.52$.

(4)

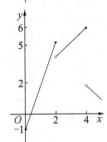

Chapter 2

Exercise 2.1

2. 2.

4. (2) 2;

(4) 2.

6. (2) 3;

(4) -3.

8. (2) -3;

(4) 3.

10. (2) 1;

(4) 3.

12. (2) 0;

(4) Does not exist.

14. (2) 1;

(4) Does not exist.

16. (2) -3.

Exercise 2.2

2. (2) $+\infty$;

(4) $-\infty$;

(6) Does not exist.

4.

x	$\dfrac{x-1}{x^2(x+1)}$	x	$\dfrac{x-1}{x^2(x+1)}$
2.9	0.05792860	3.1	0.05329814
2.99	0.05578762	3.01	0.05532465
2.999	0.05557871	3.001	0.05553241
2.9999	0.05555787	3.0001	0.05555324

6. (2) $+\infty$, vertical asymptotes at $x=5$.

8. (2) $+\infty$, vertical asymptotes at $x=1$.

Exercise 2.3

2. (2) 1;

(4) 1;

(6) No. Since $\lim\limits_{x\to 1^-} f(x) \neq \lim\limits_{x\to 1^+} f(x)$,

then $\lim\limits_{x\to 1} f(x)$ does not exist, thus $f(x)$ is not continuous at 1.

4. (2) 1;

(4) 3.

6. (2) 1;

(4) 1.

8. (2) 4;

(4) 4.

10. (2) $x=-\dfrac{1}{5}$ or 2;

(4) $x=-3$ or -1 or 1 or 3;

(6) $x=-6$ or 0 or 7.

12. (2) $(-\infty,-4)$ and $(0,2)$.

14. (2) The statement is always true;

(4) The statement is always true.

16. (2) Yes, the absolute maximum is $f(1)=1$ and the absolute minimum is $f(0)=0$ or $f(2)=0$.

18. $[-2,-1]$.

Exercise 2.4

2. (2)

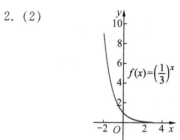

(4)

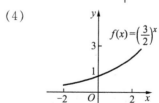

4. $x=1$.

6. (2) $I=39\%$.

8. (2) $x=\dfrac{1}{6}$;

(4) $x=0$;

(6) $x=4$.

10. (2) 25.

Since $\lim\limits_{t \to 0} V(t) = 50$ and $\lim\limits_{t \to +\infty} V(t) = 25$.

12. The medication never completely leave the bloodstream.

$$\lim_{t \to +\infty} \frac{A_0}{t^2 + 1} = 0.$$

It leaves the bloodstream after an infinite time.

Exercise 2.5

2. If, for every $\varepsilon > 0$, there exists a $\delta > 0$, such that if $0 < |u - b| < \delta$, then $|g(u) - N| < \varepsilon$.

4. If, for every $\varepsilon > 0$, there exists a $\delta > 0$, such that if $0 < |v - s| < \delta$, then $|g(v) - Q| < \varepsilon$.

6. We take $\delta = \varepsilon$.

Let us verify this.

Let $\varepsilon > 0$ be any number and choose $\delta = \varepsilon$.

Assume $0 < |x - 1| < \delta$.
Thus, $0 < |x - 1| < \varepsilon$.

Hence, $\left| \dfrac{x^2 - 1}{x - 1} \right| < \varepsilon$.

Finally, $\left| \dfrac{x^2 - 1}{x - 1} - 2 \right| < \varepsilon$.

Therefore, $\lim\limits_{x \to 1} \dfrac{x^2 - 1}{x - 1} = 2$.

8. Let $\varepsilon > 0$ be any number and choose $\delta = \varepsilon^2$.

Assume $0 < x - 4 < \delta$.
Thus, $0 < x - 4 < \varepsilon^2$.

Hence, $0 < \sqrt{x - 4} < \varepsilon$.

Finally, $|\sqrt{x - 4} - 0| < \varepsilon$.

Therefore, $\lim\limits_{x \to 4^+} x - 4 = 0$.

10. Let $M > 0$ be any number and choose $\delta = \dfrac{1}{M}$.

Assume $0 < |x - 0| < \delta$.

Thus, $0 < |x - 0| < \dfrac{1}{M}$.

Hence, $0 < x^2 < \dfrac{1}{M}$.

Finally, $\dfrac{1}{x^2} > M$.

Therefore, $\lim\limits_{x \to 0} \dfrac{1}{x^2} = +\infty$.

12. Suppose $\lim\limits_{x \to c} f(x) = L$, then for any $\varepsilon > 0$, there is $\delta_1 > 0$, such that if $0 < |x - c| < \delta_1$, then $|f(x) - L| < \dfrac{\varepsilon}{|k|}$.

Let $\delta = \delta_1$.
Assume $0 < |x - c| < \delta$.

Thus, $0 < |f(x) - L| < \dfrac{\varepsilon}{|k|}$.

Hence, $0 < |k[f(x) - L]| < \varepsilon$.
Finally, $0 < |k[f(x) - \lim\limits_{x \to c} f(x)]| < \varepsilon$.

Therefore, $\lim\limits_{x \to c} [kf(x)] = k \lim\limits_{x \to c} f(x)$.

Chapter 3

Exercise 3.1

2. (2) $-h - 2$;

(4) 3;

(6) 4.

4. (2) 6.

6. (2) $h + 5$.

8. (2) 2091.35675;

(4) 30.90675.

10. (2) $f'(x) = 0$, $f'(1) = 0$, $f'(2) = 0$, $f'(3) = 0$;

(4) $f'(x) = -2$, $f'(1) = -2$, $f'(2) = -2$, $f'(3) = -2$;

(6) $f'(x) = 3x^2 + 2x + 1$, $f'(1) = 6$, $f'(2) = 17$, $f'(3) = 34$;

(8) $f'(x) = -\dfrac{1}{(x+2)^2}$, $f'(1) = -\dfrac{1}{9}$, $f'(2) = -\dfrac{1}{16}$, $f'(3) = -\dfrac{1}{25}$.

12. (2) $\lim\limits_{h \to 0^+} \dfrac{f(0+h) - f(0)}{h} = \lim\limits_{h \to 0^+} \dfrac{h}{h} = 1$,

$$\lim_{h \to 0^-} \frac{f(0+h)-f(0)}{h} = \lim_{h \to 0^-} \frac{-h}{h} = -1.$$

Since $1 \neq -1$, it follows that $\lim_{h \to 0} \frac{f(0+h)-f(0)}{h}$ does not exist.

Thus, $f(x)$ is differentiable at $x=0$.

$(4) \lim_{h \to 0} \frac{f(0+h)-f(0)}{h} = \lim_{h \to 0} \frac{\sqrt{1+h}-1}{h} =$

0, Thus, $f(x)$ is not differentiable at $x=0$.

14. (2) $P(3)=89$, $P'(3)=0$.

Exercise 3.2

2. (2) 15;

(4) 11;

(6) 15.

4. (2) (A) $f'(x)=4x-3$;

(B) The slope of the graph of f at $x=2$ is 5, the slope of the graph of f at $x=4$ is 13;

(C) The equation of the tangent at $x=2$ is $y=5x-8$, the equation of the tangent at $x=4$ is $y=13x-32$.

(4) (A) $f'(x)=4x^3-3x^2+4x$;

(B) The slope of the graph of f at $x=2$ is 28, the slope of the graph of f at $x=4$ is 224;

(C) The equation of the tangent at $x=2$ is $y=28x-36$, the equation of the tangent at $x=4$ is $y=224x-668$.

6. (2) $S(3)=12.04$, $S'(3)=5.54$. Three months later, the total sales is 12.04 millions of dollars and increases at a rate of 5.54 millions dollars per month.

8. (2) -0.025.

10. (2) 0.

Exercise 3.3

2. (2) 12;

(4) 10;

(6) 14.

4. (2) 6;

(4) 12.

6. (2) $dy=1.4$, $\Delta y=1.461$;

(4) $dy=-15$, $\Delta y=-15.402$.

8. 60.

10. (2) The statement is not always true. For example, $y=x^2+3$.

$$\Delta y = f(1+\Delta x)-f(1)$$
$$= (1+\Delta x)^2-1=(\Delta x)^2+2\Delta x,$$
$$f'(x)=2x, \ f'(1)=2, \ dy=2dx=2\Delta x.$$

When $\Delta x=0.1$, then we get $\Delta y=0.21$ and $dy=0.2$.

Thus, $\Delta y \neq dy$.

(4) The statement is not always true. For example, $y=x^2-4x+5$.

$dy=(2x-4)dx$, $dy=0$ at $x=2$.

12. $dy=\left(\frac{8}{3}x^{\frac{1}{3}}-\frac{1}{3}x^{-\frac{2}{3}}\right)dx$.

14. $dy=-\frac{3}{32}$, $\Delta y=\frac{12-3\sqrt{17}}{\sqrt{17}}$.

16. 0.4π.

18. (2) Revenue: $-\frac{34000}{3}$,

Profit: $-\frac{40000}{3}$.

Chapter 4

Exercise 4.1

2. (2) $h'(x)=2xf(x)[f(x)+xf'(x)]$;

(4) $h'(x)=\frac{x^2[3f(x)-xf'(x)]}{[f(x)]^2}$.

4. (2) $T'(1)=\frac{5}{3}$, which means that the sensitivity of the body to the dosage at 1 is $\frac{5}{3}$;

$T'(3) = 3$, which means that the sensitivity of the body to the dosage at 1 is 3;

$T'(6) = 0$, which means that the sensitivity of the body to the dosage at 1 is 0.

6. (2) $-\dfrac{5}{2}$;

(4) $-\dfrac{3}{4}$.

8. (2) $-\dfrac{1}{2}$.

10. (2) $(uuu)' = u'uu + uu'u + uuu' = 3u^2u'$, thus $\dfrac{d}{dx}[u(x)]^3 = 3[u(x)]^2 u'(x)$.

Exercise 4.2

2. $g \circ f = x^2 - 2x + 2$;

$g \circ g = x^4 + 8x^3 + 30x^2 + 56x + 50$.

4. (2) $7(3x^2 + 5)(x^3 + 5x + 2)^6$;

(4) $-\dfrac{1}{2\sqrt{3-x}}$;

(6) $-\dfrac{24x}{(x^2 + 7)^4}$;

(8) $\dfrac{-x^2 - 5x + 3}{(x^2 + 3)^{\frac{3}{2}}(2x + 5)^{\frac{1}{2}}}$.

6. (2) $-\dfrac{1}{x^3}$;

(4) $\dfrac{2x^4 + 12x^2 - 2}{(x^2 + 3)^2}$.

8. $y = \dfrac{2}{3}x + 1$; $x = \dfrac{3}{4}$.

10. 2 or $\dfrac{2}{3}$.

12. $(4 \times 10^6)x(x^2 - 1)^{\frac{-5}{3}}$.

14. (2) $F'(A) = \dfrac{1}{2}kD^2(A - C)^{-\frac{1}{2}}$.

Exercise 4.3

2. To show it, start with $f(x_1) = f(x_2)$ and demonstrate that this implies $x_1 = x_2$.

$$f(x_1) = f(x_2),$$

$x_1^3 + 1 = x_2^3 + 1,$

$x_1^3 = x_2^3.$

Then we get $x_1 = x_2$.

So $f(x) = x^3 + 1$ is one-to-one.

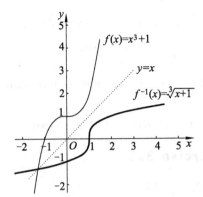

4. $f^{-1}(x) = \dfrac{1}{x - 1}$, $x \neq 1$.

6. $\dfrac{1}{3}x^{-\frac{2}{3}}$.

8. (2) $e^{3x\ln 5}$;

(4) $\dfrac{\ln(3x^2 - 4)}{\ln 2}$.

10. C_1 is the graph of e^x;

C_3 is the graph of e^{-x};

C_2 is the graph of $\ln x$.

12. $x = -1.1845$.

14. Since $0 < b < 1$, then we get $\ln b < 0$.

Since k is a positive constant, then $-k < 0$.

Let $-k = \ln b$.

Then we get $e^{x\ln b} = e^{-kx}$.

Thus $y = b^x$ can be written in the form $y = e^{-kx}$.

16. (2) $10(\lg 3.16 + 6)$;

(4) 150.

Exercise 4.4

2. (2) $y = e$.

4. Correct.

6. (2) $f'(x) = 3(2x^4 + 5x - 3)^2(8x^3 + 5)$;

(4) $f'(x) = (6x + 5)e^{3x^2 + 5x + 4}$;

(6) $f'(x) = \dfrac{6x}{x^2 - 1}$;

(8) $f'(x) = \dfrac{6x}{3+x^2}$;

(10) $f'(x) = \dfrac{6x[\ln(1+x^2)]^2}{1+x^2}$.

8. (2) $\dfrac{3}{2\sqrt{3w-7}}$;

(4) $6x(e^{x^2+1})3$.

10. He is wrong. It does not pass through the origin. The tangent line at $x = 3$ is $y = \dfrac{1}{3}x + \ln 3 - 1$, which passes through $(0, \ln 3 - 1)$.

The line tangent at $x = 4$ also does not pass through the origin. The tangent line at $x = 4$ is $y = \dfrac{1}{4}x + \ln 4 - 1$, which passes through $(0, \ln 4 - 1)$.

12. 2.2727; 0.8065; 0.4098.

14. $5000\ln 2 \times 2^{t+1}$; $40000\ln 2$; $10240000\ln 2$.

16. (2) $(\ln x)^x\left[\ln(\ln x) + \dfrac{1}{x}\right]$;

(4) $(1 - \ln x)x^{\frac{1}{x}-2}$;

(6) $(2\ln x + 1)x^{x^2+1}$.

18. $2xe^{-2x}(x^2+1)^{-2x-1}\{(x^2+1)[1 - x - x\ln(x^2+1)] - 2x^2\}$.

Exercise 4.5

2. 1.

4. $y = 2x \pm 6$.

6. $y = \dfrac{7}{\sqrt{3}}x - \dfrac{8}{\sqrt{3}}$.

8. $y = \dfrac{1}{\sqrt{3}}x + \dfrac{1}{4\sqrt{3}}$.

Exercise 4.6

2. $-\dfrac{2}{3}$.

4. $-\dfrac{3}{4}$.

6. the speed of the car is about 69.4 kilometers per hour.

8. $\dfrac{90}{16\pi}$ cm/s.

Chapter 5

Exercise 5.1

2. $f(x)$ is continuous over the closed interval $[-2, 0]$ and differentiable in the open interval $(-2, 0)$,
$$f(-2) = 0 = f(0).$$
There then exists at least one $c \in (a, b)$ such that $f'(c) = 0$,
$$c = -1.$$

4. $f(x)$ is continuous over the closed interval $[0, 9]$ and differentiable in the open interval $(0, 9)$,

Then there exists at least one $c \in (0, 9)$ such that $f'(c) = \dfrac{f(9) - f(0)}{9 - 0} = \dfrac{1}{3}$,
$$c = \dfrac{9}{4}.$$

6. Since $f(x)$ is continuous and differentiable everywhere. $f(x)$ has two roots. Then there exist x_1 and x_2 such that $f(x_1) = f(x_2) = 0$.

According to the Rolle's Theorem, there exists at least one $c \in (x_1, x_2)$ such that $f'(c) = 0$.

Thus $f'(x)$ must has at least one root.

Exercise 5.2

2. (2) The function increases in $(-\infty, -5) \cup (4, 9)$, while decreases in $(-5, -1) \cup (-1, 4) \cup (9, +\infty)$.

4. The function has a local maximum $f(0) = r$ and a local minimum $f(-r) = f(r) = 0$.

6. (2) 3;

(4) $n + 1$.

8. (2) $f(x)=\dfrac{1}{3}x^3-2x^2+C$, where

C is an arbitrary constant.

10. Assume $x_1<x_2$.

Since $f(x)$ and $g(x)$ are increasing functions, we get $f(x_1)<f(x_2)$ and $g(x_1)<g(x_2)$.

Then $f(x_1)+g(x_2)<f(x_2)+g(x_2)$, $f(x)+g(x)$ is increasing.

12. No, the condition is $f(x)>0$.

14. The critical value is $t=\sqrt{6}$ or 0; $C(t)$ increases in $(0,\sqrt{6})$ and decreases in $(\sqrt{6}, 12)$;

the local maximum is $C(6)=0.0148$ and the local minimum is $C(0)=0$.

Exercise 5.3

2. (2)(0, 3).

4. b, d, e.

6. (2) 1.

8.

x	0	1	2	3
f	$-$	$+$	$-$	0
$f'(x)$	$+$	0	$-$	$+$
$f''(x)$	$+$	$-$	$+$	$+$

10. f is concave down on $(-\infty,-2)\cup(4,+\infty)$ and concave upward on $(-2, 4)$. The x-coordinates of the inflection points are -2 and 4.

Exercise 5.4

2. (2) The absolute maximum is 1, and it occurs at $x=1$.

4. f has a local maximum at -2 and a local minimum at 3.

6. (2) $5\ln 5-5$.

Exercise 5.5

2. $+\infty$.

4. 8.

6. 0.

8. $+\infty$.

10. 3.

12. $-\dfrac{1}{5}$.

14. $\dfrac{1}{4}$.

Exercise 5.6

2. $\dfrac{\sqrt{2}+\sqrt{6}}{4}$.

4. $2\csc 2t=\dfrac{2}{\sin 2t}=\dfrac{2}{2\sin t\cos t}$

$=\dfrac{1}{\sin t\cos t}=\sec t\csc t.$

6.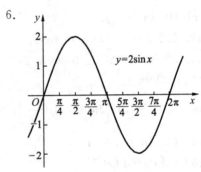

8.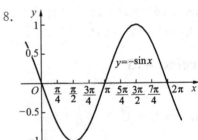

10. $\dfrac{\sin\sqrt{x}\cos\sqrt{x}}{\sqrt{x}}$.

12. $-\dfrac{\cot x}{\sin x}$.

14. $-\dfrac{\sin x\cos x}{\sqrt{1-\sin^2 x}}$.

16. $\dfrac{5}{3}$.

18. $\dfrac{4}{3}$.

20. 3.

22. Since $-1 \leqslant \cos \dfrac{2}{x} \leqslant 1$.

Then we get $-x^4 \leqslant x^4 \cos \dfrac{2}{x} \leqslant x^4$.

Since $\lim\limits_{x \to 0} (-x^4) = 0$ and $\lim\limits_{x \to 0} x^4 = 0$.

Thus, $\lim\limits_{x \to 0} x^4 \cos \dfrac{2}{x} = 0$.

Exercise 5.7

2. (2) $y = 2x - 5$.

4. $\lim\limits_{x \to \pm\infty} [f(x) - x^2] = \lim\limits_{x \to \pm\infty} \dfrac{1}{x} = 0$.

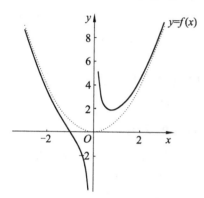

Chapter 6

Exercise 6.1

2. No, since $F'(x) = x^2 e^{\frac{x^3}{3}}$.

4. $(x \ln x - x + C)' = \ln x$ so that
$\displaystyle\int \ln x \, dx = x \ln x - x + C$.

6. $y = 40 \sqrt{t}$.

8. $f(x) = \dfrac{2}{5} x^5 - 2x^3 + \dfrac{3}{2} x^2 + C_1 x + C_2$, where C_1 and C_2 are arbitrary constant.

10. $y = 2x^2 - 3x + 1$.

12. (2) 258.133 feet.

Exercise 6.2

2. 1, above the x-axis.

4. 24.

6. (2) -6.28;

(4) -2.28.

Exercise 6.3

2. (2) 5;

(4) -460.

4. 0.

6. 1.

Exercise 6.4

2. (2) $x e^{x^2}$;

(4) $\dfrac{1}{x^2}$;

(6) $(9x - 4) x \ln x$.

4. $f(x) = 4x$.

Exercise 6.5

2. (2) $\dfrac{1}{4} \ln \dfrac{3}{2}$;

(4) $\dfrac{1}{30} (1 - 14^{10})$;

(6) $\dfrac{1}{10}$;

(8) $\dfrac{e^7 - e^3}{8}$.

Exercise 6.6

2. $x \sin x + \cos x + C$.

4. $-x^2 \cos x + 2x \sin x + 2 \cos x + C$.

6. $-\dfrac{1}{2} x \cos 2x + \dfrac{1}{4} \sin 2x + C$.

8. $2 - 17 e^{-3}$.

10. $\dfrac{16}{3} \ln 2 - \dfrac{14}{9}$.

12. $\dfrac{1}{2} (x - \sin x \cos x) + C$.

Chapter 7

Exercise 7.1

2. (2) $\dfrac{1}{6}$.

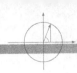

4. (2) $e^4 + e - 2$.

Exercise 7.2

2. 2.

4. 0.

6. $\approx 23.2 \ ℃$.

8. 5.

Exercise 7.3

2. 2; converges.

4. 0; converges.

6. 0; converges.

Chapter 8

Exercise 8.1

2. (2) $P_{4,5}$.

4. (2) {HHH, HHT, HTH, THH, TTH, THT, HTT, TTT}.

6. (2) {1};

(4) {1, 2, 3, 4}.

8. (2) 0.1;

(4) 0.4.

10. $\dfrac{P_{7,10}}{10^7}$.

12. $\dfrac{P_{40,365}}{365^{40}}$.

Exercise 8.2

2. 0.75.

4. (2) 0.86;

(4) 0.394.

6. (2) 0.72.

8. (2) 0.15;

(4) 0.35.

Exercise 8.3

2. (2) $\dfrac{1}{3}$.

4. (2) $F(x) = \begin{cases} 0, & \text{if } x < 1, \\ 5/14, & \text{if } 0 \leqslant x < 5, \\ 4/7, & \text{if } 5 \leqslant x < 10, \\ 1, & \text{if } 10 \leqslant x. \end{cases}$

6. (2) 1;

(4) 2.

8. (2) $F(x) = \begin{cases} 0, & \text{if } x \leqslant 1, \\ x/10, & \text{if } 0 < x < 10, \\ 1, & \text{if } 10 \leqslant x. \end{cases}$

10. (2) -1.645;

(4) 1.645;

Exercise 8.4

2. 0.7, 2.5, 2.01, 7.8, 32.16, 5.3.

4. $n = 6$, $p = 0.4$.

6. $a = 3/5$, $b = 6/5$.

8. $\dfrac{(n+1)}{2}$, $\dfrac{n^2 - 1}{12}$.

Exercise 8.5

2. (2) 0.2621.

4. $\hat{\mu} = 8.34, \hat{\sigma}^2 = 0.03^2$.

6. [61.0, 71.6].

8. $\hat{y} = 1.8999 - 0.0857x$.

Index